Introduction to Critical Care

Introduction to Critical Care

JOSEPH M. CIVETTA, M.D.

Professor of Surgery, Anesthesiology, Medicine, and Pathology
University of Miami School of Medicine;
Director, Surgical Intensive Care Unit
University of Miami/Jackson Memorial Medical Center
Miami, Florida

ROBERT W. TAYLOR, M.D.

Assistant Professor of Medicine, Baylor College of Medicine;
Director, Medical Intensive Care Unit
The Methodist Hospital, Houston, Texas

ROBERT R. KIRBY, M.D.

Professor of Anesthesiology,
University of Florida College of Medicine, Gainesville, Florida

WITH 15 ADDITIONAL CONTRIBUTORS

J. B. LIPPINCOTT COMPANY   Philadelphia
Cambridge   New York   St. Louis   San Francisco
London   Singapore   Sydney   Tokyo

Acquisitions Editor: Nancy Mullins
Indexer: Barbara Farabaugh
Production: Ruttle, Shaw & Wetherill, Inc.
Compositor: Ruttle, Shaw & Wetherill, Inc.
Printer/Binder: R. R. Donnelley & Sons

Copyright © 1989, by J. B. Lippincott Company. All rights reserved. No part of this book may be used or reproduced in any manner whatsoever without written permission except for brief quotations embodied in critical articles and reviews. Printed in the United States of America. For information write J. B. Lippincott Company, East Washington Square, Philadelphia, Pennsylvania 19105.

6 5 4 3 2 1

Library of Congress Cataloging-In-Publication Data

Introduction to critical care / Joseph M. Civetta, Robert W. Taylor, Robert R. Kirby; with 15 additional contributors.
   p.   cm.
   Includes bibliographies and index.
   ISBN 0-397-51031-4
   1. Critical care medicine.   I. Civetta, Joseph M.   II. Taylor, Robert W. (Robert Wesley), 1949–   .   III. Kirby, Robert R.
   [DNLM: 1. Critical Care.   2. Intensive Care Units.   WX 218 I656]
RC86.7.I585 1989
616'.028—dc19
DNLM/DLC   89-2734
for Library of Congress   CIP

The authors and publisher have exerted every effort to ensure that drug selection and dosage set forth in this text are in accord with current recommendations and practice at the time of publication. However, in view of ongoing research, changes in government regulations, and the constant flow of information relating to drug therapy and drug reactions, the reader is urged to check the package insert for each drug for any change in indications and dosage and for added warnings and precautions. This is particularly important when the recommended agent is a new or infrequently employed drug.

Contributors

Peter Angood, M.D.
Staff
Surgical Intensive Care and
  Trauma Unit
Montreal General Hospital
Montreal, Quebec
Canada

**Honorable Christopher J.
  Armstrong**
Associate Justice, Appeals Court
Commonwealth of Massachusetts
Boston, Massachusetts

Ned H. Cassem, M.D.
Acting Chief of Psychiatry
Massachusetts General Hospital;
Associate Professor of Psychiatry
Harvard Medical School
Boston, Massachusetts

Joseph M. Civetta, M.D.
Professor of Surgery,
  Anesthesiology, Medicine,
  and Pathology
University of Miami School of
  Medicine;
Director, Surgical Intensive Care
  Unit
University of Miami/Jackson
  Memorial Medical Center
Miami, Florida

Louise Dion, M.D., F.R.C.S.(C.)
Assistant Professor of Clinical
  Surgery and Anesthesiology
University of Miami School of
  Medicine;
Associate Director, Surgical
  Intensive Care Unit
University of Miami/Jackson
  Memorial Medical Center
Miami, Florida

**Judith A. Hudson–Civetta,
  R.N., M.S.N., C.C.R.N.**
Research Associate
Division of Surgical Intensive Care
Department of Surgery
University of Miami School of
  Medicine
Miami, Florida

**Laurence B. McCullough,
  Ph.D.**
Professor of Medicine and
  Community Medicine
Baylor College of Medicine
Houston, Texas

David B. Mishael, Esq.
Fowler, White, Burnett, Hurley,
 Banick & Strickroot
Member, Florida Bar
Member, Dade County and
 American Bar Association
Member, U.S. District Court,
 Southern District of Florida
Miami, Florida

Mary F. Murtha, R.N.
Head Nurse
Surgical Intensive Care Unit
University of Miami/Jackson
 Memorial Medical Center
Miami, Florida

S. David Register, III, M.D.
Staff Anesthesiologist and Director
Surgical Intensive Care Unit
Wilford Hall United States Air
 Force Medical Center
Lackland Air Force Base
San Antonio, Texas

Lisa Regueiro, R.N.
Staff Nurse
Surgical Intensive Care Unit
University of Miami/Jackson
 Memorial Medical Center
Miami, Florida

George L. Wallace–Barnhill, Ph.D.
Psychotherapist, Professional
 Therapy Associates
Ft. Lauderdale, Florida

Deborah Weppler, R.N., B.S.N., C.C.R.N.
Associate Head Nurse
Surgical Intensive Care Unit
University of Miami/Jackson
 Memorial Medical Center
Miami, Florida

Michael G. Wise, M.D.
Associate Professor and Director of
 Emergency Psychiatric
 Services
Department of Psychiatry
University of Texas Health Science
 Center at San Antonio
San Antonio, Texas

Ernlé W. D. Young, Ph.D.
Senior Lecturer in Medical Ethics
Stanford University School of
 Medicine;
Ethical Consultant and Director of
 Chaplaincy Services
Stanford University Hospital
Stanford, California

Mihae Yu, M.D.
Assistant Professor of Surgery
University of Hawaii School of
 Medicine;
Director of Education
Surgical Intensive Care Unit
Queens Medical Center
Honolulu, Hawaii

Preface

*I*ntensive care units (ICUs) were established from the perspective of crisis management of critically ill patients who needed specialized expertise and equipment. The first experiences reinforced the validity of this thinking. Mortality rates in coronary care units diminished as prompt treatment of life-threatening dysrhythmias prevented deaths. Observations of these patients later revealed that the life-threatening dysrhythmias were often preceded by less malignant rhythm disturbances that could be treated easily. In a similar vein, patients who developed neuromuscular paralysis and other forms of respiratory failure could be successfully ventilated in specialized respiratory care units, again changing previously lethal illnesses into manageable problems.

However, despite rapid advances in therapy, the evolution and introduction of more equipment, and new modalities of diagnosis, it became obvious that immediate or even ultimate cure was often impossible. Indeed, cure never has been always possible nor is it likely to become so.

The subsequent growth of intensive care, coming at a time of increasing focus on rising costs for all medical care, has had to include other dimensions impacting on more than just physiologic and pathophysiologic processes. Death is a reality in our ICUs, not a pathologic event. Cost consciousness has become especially and appropriately part of our daily practice. Legal, judicial, and bioethical perspectives form an increasingly important part of bedside practice. Further, the autonomy principle, emphasizing the patient's values and choices, has evolved during this same era. As the mystery of ICU medical practices diminishes due to widespread media coverage and increasing sophistication of the lay populace, the emphasis, too, on the physician's beneficence as the sole guiding principle of medical practice has diminished. Today's ICU clinicians must become increasingly knowledgeable of the content of these other dimensions and skilled in their practice.

The resulting effect of these new forces means that we can no longer maintain a restricted viewpoint, focusing upon our caring efforts solely as curative, but we must become sensitive to the need of caring for those patients who must die despite our efforts. In the words of Louis Dionne, Director of

La Maison Michel Sarrazin, a hospice in Quebec City, "We must learn to transform the failure to cure into creating a successful departure from life."

We recognize the necessity to learn far more than medicine to practice appropriately in today's ICU. In the words of an anonymous author, "As I've grown older there has been an alarming increase in the number of things I know nothing about!" Recognizing the truth of that statement, we have tried to bring together expositions about these crucial and critical aspects of daily ICU practice by physicians, nurses, psychotherapists, ethicists, judges, and lawyers. By recognizing the limitiations of current knowledge and technology, we can strengthen our human qualities. By enlarging our focus, we can fulfill important needs for our patients, ourselves, and society. We hope that this combination can decrease the stress so commonly associated with ICU practice. If we can learn successfully, ICU "burn-out" with its accompanying sense of failure can be replaced by satisfaction with an accompanying sense of pride for translating multidimensional concepts to daily bedside practice.

Joseph M. Civetta, M.D.
Robert W. Taylor, M.D.
Robert R. Kirby, M.D.

Contents

PART ONE: CONCEPTS

1 Setting Objectives: Perspectives for Care 3
Joseph M. Civetta

Selection of "Appropriate" Patients   6
Generic Goals of Intensive Care   7
Immediate Objective: Examine Societal Values   9
Distributive Justice   10
Immediate Objective: Examine Bedside Care   13
Significant Interrelationships in Critical Care   14
Conclusion   15

2 The What and When of Clinical Decision-Making   19
Joseph M. Civetta

Elements of Clinical Care   20
The Influence of Time   24
First Vantage Point: Source of Admissions   25
Second Vantage Point: Upon ICU Admission   28
Third Vantage Point: Short-Term ICU Outcome   29
Fourth Vantage Point: Continued ICU Care   30
Fifth Vantage Point: Long-Term ICU Patients   32
Last Vantage Point: Discharge from Intensive Care   33
Conclusion   34

3 Life and Death in the ICU: Ethical Considerations   37
Ernlé W. D. Young

Medical Ethics   38
Medicomoral Principles   39
Limitation or Refusal of Treatment   47
The Critical Care Team   53
Conclusion   57

4 Informed Consent 59
Laurence B. McCullough

Key Considerations to Practice Informed Consent 59
Ethical Foundations of Informed Consent 65
Special Considerations 68
Conclusion 69

5 Judicial Involvement in Treatment Decisions: The Emerging Consensus 71
Christopher J. Armstrong

The Problem 72
The Public Debate 73
The Emerging Legal Consensus 75
Conclusion 83

6 Important Legal Decisions in Critical Care 85
S. David Register

Irreversible Central Nervous System Injury/Brain Death 85
Irreversible CNS Injury Without Brain Death 88
Decision-Making for Incompetent Patients 91
Advance Directives for Patient Care 95
Do Not Resuscitate 97
Patients of Questionable Competency 98
Competent Patients 99
Withdrawal of Therapy from Minors 100
Withholding Therapy from Infants 102

7 Iatrogenesis 109
Joseph M. Civetta

Existing Status of the Patient 110
Recognition of Newly Acquired Diseases or Complications 111
Decision-Making Process 111
Diagnostic Evaluation 112
Interventions Used 113
Definitions of Outcome 114
Evaluation of Clinical Care 115

8 Avoiding Legal Problems 117
David B. Mishael

Communication Breakdowns: A Precursor to the Malpractice Claim 118
Documenting the Medical Chart 125

9 Prediction and Definition of Outcome in a Cost-Sensitive Era 133
Joseph M. Civetta

Cost Considerations 133
Definition of Outcome 134

Cost and Cost Effectiveness   136
Severity of Illness   137
Prediction and Resource Utilization   137
Cost-Containment Efforts   139
Goals for Intensive Care   140
Classification of Quantitative Indices   147

PART TWO: PEOPLE

10. Joining the Team   175
Mary F. Murtha, Lisa Regueiro

Perceptions   175
Functions of the Team   176
Organizational Factors   177
Factors Contributing to Collaboration   180

11 ICU Fellowship: Blending Science and Art   183
Louise Dion

Introduction   183
Evolution of Goals and Objectives   185
Organizing According to Tasks   186
Prioritization   187
Documentation   189
Conclusion   190

12 Getting Along in the ICU: Physician Interrelationships   191
Peter Angood

The Surgeon and the ICU   191
Members of the Team   192
Roles, Responsibilities, Freedoms, and Limitations   193
Communication   198
Uncommunicated Expectations   199
The Surgeon's Expectations of the ICU   199
Special Situations   201
Conclusion   201

13 Understanding Reactions of Patient and Family   203
George L. Wallace–Barnhill

Psychological Concepts   203
Staff Involvement With Families   206
The Patient in the ICU   209

14 Behavioral Disturbances in the ICU   215
Michael G. Wise, Ned H. Cassem

What to Do First   216
Clinical Features of Delirium   217
Is Delirium Present?   219

xii   Contents

If Delirium Is Present, What Is Next?   219
When Delirium Is Not Present   226
Conclusion   232

15 Allocating Nursing Care   235
Judith A. Hudson–Civetta

Introduction   235
Nursing Care Functions   235
Allocation of Nursing Resources   236
Conclusion   246
Appendix: Categories of Nursing Care   247

16 Preventive Care: Poorly Appreciated and Undervalued   267
Deborah Weppler, Joseph M. Civetta

Skin and Subcutaneous Tissues   268
Musculoskeletal System Considerations   275
Subtle Infectious Processes   277
Miscellaneous Conditions   283
Various Types of ICU Beds   285
Conclusion   287

17 Accepting a New Admission   289
Mihae Yu

Before Transfer   289
Admission into Intensive Care   291
Giving Report   294

Index   297

Introduction to Critical Care

PART I

Concepts

Setting Objectives: Perspectives for Care

Joseph M. Civetta

The first objective of critical care might be to decide which patients should be treated. Once, this seemed simple–choose the sickest patients. The very concept that stimulated the formation of intensive care units (ICUs) seemed to be an effective guideline for selecting appropriate candidates for intensive care. Prior to specialized care areas, and at the time when new (and expensive) equipment became available, distribution of both sick patients and scarce equipment throughout the hospital seemed inefficient in terms of efficacy and cost. Thus, ICUs were created to concentrate three critical components: the sickest patients, the highly technical and expensive equipment, and the staff with the knowledge and experience to treat the patients and use the equipment. Omitting terminal patients and those who would fare well enough in routine care areas, practitioners should have been able to select patients appropriate for intensive care *based on these medical and organizational factors.*

Today, however, there are financial, legal, ethical, moral, and religious aspects to the delivery of care, termination of life support, utilization of scarce resources, malpractice, and rising medical costs, all of which impact and, perhaps, have greater weight than "mere" patient–physician–disease interactions. To examine these interactions in today's world, we need to remember Harry Truman's words, "The only thing new in the world is the history you don't know."[1] I would like to start with the implicit contract between society and the medical profession to see why recent technological changes have caused conflict among these frames of reference which previously seemed free of major incompatibility.

The Edwin Smith Surgical Papyrus is, perhaps, the oldest existing medical document.[2] It was scribe-copied about 1600 B.C.E. from a document possibly written 5,000 years ago. It is a collection of 48 case descriptions, classified by three different verdicts, the term used to describe the diagnosis: (1) "an ailment which I will treat"; (2) "an ailment with which I will contend"; or (3) "an ailment not to be treated." Thus, in the earliest of medical documents, physicians were cautioned to recognize those ailments which were beyond their curative powers, ailments not to be treated. I believe that one of the problems today is that we have stopped identifying these ailments and separating them from the ones we should treat. We have substituted what

Ronald Preston calls aspirational heroism—a belief that science and technology should defeat disease and death.[3] This is not true. Bulkin and Lukashok succinctly expressed the result of this belief: Viewing death as unnatural causes us to confuse our inability to cure with failure.[4] If we could recognize an ailment that "ought not be treated" because it cannot be treated successfully, we would realize that the term "life support" in such a case is inaccurate: continued intervention can only prolong dying, not support life. However, this distinction is not always clear and certainly is not fully accepted by either the medical profession or society in general.

Because society can only be expected to resolve these complex and interrelated issues over time, and although the situation for us today is serious and even baffling, it is not hopeless. As we attempt to select admission criteria for the proper use of the ICU, we must depreciate the current focus on money and medicolegal considerations, notwithstanding their considerable visibility and impact. We must remember Fein's important observation, "We live in a society, not an economy."[5] Unfortunately, continually rising costs for medical care have been cited as the reason to institute major changes in health care financing; these now have an impact on the delivery of care. Moreover, there is a growing tendency to try to exclude patients from the ICU based on what I believe to be an incomplete appraisal of the role of intensive care in today's hospital environment.[6–8] There is also an ominous spectre to this emphasis on rising costs: cost containment, if poorly conceived and implemented, will reduce the access to care as well as the quality of care, yet fail to achieve true savings. Opinions are quite divergent with respect to the directions which should be taken. Proponents of prospective payment systems, such as diagnosis related groups (DRG) now used by Medicare, believe it will solve many of the ills attributed to cost-based reimbursement. Richard Schweiker, the former Secretary of Health and Human Resources, said to Congress that a DRG-based system will provide hospitals with an incentive to improve efficiency, establish Medicare as a prudent buyer of hospital services, reduce the administrative burden on hospitals, and yet, still will assure beneficiary access to quality health care.[9] We should note that the DRG system was not designed as a tool for reimbursement, and no one has outcome criteria to assess the effects of the system, especially with regard to intensive care.

All eyes focus on the fact that medical costs are increasing in general. Even after 4 years of concerted efforts, medical costs rose at a 7.5% annual rate in 1986 whereas the overall inflation rate had fallen to below 2%. At the same time, all eyes focus on the spectacular successes achieved in transplantation even though costs for an individual patient in our hospital actually exceeded $1,000,000 for the hospitalization for the transplantation. George Orwell's major error in *1984* was not in predicting the *type* of future but in attributing the *cause* of the changes to direct governmental intervention.[10] Many of the changes have occurred without obvious "Big Brother" control. Many Newspeak concepts, if not the words, are with us today. For instance, the term "doublethink" referred to the developed ability to hold two contradictory ideas in the mind at the same time and not notice that they were diametrically opposed. Thus, it does not seem contradictory today to expect to lower costs and to introduce better and more expensive forms of effective therapy at the same time. We must await society's realization that this is a problem which must be addressed, will not go away, and, if medical science is to continue to discover, refine, and improve therapy, the conflict between the desire to lower costs and to improve care will actually become more acute.

Although improved efficiency could have been considered an initial realistic method to decrease spending, true improvements in care which may be costly must be factored into the overall equations. Stern and Epstein wrote that although DRGs have a moderate chance of decreasing total health care costs, they were also likely to have deleterious effects on the quality of patient care and on the access to care.[9] Jerry Avorn in an essay entitled, "Benefit and Cost Analysis in Geriatric Care–Turning Age Discrimination into Health Policy" noted that, "Until a century ago, medical therapy was, for the most part, both cheap and useless, thereby posing no great problems of distributive justice. Quite the opposite is now the case. The remarkable progress of biomedical technology since World War II has made it possible for physicians to keep sicker and sicker patients alive longer and longer at greater and greater costs."[11] Apparently, he viewed this as true medical "progress."

We face the problem most acutely in the ICU where we have learned that terms such as "sicker" and "alive longer" carry implications unknown in prior human history. Patients may enter an unprecedented state of prolonged dying, a period lasting from days to weeks to months and even years, if we maintain careful attention to numerous details of bedside care and continue measures often termed "life support." The transition from life to death, especially when artificially lengthened and almost "frozen in time," can make it difficult for us to decide when a patient is just sick enough to be in the ICU with a potential to survive following treatment or so sick that the natural progression to death occurs even if delayed or prolonged by our perhaps poorly termed "life support" techniques.

Even the term "alive" no longer is simple in concept. We value both the sanctity of life and the quality of life. Before we intervened to create this unprecedented dying state, there were few occasions in which the two societal values relating to life came in conflict. For the most part, the period of dying was mercifully short, and prolonged vegetative states were more curiosities because of their rarity than a matter of major medical or societal concern. This is no longer the case, and society–and all members of society, that is, individuals as patients, lawyers, judges, physicians, and nurses–are often perplexed, anguished, and confused. Edgar Allan Poe, the master of horror stories, wrote, "The Strange Facts in the Case of M. Valdemar" in 1845.[12] In the story, "Mesmerism" was used in a patient at the moment of death. The patient remained suspended in this state for months. It makes chilling reading today, mesmerized as we are by the analogous situation in the ICU. It will take time, once again, for resolution.

These issues are addressed in more detail in Chapters 3, "Life and Death in the ICU: Ethical Considerations," and 6, "Important Legal Decisions in Critical Care." It is fitting that these chapters approach the problem differently. Dr. Young proposes concepts to resolve (or at least reduce) the conflict between quality-of-life and sanctity-of-life decisions. Dr. Register presents a striking view of the variations in response which have already been rendered by judicial or legislative action, and he presents the viewpoints of those less comfortable with the societal tendency toward "quality of life" decisions. The societal confusion is more understandable, Dr. Thomas Starzl discussed (in a recent conference I attended), given the jolt to the definitions of life and death, unquestioned and undisturbed throughout all of human history until 30 years ago. Cessation of vital signs (cardiac activity and breathing) was a sign of death. Now it is often termed cardiac arrest and after prompt resuscitation, indeed, these patients are not dead, but are functioning, active members of society. On the other hand, cardiac and respiratory activity no longer necessarily signify life. The concept of brain death, stimulated by successful human organ transplantation, has now evolved and achieved both medical and legal status.

All of these deliberations and changes superimposed on the unfortunate restricted focus upon rising costs which, forgetting Fein's observation, seem to view economics as the sole important driving force to determine the delivery of medical care, cannot delay us from setting objectives for critical care today. We must delineate goals for intensive care, understand the limitations of present care, examine the process of bedside care, adjust our functioning to conform with the hospital's goals and resources, and finally, remain congruent with overall societal values. It is likely, therefore, that a simple list of admission and discharge requirements would be both infeasible and untenable.

SELECTION OF "APPROPRIATE" PATIENTS

Life was simpler when we believed that we could characterize patients as too well, too sick, and just right for intensive care. In this conception, a patient was an appropriate candidate for intensive care if the illness was deemed too severe for care in a routine hospital area (death could be predicted) and *the illness was likely to respond to treatment in the ICU.* Unfortunately, few disease states and even fewer patients meet those criteria such that there is unequivocal evidence of the efficacy of intensive care.[13] However, for the sake of discussion, one could then distinguish two other classes of patients, those whose illness was known to be terminal or was so severe that death was likely even after treatment in the ICU and patients who were likely to survive even if "deprived" of the benefits of intensive care. This classification system fails to recognize that these distinctions are not always possible and not necessarily desirable. While "terminal" patients would experience little benefit from the ICU, neither clinicians nor patients and their families usually want ICU admission. Although 80% or more of patients in the United States presently die in hospitals, and many patients with terminal illnesses are readmitted to the hospital primarily to die, the motivating force is not one last ditch effort to avoid death but rather comfort for the patient and relief of stress on the family. Patients with acute devastating illness, even if admitted to the ICU, usually have a prompt fatal outcome. Resource utilization is not a problem and efficient, rapid, crisis-oriented care can and does produce the dramatic success idealized if not exactly typical of intensive care. Exclusion of the patient "too sick" has little salutary effect in terms of treatment goals and essentially no impact on resources, less than 1% of patient-days.[14] In fact, in order to choose all the appropriate patients, we must, by design, broaden the admission of criteria, thus including patients who ultimately might be deemed "too sick" because of our inability to select only the appropriate patients. In like manner, we often extend our selection process to include patients who may be considered "too well" for intensive care. Some have proposed that patients be excluded if the risk of mortality or morbidity is low or if the need for treatment is low.[6-8] Conceptually, this too might be considered reasonable but only from a very restricted viewpoint. Any changes in current policy, if undertaken because of financial constraints, should have a significant potential benefit to justify the attendant risks which are at least implicit in excluding currently admitted patients from the ICU. In one study, if the estimated probability of needing ICU-type treatment was 10% or less, the intensive care admission would be considered unnecessary.[6] Given the present hypersensitive medicolegal scrutiny, particularly blurring the distinction between bad outcome and negligence, it seems hard to believe that the negligible financial saving of a single day's observation in the ICU is likely to be considered a justifiable defense for the refusal to admit such patients, should a complication needing treatment develop in an excluded patient. While unnecessary admissions are clearly wasteful, an analysis of the risk of complications proposed by the Consensus Development Conference weighted two distinct factors: the risk of complication and likelihood of successful treatment.[13] Clearly, patients at a markedly increased risk deserve the observation currently available only in ICUs. If equivalent treatment of a developed complication can be reasonably expected in both routine care areas and the ICU, no advantage to ICU admission can be postulated. However, when delay in diagnosis or treatment can be predicted from the staffing and equipment levels currently available in a given hospital's routine care areas, ICU admission would seem warranted. After all, if ICUs were created by clustering expensive equipment and knowledgeable and experienced personnel, we must consider what was left behind: routine care areas without extra equipment and staffed by persons neither trained nor experienced in the management of problems now routinely confined to the ICU. In fact, this effect on routine care areas was considered to be one of the detrimental effects of the development of ICUs.[13]

GENERIC GOALS OF INTENSIVE CARE

We need a different perspective, a qualitative basis for categorizing patients depending on the generic goals of intensive care.[15] These categories were developed to distinguish patients from routine postoperative surgical patients but, in general, applied to all "specialty" ICU patients as well. The three categories are: monitoring/observation; extensive nursing requirements; and constant physician care. Patients are considered appropriate candidates for ICU admission for "just" monitoring and observation even if they are physiologically stable. These patients must have a recognized risk of complications and should be admitted when the likelihood of recognition and successful treatment is higher in the intensive care setting. The focus on cost containment has not been confined to the ICU. In fact, ICU staffing levels and equipment have generally been affected far less than in many other areas of the hospital. The reality is even worse; with a nationwide nursing shortage and crisis, both ICUs and routine care areas often have fewer nurses working than the number of positions allocated or planned staffing level.

Intensive monitoring and observation were never particularly easy or effective in routine care areas; after all, one of the earliest forms of intensive care in this country, the coronary care unit, was created to correct this deficiency. Monitoring and observation with early institution of effective treatment for simple, premonitory dysrhythmias have been well documented to reduce mortality. However, we must address the issue of monitoring and observation quantitatively as well as qualitatively. The patient:nurse ratio is 12:1 during the night shift in our regular hospital care areas. Allowing time for necessary administrative functions and his/her physiologic needs, the nurse has less than 30 minutes per shift available for any individual patient. This staffing pattern was designed *because* patients needing intensive observation and monitoring are now admitted to the ICU. Should these patients now be excluded from the ICU, the hospital will have to increase its staffing in the general care areas to provide the required monitoring and observation. This may be accomplished by establishing intermediate care areas or "overnight recovery rooms";[16] in practice, the same patients must be provided increased nursing surveillance outside the ICU. The particular "solution" is not the issue. Increased staffing and more equipment will be necessary to create the monitoring/observation environment, no matter where it is located or what name is used. Thus, the advantages of concentration underlying the initial conception of the ICU will be lost; the ICU will still be necessary for its other patients and the overall net result will be increased total hospital costs rather than the savings projected from the restricted viewpoint based on the likelihood of interventions. Monitoring/observation patients belong in today's ICU. Finally, medical coverage of these newly created areas will be deficient or lacking; this fact is commonly overlooked when administrators focus only upon physical space, beds, and nursing staff.

The same limitations apply to patients who need extensive nursing requirements. Frequent position changings, complex dressings, intake and output measurements, laboratory testing, and a myriad of additional nursing tasks are beyond the capabilities of the small nursing contingent now assigned to large care areas. The measures designed to improve efficiency which have been enacted over the past years clearly eliminated both the type and number of personnel necessary to accomplish these tasks; this was reasonable since these capabilities were included in the ICU as a part of the overall design. These patients make up approximately 60% of our patient population but are a most important focus for more than mere numbers.[17] These patients are generally physiologically stable; using most indices of severity, they were neither very sick nor very well. They constitute a large percentage of the daily ICU population for the following reasons. Patients in the monitoring/observation class may be discharged within a day or two and no longer need be considered. Patients requiring constant physician care, 10% to 20% of our population, can only stay in this category for a short period of time; thereafter, the acute abnormalities are resolved successfully, in which case they commonly enter the large extensive care category or, if therapy has been unsuccessful, these patients die. Although these remaining patients, the extensive care group, may be physiologically stable, careful monitoring and observation are always necessary. The complexity and frequency of nursing tasks that exceed the reasonable expectations of time available in general nursing units are the motivating force behind ICU admission. These patients remain in the ICU for extended periods and are subjected to many complications related to the primary admitting diagnosis, subsequent failure of initially functioning organ systems, especially related to the interrelationships among sepsis, immune function, and nutritional state, all of which create demands on nursing resources. Patients needing extensive nursing care must also be admitted to the ICU.

The third group is characterized as the patients requiring constant physician care. They are physiologically unstable, and physicians and nurses must remain at the bedside reacting to changes and implementing, validating, and refining further therapy. They conform to the popular image of intensive care because of the elements of high technology, rapid but efficient activity, crises, and perhaps, dramatic successes. There is no problem in the selection of these patients for ICU admission. Yet, even in these circumstances, once this acute stage passes, as it must, the reality includes other elements as well, such as the nearness of death and illnesses lasting months—because it is rare that the devastating illness resulting in their initial classification can resolve rapidly. It is this form of intensive care, prototypical in initial concept, that must now evolve beyond crisis orientation in both medical and nonmedical areas to develop consonance with evolving societal values.

IMMEDIATE OBJECTIVE: EXAMINE SOCIETAL VALUES

I believe that we must strive today to attain two immediate objectives for our patients and society as well as for ourselves. To do so, we must personally address the issue of the relationship between society's values and the goals of medicine, and secondly, we must examine our daily bedside practice to learn exactly what we have been doing. The relationship between the goals of medicine and societal values is developed in Chapter 3. Briefly, the goals of medicine, the preservation of life and the alleviation of suffering, are respectively derived from societal values of both the sanctity and quality of life. Today these two societal values are often in conflict. Because the passage from dying to death may almost be "frozen," resolution of the conflict becomes necessary. Prior to life support, death rapidly occurred, and there was no real problem. Of course, the conflict existed; however, it was so rare or short-lived that nothing needed to be done about it. Resolution did *not* occur; however, the conflict *disappeared* with the death of a patient. However, now we must make a choice. There seems to be an increasing recognition of these conflicts and a growing tendency to evaluate quality of life both within the medical profession and society in general. When there is objective medical evidence in an individual case that the disease is irreversible, and if we feel confident that this information is truly perceived and understood by the patient or family (in the case of an incompetent patient), we can more easily accept their choice which is the third element of informed consent. We will also feel more confident if we have either direct or indirect evidence (from the family) of the patient's values and wishes regarding quality of life decisions. Thus, we can align our goals of care with societal values for this patient both before and after our recognition that further medical care will be fruitless, that is, the patient's condition is irreversible. Up to this point, care is appropriately devoted to cure. Our therapeutic efforts can be successful, and we should strive for the preservation of life in concert with the societal value of sanctity of life. When our care cannot achieve cure, it is all too easy to sense failure and frustration but we actually have new and important goals for our caring efforts. Armed with conclusive knowledge of the irreversibility and specific information relating to this patient's perceived view of the quality of life, our continued care aligns the alleviation of suffering with the societal value of the quality of life. Pain and anxiety should be relieved, of course, but we must extend the concept of the alleviation of suffering to include efforts to aid the patient and family in adjusting to the nearness of death. When cure cannot be achieved, dying should not be prolonged with technology. If life cannot be extended with dignity and purpose, meaningless prolongation of dying is the inevitable outcome. This costly and ineffective utilization of resources during a patient's dying is neither necessary nor desirable for medicine, the patient, or society. This is my personal view, but I offer it for evaluation along with the views and projections of others (see Chap. 6). It is important to recognize that we live in a period of reevaluation and change. We must strive to understand all the potential consequences of this yet unresolved process.

DISTRIBUTIVE JUSTICE

Critical care today requires a focus beyond the needs of a specific patient and must encompass the total number of patients who could be considered eligible for care, given the number of available beds. Since the beds are so expensive, it is clear that the hospital cannot afford to maintain an excess of beds with available staffing to accommodate emergency admissions. However, since emergency admissions—though not the timing—are predictable, should all the existing care have already been allocated, some decision will have to be made to distribute resources in an ethical manner.

At the outset, however, it is important to remember that although the *problem* needs a solution, the *solution* may be effected step-by-step so that, in reality, no patient is deprived of necessary care. This process, however, usually requires creativity, cooperation, and a great deal of work to bring to a successful conclusion. In fact, a good portion of the day in many ICUs (mine included) is spent in just this fashion. The physical process of discharge can be accelerated (often hours elapse before the "recipient" bed on the floor can be emptied, while waiting for a family member to pick up a patient, or medications to be ready); the bed must be changed, the room must be cleaned, creating delays in waiting for housekeeping, actual transfer may be dependent on transport personnel, the personnel on the floor may wish to wait until after shift report, and so on. Other possible solutions include special duty nurses provided for patients who might require extra monitoring outside the unit, another ICU may temporarily "loan" a vacant bed, overnight care may be provided in a recovery room in place of ICU admission, extra nursing personnel may be enticed to work overtime or give up a day off, nursing personnel may be added to the unit's staff temporarily from another ICU, from the floor, supervisory personnel, or an agency, and even physicians have been recruited to provide independent and dependent nursing role functions. Using overtime or "day off" personnel, though sometimes necessary and possible, is a major factor in increasing the stress of daily ICU life since these crises, that is, more patients than can be cared for by the available assigned nursing staff, occur regularly because staffing cannot be predicated on the peak requirements. Continuously asking for double shifting and working on days off have been mentioned as factors leading to "burn out" or an inner pressure to resign from a position previously highly desired.

Unfortunately, no matter how creatively and diligently the participants work, new patients will arrive when all beds are full and all the temporizing measures have been exhausted. This serious problem has existed for the last 20 years despite the incredible expansion of the number of ICU beds during that era. In terms of the ethical principle of distributive justice, one method commonly and effectively used is "first come, first served." Care is apportioned to appropriate candidates seeking admission; these patients may continue to receive care until their outcome is determined. This seemingly simple principle was confounded during the evolution of critical care through the creation of the unprecedented prolonged dying state (see Chap. 2, "The What and When of Clinical Decision-Making"). The difficulty in making such choices was examined by the National Institutes of Health Consensus Development Conference on Critical Care Medicine in 1983.[13]

> It is not medically appropriate to devote limited ICU resources to patients without reasonable prospect of significant recovery when patients who

need those services and who have a significant prospect of recovery from acutely life-threatening disease or injury are being turned away due to lack of capacity. It is inappropriate to maintain ICU management of a patient whose prognosis has resolved to one of persistent vegetative state, and it is similarly inappropriate to employ ICU resources where no purpose will be served but a prolongation of the natural process of death.

These statements, I believe, are of great help in focusing attention on this difficult problem. However, some major difficulties remain; for instance, it is extremely difficult to define "without reasonable prospect of significant recovery" in most clinical situations. The actual numbers of patients who can be certified as brain dead are limited, and usually, because of the urgent need for rapidly harvesting organs, such determinations are made rapidly. Most of the prognostic indices lack the accuracy to make such a definitive diagnosis; indeed, if the data were present already, prolongation of dying would have been terminated so that the bed would have been available when the new patient arrived. It is also most difficult to develop consensus about a definition of "reasonable prospect." In our ICU, I poll the assembled residents, students, nurses, and other personnel during rounds about once a month concerning their desires to treat given certain mathematical probabilities of success. By starting at 1 chance to survive in 10 and 1 chance in 1,000,000, I can usually find full agreement to treat in the first and full agreement to stop treatment in the second case. Everyone also usually agrees not to treat if the probabilities of success are 1 in 100,000 or 1 in 10,000. There are some, nearly every rotation, who would wish to continue treatment if there were 1 chance in 1000 of success. At the same time, there are always individuals who would be willing to stop treatment if the chance of success were 1 in 100. Until more accurate predictors are available and until there is a consensus concerning "reasonable prospect," the problem will continue. Society seems to be wrestling with this problem today, having finally reached reasonable consensus concerning brain death (most, but not all states, now have statutes).

An even more difficult problem concerns distribution of limited care when the differences in outcome are only of degree, that is, when a patient with a 70% expected rate of recovery is compared to a patient with, perhaps, only *a realistic* 5% chance of survival. At the present time, it would seem that the only acceptable solution is to find an alternative rather than be confined to just an either/or choice as described. Some temporizing measure may be possible, perhaps until another patient recovers sufficiently for discharge or dies. The alternatives listed before, by the way, do not reflect all possible solutions. This exposition is not intended to resolve or solve the problem of limited resources and excessive demand. Rather, temporizing measures, creative thinking, extra effort, and cooperation will be necessary. This one problem has occupied more of my own professional life as an ICU director than any other. I see no reason to believe it will either be solved or even ameliorated in the immediate future.

IMMEDIATE OBJECTIVE: EXAMINE BEDSIDE CARE

Notwithstanding our present inability to predict accurately either the ultimate legal or ethical standing to be given to the "quality of life" viewpoint and the problem of distributive justice, we still must examine what we are doing today. I believe that many of our practices and habits increase costs but have no discernible effect on outcome.[17] Our high level of activity can be mistakenly interpreted as evidence of productivity. If this is true, then we can find and eliminate those elements which are unnecessary; we can, thus, alter practice without effecting the fundamentally necessary and important care functions. Francis Moore quoted E. D. Churchill who once made an analogy between the conduct of military operations and the conduct of surgical operations.[18] Churchill said that you must have a lot more of everything available than you will ever use to avoid disaster. Perhaps, in our overly enthusiastic application of high technology in medicine over the last years, a subtle error crept in so that his observation has been interpreted to mean that you *must use* everything available to you *all* the time to avoid disaster. We savor the term "the art of medicine" sometimes, I believe, to hide our ignorance of the logical steps hidden in the clinical decision-making process. We must achieve a better understanding of our clinical practice so that we can weed out the unnecessary from the necessary, preserving the quality of care and diminishing costs at the same time.

A crucial issue, however, is the ultimate effect of reducing costs in one part of an entire economic system. Francis Moore recently described surgical streams in the flow of health care financing, using a complex six-level model, tracing money invested in health care through our society.[18] He pointed out that attention is often mistakenly focused on just the budgets of the care providers and the expenditures of hospitals for hiring and buying. He later traces these dollars back into the general economy through the distribution of funds as investments, taxes, living expenses, and the income of vendors. Finally, all funds return to their source, the national economy, reposing in national wealth, government, and disposable income. Do efforts directed at improving efficiency in one sector indeed result in true savings? I believe that improved efficiency can occur when considered from the standpoint of the effects of our repeated interventions. I was stimulated by the observations of Eugene Robin who described four types of harm which result from unnecessary measurements and interventions.[19] All of these will be diminished when we weed out unnecessary activity from the truly important care functions. They include technical errors in the laboratory; an intervention based on an erroneous report may lead to direct harm. The second group is iatrogenic harm, which represents physical injuries to patients resulting from invasive procedures selected or performed inappropriately. Robin named a third category, iatrodemics, which he defined as the epidemic of systemic misdiagnosis or mismanagement of patients caused by the poor application of science or technology to patient management. This can be more simply stated as interpretive errors which lead to incorrect decisions. Finally, he described the fourth category which he called "informational overload," or too much information leading to a distortion of the correct identification and selection of proper priorities.

The improved efficiency of the utilization of resources and a better focus for the care of patients who are dying are both objectives attainable today. Diminishing unnecessary activity will both decrease complications and have salutary effects. Having more time to be with patients and their families will decrease our sense of failure and fulfill the important goal of caring. Physicians and nurses can return to thinking, assessing, and decision-making instead of frenetically ordering, reacting, and intervening which, I believe, accurately describes informational overload created by undue emphasis on high technology. In this way, we can respond to Fuch's exhortation that physicians consider the possibility of contributing more by doing less.[20] In responding, however, we must never forget that the societal, not merely economic, impact of medical care is our principal consideration. We must first contribute more by achieving a greater understanding of the medical care process. Only then can we know how to do less at the beside. We *can* and must distinguish between costly quality and high quality–they are not necessarily synonymous.

SIGNIFICANT INTERRELATIONSHIPS IN CRITICAL CARE

Objectives for critical care are more complex than the selection of patients for admission. Even this admission process is no longer a simple task, dependent on our skills as practitioners to recognize different degrees or severities of illness. Of course, this information is fundamental to the practice of intensive care. It is clear that the crisis orientation to disease no longer is the most significant feature of intensive care practice. At the risk of oversimplification, intensive care reflects interrelationships including (but not limited to): the patient and disease; the physician; the nurse; and the hospital. We will consider these interrelationships in greater detail for, I believe, they are of fundamental importance to understand the true meaning and value of intensive care. We must consider the position and function of the physicians assigned to the ICU (see Chap. 11, "ICU Fellowship: Blending Science and Art") and their relation to the patient's admitting or operating team (see Chap. 12, "Getting Along in the ICU: Physician Interrelationships"). The distribution of authority and responsibility within the ICU team will vary by hospital but certain observations related to level of experience and expectations for performance may facilitate both education and improved care. Shared responsibility is sometimes easy. In such cases, most often, a standardized plan and agreement exist ahead of time. When difficulties occur, it is common to "point fingers." The easiest direction to point, of course, is away from one's self. It is more likely, however, that problems arise in situations where there are no clear-cut answers. Deprived of a scientific basis for decision-making, we rely on bias and personality factors which end up having a more important role in deciding "who wins" than they should.

Everyone must enter the ICU for the first time and the "newcomer" must learn to join the team. Tribal customs are part of our human heritage; the ICU is no different. There are reasons, however, for testing: the "right" answers relate more to attitude and willingness than scientific or objective information (see Chap. 10, "Joining the Team"). The newcomer must also learn how previously learned habits, such as order writing, affect the functioning of the unit. Standing orders and policies are not intended to harass but are based on analyzed experience to effect continuity of care in an environment and for a work force that is constantly changing (see Chap. 15, "Allocating Nursing Care").

The patient and the family wrestle with a severity of illness and uncertainty of outcome that is often difficult to grasp. The approach to societal values and medical goals must undergo constant reevaluation. The legal and ethical implications of informed consent in the ICU are different from the circumscribed and controlled circumstances outside the unit, for instance, for contemplated elective surgery (see Chap. 4, "Informed Consent"). Despite every effort to transmit information to the patient and family, we are often perplexed at their reactions. Although an event such as death may be anticipated, the impact cannot, and adjustment can occur only after the fact. It is safe to say no matter how preparation is undertaken, the magnitude of the impact and its ramifications can never be accurately predicted by the care givers or the patient and family. We can do a great deal to ease the patient's and family's period of adjustment (see Chap. 13, "Understanding Reactions of Patient and Family," and Chap. 14, "Behavioral Disturbances in the ICU"). Finally, even though we may be replete with knowledge and technical skills as well as armed with information related to these other determinants of intensive care, our initial contact with the new patient will be facilitated if we have a suitable mental framework (see Chap. 17, "Accepting a New Admission").

CONCLUSION

It is a common axiom that to learn about the future we must often return to a study of the past. Instead of a restricted focus on technology in intensive care, we must reemphasize the marvelous therapeutic quality of the physician/patient relationship, the principle tool possessed by our predecessors. Medical "success" needs human dimensions to achieve fulfillment and be sustaining for both patient and staff. For the patient who survives we can make the experience less fearful. Indeed, we must remember that patients often completely "forget" their stay in the ICU, even though we can remember many "rational" conversations. Denial, the mind's defense against memories which cannot be tolerated, is most powerful. We need to remember how helpless the patient must feel. A sympathetic approach will help, but we should strive to diminish their dependency when possible by giving them some control (see Chaps. 13 and 14). For the dying patient, we will supply the only needs which matter and can be met, an easing of the lonely, frightening, and often painful transition to death. For society, we will preserve the scarce resources. For ourselves, as professionals, we will better understand the art of medicine and for ourselves, just those members of the human race who happen to have chosen medicine as a profession, we can more confidently approach the future, secure in the knowledge that our human qualities are society's greatest medical resource.

REFERENCES

1. Miller M: *Plain Speaking: An Oral Biography of Harry S Truman.* New York: Berkeley Publishing Group, 1973
2. Hook D: The Edwin Smith Surgical Papyrus. *Bull Cleveland Med Library Assoc* 1973; 20, 23
3. Preston RP: *The Dilemmas of Care: Social and Nursing Adaptations to the Deformed, the Disabled and the Aged.* New York: Elsevier, 1979
4. Bulkin W, Lukashok H: Rx for dying: The case for hospice. *N Engl J Med* 1988; 318, 376
5. Fein R: On measuring economic benefits of health programmes. In: McLachlan G, McKeown T (eds): *Medical History and Medical Care: A Symposium of Perspectives.* 179. London: Oxford University Press, 1971
6. Fogel R: United States General Accounting Office. Medicare: Past overuse of intensive care services inflates hospital payment. In *Report to the Secretary of Health and Human Services,* GAO/HRD-86-25, March 1986
7. Knaus WA: When is intensive care inappropriate? New "prognostic" measures provide answers. *Hospital Medical Quarterly* 1986; 14
8. Henning RJ, McClish D, Daly B, et al: Clinical characteristics and resource utilization of ICU patients: Implications for organization of intensive care. *Crit Care Med* 1987; 15:264
9. Stern RS, Epstein AM: Institutional responses to prospective payment based on diagnosis related groups: Implications for cost, quality, and access. *N Engl J Med* 1985; 312:621
10. Orwell G: *1984,* New York. Harcourt Brace Jovanovich, 1949
11. Avorn J: Benefit and cost analysis in geriatric care: Turning age discrimination into health policy. *N Engl J Med* 1984; 310:1294
12. Poe EA: The Facts in the Case of M. Valdemar. In Hubbard A (ed): *The Book of Poe.* New York, Doubleday, Doran & Co, 1934
13. Critical Care Medicine, Consensus Development Conference Summary, National Institutes of Health 1983; 4(6)
14. Civetta JM, Hudson–Civetta J, Nelson LD: Costly care: Data problems and proposing remedies (abstract). *Crit Care Med* 1985; 202: 524
15. Civetta JM: The inverse relationship between cost and survival. *J Surg Res* 1973; 14:265

16. Teres D, Steingrub J: Can intermediate care substitute for intensive care? *Crit Care Med* 1987; 15:280
17. Civetta JM, Hudson–Civetta JA: Maintaining quality of care while reducing charges in the ICU: 10 ways. *Ann Surg* 1985; 202:524
18. Moore FD: Surgical streams in the flow of health care financing. *Ann Surg* 1985; 201:132
19. Robin ED: A critical look at critical care. *Crit Care Med* 1983; 11:144
20. Fuchs VR: A more effective, efficient, and equitable system. *West J Med* 1976; 125:3

The What and When of Clinical Decision-Making

2

Joseph M. Civetta

*O*ur earliest exposure to clinical decision-making probably occurs when we are taught as medical students to construct a differential diagnosis at the end of the initial history and physical examination. At that time, the quality of our efforts was often judged by the length of the list, a rather superficial, quantitative index. Although this served a useful purpose, to link the patient's signs and symptoms with the previously memorized lists of signs and symptoms associated with various disease processes, prioritization may not have been an initial requirement. Thereafter, learning the prevalence of disease states, we might have prioritized our list in terms of the frequency of occurrence. This application of Willy Sutton's law was efficient in concentrating our attention to the most likely possibilities. Willy Sutton, the often captured bank robber, was once asked why he continued to rob banks. His answer was, "That's where the money is." While frequency is important, in certain "crisis" situations in the intensive care unit (ICU), reversibility (especially with mechanical problems) must be placed at the top of the list. For example, hypoxemia caused by a disconnected ventilator can be–and must be–rapidly reversed if it is detected; it will only be detected in time if it heads the list of possibilities. Hypoxemia due to acute respiratory diseases may be more common but reversible entities should be considered first.

Later, as we became more familiar with a diagnostic evaluation, we may have learned to construct decision trees or to proceed through the list of potential diagnoses using algorithms. Thus, bleeding in a postoperative patient can be divided into surgical and nonsurgical causes, and nonsurgical bleeding can be analyzed in terms of defects in primary and secondary mechanisms of coagulation. This approach, too, is useful at the beginning of the process of clinical decision-making. However, neither the list of differential diagnoses nor even a set of complex algorithms can fully capture the essence of clinical decision-making in intensive care because decision-making is a process which evolves through the accumulation of additional information and is influenced by the passage of time. It cannot, therefore, be adequately portrayed at a single instant or in a single representation any more than a single picture of the start or even the finish of a race can convey the essence of the race from the moment after the start to the moment before the finish. Clinical decision-making must be a process of many steps based on elements gathered over time. Some of the information must be gleaned from the past, providing the basis of decisions made in the present and forming the framework for plans for the future. The process can be viewed from separate vantage points during the passage of time to assess the objectives of therapy and the results attained. Reevaluations are necessary and desirable as the perception of the patient's illness evolves, resulting in realistic appraisals at each succeeding stage. These two determinants of decision-making coalesce to form a continuously changing perception in the mind of the clinician. Elements are added and deleted, augmented and subtracted, weighted or discounted, appreciated or unrecognized, or incorrectly assessed. It is no wonder, in this ever-changing and poorly delineated process, that we consider clinical decision-making to be a part of the art of medicine. Because of these changes and uncertainties, we may feel that clinical decision-making is not science. Rather, it bespeaks the necessity to learn more about the process so that decision-making, once identified and understood, can be synthesized into a cohesive whole, thus providing a scientific basis. First, however, we must describe and analyze the elements in clinical care and the sequence of vantage points over time.

ELEMENTS OF CLINICAL CARE

Analysis of clinical care can distinguish the following elements: the health care status of the patient; newly acquired diseases and complications; selection and sequencing of the diagnostic evaluation; an assessment of the likely effects of therapy; a clinical decision (identification of the problem and selection of therapy); short-term and long-term objectives; changes in the diagnosis and therapy influenced by acquisition of new information; and definition of outcome.

HEALTH CARE STATUS OF THE PATIENT

General demographic information such as sex, age, and other socioeconomic variables are available but provide limited insight into the management of a unique, individual patient. Usable knowledge concerning the impact of preexisting chronic disease states is at a rudimentary stage in intensive care. Although we know that an elderly patient with diabetes, hypertension, and arteriosclerosis may tolerate surgery poorly, we do not have the ability to quantitate either the degree of functional impairment or the subsequent effect on total health status. The data are only qualitative and do not have discriminatory ability.[1,2] Individual variation is so great and objectives for therapy differ according to the perception of the physician and the desires of the patient so that this information presently is of little value to aid even the selection of patients who are appropriate for admission to the ICU. However, such qualitative assessments may help in the selection of patients for preoperative invasive monitoring.[3,4] In patients who are considered at high risk, this qualitative judgment is often satisfactory even if strict quantitation is not possible.

NEWLY ACQUIRED DISEASES AND COMPLICATIONS

Because of the tremendous variability among patients who appear to have similar disease states and the large number of specific circumstances that occur infrequently, quantitative methods of ascertaining the impact of acquired diseases and complications cannot be used to predict outcome in an individual case. Numerous scoring systems have been devised and are discussed more extensively in Chapter 9, "Prediction and Definition of Outcome in a Cost-Sensitive Era." This failing is not inherent in the studies themselves or because of limited data collection but, rather, the multifactorial impact of known, expected, and unexpected happenings may preclude a predictive model of sufficient validity to use in an individual case. In general terms, these indices easily separate the easily separable, that is, patients who are healthy and have low expected mortality are usually predicted to survive, whereas patients with profound physiologic derangements in many organ systems usually die. However, quantitation in these instances has little to offer in clinical decision-making because results are equally predictable to experienced *and* inexperienced clinicians.[5,6] Patients not clearly separable by clinical decision-making unfortunately fall into the area of overlap between survival and death of the predictive indices.[7] However, it may be more important to recognize the determinants of outcome at different stages in the patient's ICU course; this matter is discussed as the basis for the temporal vantage points.

Low prevalence-high impact discriminators have usually been identified in multivariant analyses (*e.g.*, oliguric renal failure and coma).[8] Today, it may be more important to understand the high prevalence factors which result in high resource utilization even if they have a low impact on outcome because they may greatly contribute to cost without a demonstrable effect on outcome.

SELECTION AND SEQUENCING OF THE DIAGNOSTIC EVALUATION

There is a vast and ever-increasing number of potentially useful diagnostic tests. Particularly in intensive care, many of these tests may be used repetitively. Often the explosion of utilization has been glibly attributed to a better awareness on the part of physicians and nurses to use these tests of proven superiority to traditional history-taking and physical examination. However, the proper timing, sequence, and repetition of diagnostic testing have not been assessed by outcome criteria. Given the absence of a scientific basis for selection of initial and subsequent laboratory testing, methods have been devised and tested to control laboratory testing.[9] Interestingly, more than half the tests could be eliminated in patients with the same severity of illness in the same proportions without affecting the time spent in the ICU or survival. These guidelines (see Chap. 9, "Prediction and Definition of Outcome in a Cost-Sensitive Era") should encourage further scrutiny in both the selection and sequencing of subsequent testing. In terms of efficiency, many tests are often selected initially. This removes the possibility of omission, and may be justified to speed both diagnosis and management. It may be far cheaper and certainly faster to order a $50 specific laboratory test in all patients at the same time or in place of a cheaper screening test, even if half the group would be eliminated by the screening test, *if* simultaneous testing could eliminate an extra day of ICU care in the other half. Thinking rather than automatic behavior is the key to eliminating unnecessary testing, without creating unnecessary delays.

AN ASSESSMENT OF THE LIKELY EFFECTS OF THERAPY

We must constantly evaluate the possible forms of therapy in terms of the projected benefits and risks inherent in the therapy itself and as influenced by the patient's current health status and disease state. Of perhaps greater importance in the ICU is the distinction between "therapeutic" interventions and "manipulation." Therapy implies a chance for cure, which means there must be evidence linking an improved outcome to the application of this remedy. It is for this reason that prospective randomized trials are considered to be a proper method of evaluating new forms of therapy. On the other hand we might consider "manipulation" as the minute-to-minute response to abnormalities in physiologic variables based on a constant stated or unstated desire to return as many to the normal range in as short a period of time as possible (at least in time for morning rounds). Orders to keep the pulmonary artery occlusion pressure between 16 and 18 mm Hg or to maintain the serum potassium concentration at 4.0 ± 0.3 meq/liter are never actually written or intended but seem to be discernible bedside habits which I have observed in many ICUs (including mine) which have no effect on outcome and result only in increased costs and poor utilization of both nursing and laboratory personnel. Unfortunately, this form of "manipulation" is standard practice. We all were trained this way, but must fight against continuing this practice.

A CLINICAL DECISION

After assessing the patient's health status, recognizing newly acquired diseases or complications, selecting the proper diagnostic tests and their sequencing, and evaluating the potential forms of therapy, a discrete clinical decision is necessary. In fact, this decision, seemingly central and fundamental to care, is rarely evident in the medical record. Progress notes contain observations and data; rarely are impressions and judgments delineated clearly.[10] If the preceding four elements are analyzed and synthesized, the art of clinical decision-making will have been replaced, at least in part, by science. To the degree that this process has not been completed in the minds of the clinician, we may expect that the medical record will lack evidence of the decision-making. Conversely, we can view the current emphasis on adequate documentation as an additional force serving to stimulate clinical decision-making (see Chap. 8, "Avoiding Legal Problems").

SHORT-TERM AND LONG-TERM OBJECTIVES

It is important to identify our expectations for treatment. We must also recognize that immediate objectives may be attained without the desired long-term effect. For instance, a patient in shock may be profoundly hypovolemic. Volume expansion is selected and implemented. The hypovolemia may be corrected and, indeed, cardiac function may improve. Much later, the patient may develop sepsis and die. The short-term objectives were correctly identified and attained through the process of clinical decision-making. The failure to achieve long-term success should not necessarily be construed as evidence of improper decision-making. Recently, invasive monitoring has been criticized[11] because these important limiting interrelationships were not perceived. The failure to obtain a long-term objective should not be used as criticism of a technique that may only be directed at short-term objectives, such as improvement in cardiac function. The evolution of objectives is also part of the temporal framework of clinical decision-making.

ACQUISITION OF NEW INFORMATION

The changing nature of the decision-making process reflects the effects of diseases during evolution, changes created by the introduction of therapy, and the subsequent development of other complications. Thus, it is necessary to acquire new information and reassess both the choice of diagnosis and the effects of therapy. The continually updated decision will also be influenced by the passage of time and the selection of objectives appropriate to the evolved state of illness and response.

DEFINITION OF OUTCOME

Immediate results are gratifying but infrequent. Crises commonly reflect acute cardiorespiratory and oxygen transport problems. Clearly, initial success may not be sustained, and death may occur in the ICU or even after discharge. However, an evaluation of long-term outcome must form part of the process of initiation of therapy even in cases characterized as crises. Even in cases of cessation of cardiac activity, there are two immediate diagnoses possible: cardiac arrest or death of the patient. If a judgment is made that the patient died, clearly, cardiopulmonary resuscitation would be inappropriate. We must incorporate long-term objectives into early decision-making.

It is difficult, at times, to comprehend or formalize the "benefits" of critical care. Survival in patients who otherwise would die is one, and quite a limited, criterion of evaluation. Patients may have improved quality of life, referenced to the state of acute illness and *not necessarily* the prior state of health. Life may be extended but it may not be the same life expectancy as before the onset of the catastrophic illness. The benefit depends in large part upon the patient's perception of the value of the resulting quality and duration of life, relative to that which was associated with the worst state in the ICU, not life prior to the onset of the illness.

We cannot delay current clinical decisions awaiting future improvements reflecting advances in the science of decision-making. Rather, an understanding of the elements which must be synthesized will lead us to a more thoughtful and disciplined approach. We must also step back and evaluate the process itself once it has been completed. Too often, under pressure to move forward to the next urgent case, we neglect to evaluate the flow of decision-making. Even mortality and morbidity conferences tend to focus on specifics rather than process. Clarity of understanding, improved communication, and better documentation in the medical record are immediate, obtainable objectives.

THE INFLUENCE OF TIME

Many methods have been proposed to assess severity of illness and risk of death or outcome variables such as sepsis or other complications. The groups studied include trauma patients, all ICU admissions, elective surgical candidates, patients for cancer surgery, and patients given a preoperative nutritional assessment. Parameters were found to be effective in prediction for each specific group of patients. Although it had been hoped that the vast mass of data, when subjected to proper statistical techniques in sufficient quantities, would quantify the degree of illness and predict the likelihood of recovery prospectively, these expectations have not been realized.[12] While it was hoped that precise mathematical models could replace the uncertainties of clinical judgement, this prior uncertainty reflected that outcome is often determined by the unpredictable occurrence of catastrophic events, development of new illnesses or complications, iatrogenic events, and, especially, ultimate failure of organ systems functioning early in the patient's course. These same events must affect the reliability of all mathematical predictive systems.

However, we can still examine the predictive indices or scoring systems to extract the important elements at each temporal vantage point. Combined with the elements of the clinical care process, we can focus our attention on the relevant physiologic processes which have the greatest effect on survival at that vantage point (Table 2-1). In this way, clinical decision-making is concerned with appropriateness of therapy given the existing circumstances for *this* patient at *this* point in the illness. We must consider decision-making in the context of effecting a balance between the probable effects of disease and the wishes and values of the patient. Algorithms describing the disease apart from the patient can only give an incomplete picture.

TABLE 2-1.   Clinical Decision-Making—The Influence of Time

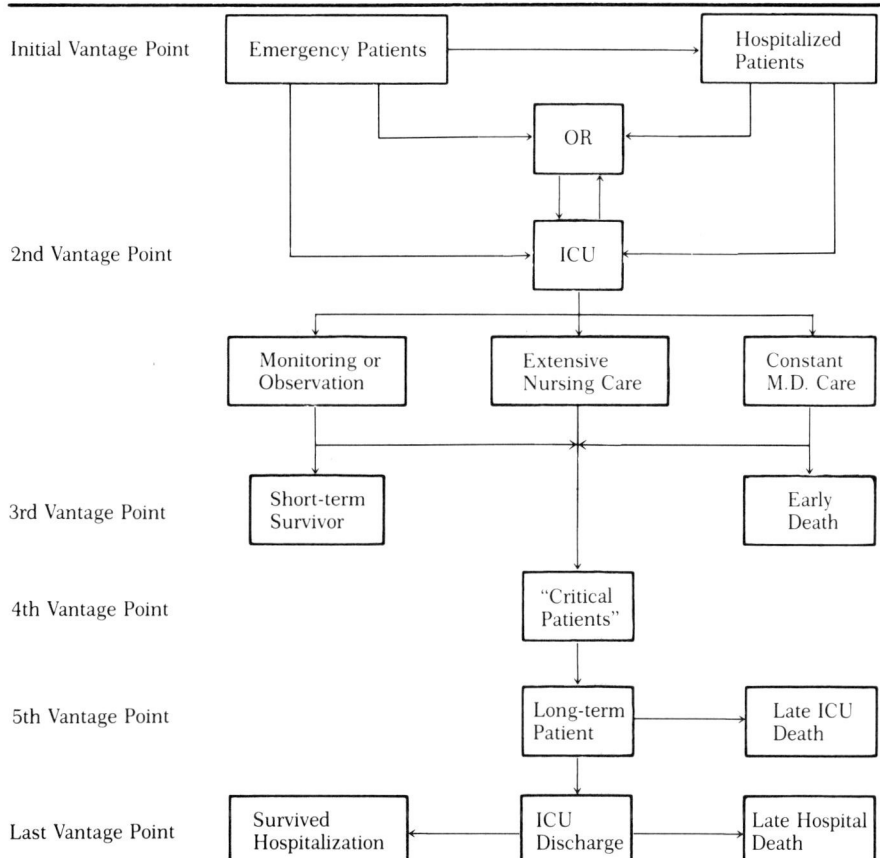

FIRST VANTAGE POINT: SOURCE OF ADMISSIONS

We should consider patients admitted from emergency and elective sources separately. Emergency patients have a higher mortality rate and serve to draw our special attention because of their initial acuity; thus, the important parameters to help decision-making are usually related to cardiorespiratory integrity. Further, little may be known or there may be little time to amass other relevant information. In contrast, elective (usually surgical preoperative) patients are in a stable state even if chronic illness is present; further, their course will be based on the capacity to withstand future physiologic stress (physiologic reserve) rather than the capacity to respond to existing stress which characterizes the emergency patients.

The greatest wealth of analyzed data exists for the multitrauma patient. Many scales have been developed primarily for the purpose of triage within trauma systems. They usually rely on simple measurements to be performed by paramedics or other non-physicians. The scores include the Triage Index,[13]

Trauma Score,[14] Trauma Index,[15] Illness–Injury Severity Index or IISI,[16] and Circulation, Respiration, Abdomen, Motor, and Speech (CRAMS).[17] The number of variables, therefore, is relatively small and there is considerable overlap as seen in Table 2-2. These factors are important because the multicellular organism depends on integrated function of the cardiorespiratory system to transport oxygen from the environment to the individual cells. Thus, both cardiac and respiratory functions are necessary components as are end-organ functions, particularly the central nervous system. In analyzing the results of 2000 patients categorized by the Trauma Score, there is a clear relationship between the expected mortality and degree of abnormality.[14] We can judge severity and design our interventions based on this assessment. For instance, patients with pulmonary contusion or flail chest present with disorders in the respiratory components and need continuous positive airway pressure or mechanical ventilation. Patients with multiple fractures may suffer cardiovascular instability and manifest significant bleeding. The closed-head injury will cause derangement of the neurologic components necessitating careful monitoring of the evolving neurologic status.

With respect to other types of emergencies such as gastrointestinal

TABLE 2-2. Components of Trauma Scoring System

COMPONENT	INDEX
Respiratory system	Trauma Index, Illness–Injury Severity Index, CRAMS
Expansion	Triage Index, Trauma Score
Rate	Trauma Score
Cardiovascular	Trauma Index
Blood pressure	Trauma Score, Illness–Injury Severity Index
Pulse	Illness–Injury Severity Index
Central nervous system	Trauma Index
Eye opening	Triage Index, Trauma Score
Motor response	Triage Index, Trauma Score, CRAMS
Verbal response	Triage Index, Trauma Score, CRAMS
Level of consciousness	Illness–Injury Severity Index
Perfusion	
Capillary refill	Triage Index, Trauma Score, CRAMS
Skin color	Illness–Injury Severity Index
Other*:	
Age	Illness–Injury Severity Index
Mechanism of injury	Illness–Injury Severity Index
Region of injury	Illness–Injury Severity Index, CRAMS

* Age, mechanism, and perhaps other factors of injury used in combination with Trauma Score and others for purposes of triage.

inflammation, obstruction, or perforation, distribution of patients within a community has not yet been seen as a problem; no similar triaging instruments exist. However, similar types of abnormalities in cardiorespiratory integrity and end-organ function exist. For instance, the decision for urgent operation in patients with bowel obstruction and metabolic acidosis is made because of the derangement in cellular oxygen utilization suggestive of ischemic or infarcted bowel.

Although elective patients usually have stable cardiorespiratory function and oxygen transport before surgery, some of these functions, as well, will be incorporated into decision-making in the postoperative period. However, of greater interest are descriptors of organ system function and physiologic reserve. Using similar statistical methodology to the evolution of trauma triage instruments, various measures of nutritional status as predictors of both sepsis and mortality have been tested. Some of the components also reflect hepatic function. Since multiple organ system failure and sepsis are common clinical syndromes in patients who die after elective surgery, again, it is not surprising that these indices tend to be relatively similar and reasonably simple in construction. Three representative instruments are the Prognostic Nutritional Index,[18] Hospital Prognostic Index,[19] and Sepsis-Related Mortality.[20] The components used are listed in Table 2-3. It is interesting that of all the complex measurements of immune response and hepatic function possible, serum albumin levels and delayed-type hypersensitivity skin test response were found to be important predictors in all three instruments; the less reactivity and the lower the albumin, the higher was the risk of complications, sepsis, and mortality.

Patients considered to have compromised hemodynamic function are often admitted to the ICU preoperatively for invasive hemodynamic monitoring and assessment of the physiologic reserve of the cardiovascular system. Creation of the physiologic profile also incorporates measurements used in the prehospital trauma score. However, the data base also includes other

TABLE 2-3. Components of Nutrition–Immune Function Prognostic Instruments

COMPONENT	INSTRUMENT*
Triceps skin fold	PNI
Albumin	PNI, HPI, SRM
Transferrin	PNI
Delayed hypersensitivity†	PNI, HPI, SRM
Sepsis/cancer†	HPI
Age/sex	SRM

* Common elements in three prognostic instruments: PNI = Prognostic Nutritional Index[18]; HPI = Hospital Prognostic Index[19]; SRM = Sepsis-related mortality.[20]
† Definitions of delayed hypersensitivity and value assigned to diagnoses are different, although the categories are similar.

TABLE 2-4. *Physiologic Profile: Measured Parameters**

CARDIOVASCULAR	RESPIRATORY
Cardiac output	Hemoglobin
Systematic arterial pressure	Inspired O_2 tension
Heart rate	Arterial O_2 tension
Pulmonary arterial pressure	Arterial CO_2 tension
Left ventricular filling pressure	Arterial O_2 saturation
Right ventricular filling pressure	Venous O_2 tension
Height and weight	Venous O_2 saturation

* Parameters obtained by direct measurements including intravascular pressures and blood gases (requires pulmonary artery catheterization).

parameters of cardiorespiratory function which require invasive monitoring (Table 2-4). These are also used to calculate oxygen transport and utilization parameters which together form the basis of the decisions at the first vantage point.

In addition to this assessment of baseline function, a step-wise approach to analysis of physiologic reserve has also been used.[3] *Step 1.* If patients are considered to have compromised hemodynamic function, invasive monitoring is used preoperatively. *Step 2.* If there is evidence of inadequate baseline function, such as decreased cardiac output or left ventricular stroke work, increased oxygen extraction, or inadequate oxygen delivery, augmentation of ventricular function using preload, manipulation of after-load by vasodilators, and augmentation of contractility may be attempted. *Step 3.* If none of the above measures can improve function and oxygen delivery remains diminished, the risk of developing cardiac complications and potential mortality is considered to be extremely high. However, 95% of patients can be rendered suitable candidates for the intended surgery using this approach.[3,4]

Deterioration in clinical status may occur in the hospitalized patient. The parameters of sudden clinical deterioration necessitating emergency intensive care admission usually are related to similar cardiorespiratory and oxygen transport values in other emergency patients.

SECOND VANTAGE POINT: UPON ICU ADMISSION

Patients admitted to the ICU have one factor in common, an increased risk of mortality. Thus, in our process of clinical decision-making, we must examine the factors correlated with mortality. We will find that the majority of predictors based on mortality use measurements common to critically ill patients.

Patients may be received directly from surgery or the emergency room because of existing instability or the likelihood of postoperative complications. Furthermore, patients can be directly admitted to prepare for both elective and emergency surgery using the ICU appropriately to assess and correct preexisting physiologic abnormalities so that the surgical procedures can then be performed more safely. Although the specific disease, the patient's physiologic reserve, and the presence of chronic diseases may all complicate the evaluation of the overall degree of illness in an individual patient, the most important components which influence immediate survival again reflect cardiorespiratory function and oxygen transport. On the other hand, in patients without major acute physiologic derangements, parameters reflecting the immune system, liver, kidneys, and nutritional state have the best predictive value and, therefore, are of more use in the clinical decision.

THIRD VANTAGE POINT: SHORT-TERM ICU OUTCOME

The relationships among mortality rate, duration of intensive care stay, and severity of illness are complex. In surgical ICUs, a significant number of patients are admitted for monitoring/observation and have short ICU stays. A small number of patients are so critically ill that they die despite all efforts within the same short time frame. The mortality *rate* for short-term ICU admissions is low since it reflects the relatively few patients who die and the large number of the monitoring/observation patients who live. Clinical decision-making is relatively easy for both groups: little needs to be done for the monitoring/observation group and everything must be done for the most critical group, but usually it is only possible to intervene for a short time.[21] The mortality rate for patients who have long ICU admissions is much higher, commonly approaching 50%.[22] One might mistakenly conclude that long ICU admissions correlate with a higher severity of illness. This is not true because the short-term ICU admission group actually contains the patients with the most severe illnesses. The long-term group is the most problematic especially to differentiate between what we want to do (a lot) in order, somehow, to achieve success and what we should or must do, which may be much less or even, at times, nothing. Our sense of urgency to effect outcome may not be satisfied, but our actions will be appropriate.

We must distinguish between the aphorism of our training focusing on crisis orientation, "Don't just stand there, do something" and, when we realize that death is inevitable, "Don't just do something, stand there." Decision-making becomes all the more difficult when dealing with these in-between patients. Collection of information from both medical and patient-related sources must continue to allow reassessment and reappraisal of both risks and benefits. The longer the illness and the graver the prognosis, the less medicine has to offer and the greater the weight should be given to the patient's choice based on personal values (see Chap. 4, "Informed Consent").

Most patients admitted for monitoring/observation do not and should not develop complications; therefore, the following day they are safely discharged to routine care areas. This decision is usually easy. In a certain number of cases, however, problems will develop; these patients may then require an increased level of nursing and physician care as well as an increased duration which also correlates with higher costs.[21] Patients with the highest degrees of abnormal cardiac, respiratory, and oxygen transport function will have not only a high mortality rate but also a short duration of intensive care before death occurs. Clinically, these patients are clearly the most severely ill and not surprisingly are so judged by predictive instruments. Therefore, we must determine the basis of the indices which can distinguish short-term survivors from early deaths. We can then focus on the identified components to direct our decision-making.

The Acute Physiology Score and Chronic Health Evaluation (APACHE) was introduced in 1981.[2] Initially, 34 physiologic measurements were obtained from the patient's clinical records; additionally, a four-category designation of preadmission health status was made. More recently, the APACHE II was developed, which was compressed to 12 routine physiologic measurements plus age and previous health status.[23] The Therapeutic Intervention Scoring System (TISS) assigned point values in a similar fashion to APACHE but to interventions rather than physiologic abnormalities.[24] Patterns of evolving cardiorespiratory function in surviving and nonsurviving patients were the basis of a third instrument.[25] While the two previous indices had subjective weights assigned to the variables, actual measurements form the basis of the third predictive system. Finally, simple variables available at the time of admission were analyzed mathematically to form the basis of the fourth instrument.[8] Except for the complete listing of therapeutic interventions in TISS, the other three instruments contain approximately 12 individual components; seven of them appear in at least two, and four of them appear in all three instruments (Table 2-5). This similarity underscores the fundamental biologic necessity for delivery of oxygen and cellular utilization. The fact that these parameters are few and have important statistical value support the need for early and intense monitoring of cardiorespiratory function as well as oxygen transport. These parameters, then, will be included in the diagnostic testing; the values serve as the basis of the selection of interventions. Reassessment in terms of short-term objectives will be based on the demonstrated response to the chosen intervention.

FOURTH VANTAGE POINT: CONTINUED ICU CARE

Since outcome has already been decided for patients with the least and most degrees of severity, the ICU now contains patients midway along the severity spectrum.[21] Mortality rates will be higher and, of course, halfway along the severity spectrum the mortality rate should be 50%, because the severity spectrum starts with patients with the least degree of illness (the mortality rate approaches zero) and as a continuum extends to the most severe, those with lethal illnesses (with mortality rates approaching 100%).

These patients may also be considered "critical." The distinction between those patients who will live and those who will ultimately die is impossible to achieve on admission; time and intervention will both be

TABLE 2-5. *Common Elements in Acute Severity Indices*

ELEMENT	INDICES
Cardiovascular	
Blood pressure	APACHE II, TISS, CRV, MLR
Heart rate	APACHE II, TISS, CRV, MLR
Cardiac output	TISS, CRV
Respiratory	
Arterial oxygenation	APACHE II, TISS, CRV, MLR
Neurologic function	APACHE II, TISS, MLR
Oxygen transport	
Hemoglobin	APACHE II, CRV
Bicarbonate/*p*H	APACHE II, TISS, CRV, MLR
Renal function	APACHE II, TISS, MLR

* APACHE II = Acute Physiology Score and Chronic Health Evaluation, Knaus[23]; TISS = Therapeutic Intervention Scoring System, Cullen[24]; CRV = cardiorespiratory variables, Shoemaker[25]; MLR = multiple logistic regression, Lemeshow[8]. Note that TISS reflects therapeutic interventions chosen to affect listed variables.

necessary to achieve resolution or separate these groups. Decision-making is both more difficult and more necessary. "Critical" in this context should be used to underscore the need for effective intervention and the realization that such intervention does not produce immediate results; rather, a successful outcome can only be determined after a considerable investment of time. In a study of long-term patients, the average duration of stay was approximately 3 weeks in both patients who ultimately lived and died.[21] If resolution took this length of time, it is clear that the initial physiologic state must have been similar in both groups. When APACHE II and TISS were calculated repetitively, statistical separation of those who ultimately survived from those who died was only possible after 2 weeks of applied interventions. Since these patients are midway along the severity spectrum and since outcome was not determined for weeks, it is clear that indices designed to assess patients early in their course and heavily weighted to cardiorespiratory and oxygen transport parameters cannot characterize the events which ultimately determine outcome in this small subgroup (7% of total) of patients. On the other hand, these patients used 35% of the total patient days of care. Decision-making is a long and arduous problem balancing benefits and resource utilization. A predictive index must be based on data available at the time it is calculated. The events that actually determine outcome, evolution of the illness, unforeseen illnesses or complications, and especially, failure of organs functioning earlier, have not yet been "predicted"; decision-making depends on constant data gathering and reappraisal. The ICU patient is not like a train with both destination and direction fixed by the tracks. Rather, the patient's course must be "driven" by clinical judgment much as a car is guided through traffic and around obstacles.

FIFTH VANTAGE POINT: LONG-TERM ICU PATIENTS

Obviously, resource utilization is an important focus, but we must remember that our decision now must include what *not* to do as well as what to do. The long-term patients are midway along the severity spectrum and survival rates approximate 50%. We must continue to treat these patients since we recognize that the degree of physiologic abnormality, using our best quantitative methods, is not particularly high nor is there any accurate way of predicting outcome. The uncertainty of outcome affects the patients, their families, and the ICU staff. Since oxygen transport and cardiorespiratory parameters are not grossly deranged, it should be clear that usual ICU interventions, such as cardiovascular monitoring/interventions and ventilatory support, have little to offer these patients. We must remember that we have little true treatment to offer when renal, hepatic, and immune function deteriorate despite maintaining cardiorespiratory function and nutritional support.

We must temper our desire to use the "technological imperative," that is, to use continually everything in the therapeutic armamentarium until the moment of death. We must also recognize the impact of the uncertainty of outcome on the patient and family as well. Our desire to restore health to all of our patients must face the reality that nearly 50% of these patients ultimately die. Rather than view this as failure, we must include a new factor in our decisions, a perspective based on achieving good from our medical interventions in all cases.

We must remember that there are two principles or goals of medical care (see Chap. 3, "Life and Death in the ICU: Ethical Considerations"). The first, which is consonant with the primary goal of intensive care, is the preservation of life. The second, more important in these patients, is the alleviation of suffering. As prognosis worsens, we must make decisions to strive for the alleviation of suffering and, again, depart from the illness-based algorithm approach which concentrates only on diagnosis and treatment.

Based upon the realization that death is an increasingly likely possibility in the long-term patients, and recognizing the limitation of early physiologic assessors for differentiating between patients who ultimately live or die, we must look to more basic and fundamental biologic processes, such as methods of quantitating protein metabolism and immune function. They can reflect the ability of the host to heal and resist sepsis as well as reveal vital organ system function; these are often the capabilities which differentiate success from failure in prolonged and critical illness. The multiple organ failure syndrome is seen to have a metabolic basis in substrate–energy failure.[26] Many, if not most, of these long-term patients have primarily or secondarily developed the sepsis syndrome. Analysis of long-term patients who survived and died showed significant differences [27] such that patients who later succumbed could be identified more than a week before death with a high degree of certainty (Table 2-6). Note that many of these variables occur as a

TABLE 2-6. Surviving and Dying Septic Patients: Discriminators and Nondiscriminators

DIFFERENCES	NO DIFFERENCES
Urea	pH
Lactate	Pa_{O_2}
Z* nonessential amino acids	Systematic blood pressure
α-Aminobutyrate	Heart rate
Glucagon	Respiratory rate
Z valine	
Z aspartate	
Z glutamine	
Glucose	

(Adapted from Moyer[27])
* Z = fractional concentration of total group of amino acids rather than absolute amount of particular listed component. Note that common components used in early predictors were of no value in these patients.

result of the failures in substrate metabolism, including increased urea, lactate, and glucose. However, the differences presently serve only to underscore the fundamental defects in metabolic pathways that are beyond our capacity to influence. The majority of the parameters that have been found to be discriminatory in these patients are not related to acute cardiorespiratory dysfunction nor to the types of bedside assessment which were so prevalent in the early predictors and are deemed so responsive to active early ICU treatment. Our decision-making now has a different tone, direction, and even destination, at times.

We must redirect our efforts from the common technological ICU procedures to measures to alleviate the patient's suffering as we support the patient and await resolution based on the patient's ability to restore normal metabolic processes or, if this is impossible, to succumb ultimately. We must maintain efforts. We must continue our support. But we also have an equal imperative to avoid unnecessary manipulations which cannot influence the outcome and can only prolong dying, increasing stress to patients and families, and draining already limited ICU resources.

LAST VANTAGE POINT: DISCHARGE FROM INTENSIVE CARE

Our last, important clinical decision is made to effect discharge from the ICU. One might believe that if discharge were delayed until all major physiologic abnormalities had been resolved, patients would continue their recuperation in a routine hospital area and be discharged. However, 20% of the deaths in our ICU population occurred in the period between discharge from the ICU and hospital discharge. Because we rarely discharge dying patients to the floor, these deaths occurred in patients considered well enough to be discharged with an expectation of survival, yet they died during their subsequent hospitalization. Thus, the decision for discharge is not easy, even given resolution of the acute physiologic abnormalities prompting admission. Certain problems, the late dysrhythmia or pulmonary embolism, may develop *de novo*. However, respiratory arrest soon after ICU discharge in a patient treated for respiratory failure may represent a poorly formulated decision. Our decisions must incorporate more than an appraisal of the risk of death. Many patients survive hospitalization only to be permanently placed in nursing homes or to undergo chronic hospitalization for severe physical and mental impairments. Thus, social and societal parameters must enter our decision-making process and, at this stage, are more important than physiologic measurements. This has important implications for our care. Once again, high technology and repeated measurements, which are often important when significant physiologic abnormalities are the immediate determinants of outcome, must be restrained. Our decisions must be guided by an understanding that our role in caring for the patient may have to focus on a process of educating the patient and family with respect to short- and long-term prognosis. This direction will vary according to the stage of the illness and the likelihood of successful outcome (see Chap. 4, "Informed Consent"). In general, the higher the expected mortality rate or the greater the change in quality of life, the more important it is to provide this information in a sympathetic and understanding way so that the patients or, in the case of incompetent patients, the family, can properly exercise its autonomy to choose the course most consistent with the patient's values. It is important to preserve the patient's desires with regard to quality of life, but because the chain of events can rarely be foreseen ahead of time, we should explore these issues before hospitalization or operation whenever possible. This is especially relevant when we are dealing with elderly patients with chronic diseases and specific diagnoses which have low success rates, such as carcinoma of the stomach or lung. We should recognize that information concerning quality of life that would be vital to know during prolonged illness is often unobtainable at that time. We must, therefore, include such deliberations in our preoperative evaluation, giving these patients the opportunity to consider their feelings about quality of life. In this manner, when the "critical" patients pass on to the long-term ICU stage and reach the point of consideration of discontinuation of interventions so as to shorten the dying process, consensus will already be present among the patient, family, and physicians. The burden of decision will not be placed on distressed family members, quasi-incompetent patients, nor well meaning but, perhaps, poorly informed physicians.

CONCLUSION

We often feel uncomfortable with the uncertainties of clinical judgment, long described as one of the arts of medicine. In our highly technological society and the environment in today's ICU, we hoped that this uncertainty could have been dispelled by analyzing the massive data base accumulated. All numerical indices have approximately a 15% misclassification rate for survival or death.[12] Interestingly, this is essentially the same rate as reported for prospective analyses of clinical judgment.[5,6] Thus, quantitative instruments have not supplanted clinical judgment nor improved it. Clinical judgment should not be dismissed with its categorization as part of the art of medicine but we should recognize that the expression of the art is as dependent on education and experience as music, theatre, and painting. We must concentrate on learning the fundamentals to improve our technique as artists. I believe that the fundamentals are captured in the elements of the clinical care process and the components of the predictive indices. The important determinants, when viewed from different vantage points during the ICU stay, are few in number and remarkably consistent among different instruments. We can, therefore, learn to focus on these elements as we try to characterize a particular patient's outcome. When the possibility of death increases, however, we must learn to restrict useless interventions and focus on caring for the patient and his family. Our time should be spent in communication, explanation, and clarification rather than ordering new drugs, tests, or procedures. Patients seek medical *care,* not necessarily expecting *cure.* Technology, including intensive care, can then be seen as a method to enhance our clinical judgment when appropriate, but we should not look to technological solutions for social and societal issues which are especially important in prolonged ICU care. Effective clinical decision-making, at this point in time, still depends primarily on the processor, a knowledgeable and caring physician.

REFERENCES

1. DelGuercio L, Cohn JD: Monitoring operating risk in the elderly. *JAMA* 1980; 243:1350
2. Knaus WA, Zimmerman JE, Wagner DP, et al: APACHE—acute physiology and chronic health evaluation: A physiologically based classification system. *Crit Care Med* 1981; 9:591
3. Orlando R, Nelson LD, Civetta JM: Invasive preoperative evaluation of high risk patients. *Crit Care Med* 1985; 13:263
4. Shibutani K, Del Guercio LRM: Preoperative hemodynamic assessment of the high-risk patient. *Semin Anesth* 1983; 1:231
5. Rodman GH, Etling T, Civetta JM, et al: How accurate is clinical judgement? *Crit Care Med* 1978; 6:127
6. Civetta JM, Caruthers–Banner TE: Does clinical judgement correctly allocate surgical intensive care? *Crit Care Med* 1983; 11:236
7. Civetta JM: Determinants of Survival. In Brennan MF (ed): *Pre and Post Operative Care Manual,* developed by the American College of Surgeons and Scientific American Medicine (in press)
8. Lemeshow S, Teres D, Pastides H, et al: A method for predicting survival and

mortality of ICU patients using objectively derived weights. *Crit Care Med* 1985; 13:519
9. Civetta JM, Hudson–Civetta JA: Maintaining quality of care while reducing charges in the ICU: 10 ways. *Ann Surg* 1985; 202:524
10. Weed LW: *Medical Records, Medical Education, and Patient Care: The Problem-Oriented Record as a Basic Tool.* Chicago, Year Book Medical Publishers, 1970
11. Robin ED: Death by pulmonary artery flow-directed catheter: Time for a moratorium? *Chest* 1988; 92:727
12. Kirby RR, Civetta JM: Critical care outcome. In Brown DL (ed): *Risk and Outcome in Anesthesia*. Philadelphia, JB Lippincott, 1988
13. Champion HR, Sacco WJ, Hannon DS, et al: Assessment of injury severity: The triage index. *Crit Care Med* 1980; 8:201
14. Champion HR, Sacco WJ, Carnazzo AJ, et al: The trauma score. *Crit Care Med* 1981; 9:672
15. Ogawa M, Sugimoto T: Rating severity of the injured by ambulance attendants: Field research of trauma index. *J Trauma* 1974; 14:934
16. Bever DL, Veenker CH: An illness–injury severity index for non-physician emergency medical personnel. *EMT J* 1979; 3:45
17. Gormican SP: CRAMS scale: Field triage of trauma victims. *Ann Emerg Med* 1982; 11:132
18. Buzby GP, Mullen JL, Matthews DC, et al: Prognostic nutritional index in gastrointestinal surgery. *Am J Surg* 1980; 139:160
19. Harvey KB, Moldawer LL, Bistrian BR, et al: Biological measures for the formulation of a hospital prognostic index. *Am J Clin Nutr* 1981; 34:2013
20. Christou NV: Predicting septic related mortality of the individual surgical patient based on admission host defense measurements. *Can J Surg* 1986; 29:424
21. Civetta JM, Hudson–Civetta J: Costly-care: Data, problems and proposing remedies. *Crit Care Med* 1986; 14:357
22. Civetta JM: The inverse relationship between cost and survival. *J Surg Res* 1973; 14:265
23. Knaus WA, Draper EA, Wagner DP, et al: APACHE II: A severity of disease classification system. *Crit Care Med* 1985; 13:818
24. Cullen DJ, Civetta JM, Briggs BA, et al: Therapeutic intervention scoring systems: A method for quantitative comparison of patient care. *Crit Care Med* 1974; 2:57
25. Shoemaker WC, Pierchala BS, Chang P, et al: Prediction of outcome and severity of illness by analysis of the frequency distribution of cardiorespiratory variables. *Crit Care Med* 1977; 5:82
26. Siegel JH: Cardiorespiratory manifestations of metabolic failure in sepsis and the multiple organ failure syndrome. *Surg Clin North Am* 1983; 63:379
27. Moyer E, Cerra F, Chenier R, et al: Multiple systems organ failure: VI. Death predictors in the trauma–septic state—the most critical determinants. *J Trauma* 1981; 21:862

Life and Death in the ICU: 3
Ethical Considerations

Ernlé W. D. Young

Our contemporary technological ability to preserve and extend life in the intensive care unit (ICU) is almost awesome. Certainly, it is impressive. But for a minority of patients, those whose lives can no longer be extended but whose dying can only be prolonged, the technology of the ICU has come to have more sinister and frightening connotations. What most people dread, more than death itself, is an inevitable process of dying meaninglessly and agonizingly protracted by artificial means. There are times when the instruments of healing become the tools of torture. There are situations in which the benefits of intensive care medicine are far outweighed by the harms inflicted in attempting to realize them. There are moments when death ought not to be resisted and fought back as an enemy, by any and all means possible, but rather ought to be welcomed and embraced as a friend. And I am concerned that these times will not be discerned, these situations will remain unrecognized, these moments will be missed.

There are good grounds for this uneasiness. Sometimes it seems that there is an overwhelming fascination—even infatuation—with the toys of technology, which prompts intensivists unconcernedly to play with them, in circumstances of life and death too momentous for mere games. And often intensivists are genuinely concerned that if they do not do everything possible for their patients, unquestioningly and unremittingly, they will later be sued. The defensive practice of medicine is an inevitable corollary to the litigious nature of American society.

Fortunately, some of the court cases to be mentioned later in this chapter have served substantially to alleviate physicians' legitimate concerns about possible malpractice litigation. There are now some good legal precedents for at times *not* doing everything that it is possible to do. Also, the American Medical Association and the American Bar Association are beginning to look for alternatives to malpractice litigation to compensate and redress aggrieved consumers. However, these investigations are still in their early stages, and the problem has not yet been resolved.

In addition to the technological imperative and the fear of malpractice litigation, a third factor motivates intensivists to cross the line between extending life and prolonging death in sometimes inappropriate fashion. It is a lack of skill in ethical decision-making, especially when those involved in the decision-making process are many and speak with different voices. In the ICU of a modern medical center, ethical decision-making may involve not only the patient and the primary (community) physician, but also the family, the director of the intensive care unit, the house staff, the nurses, the respiratory therapists, the social worker, the chaplain, the ethics consultant or committee, and the hospital's legal counsel. This complicates things extraordinarily. It is far simpler not to make any decision at all; yet not to decide is itself a decision. And in the circumstances we are now considering, it is one that can have dire consequences for the patient.

MEDICAL ETHICS

Courses in medical ethics, now being offered in almost every medical school, attempt to remedy this lack of skill. In order to describe the function of medical ethics in this regard, it may be useful to begin by briefly considering the meaning of three other related terms: "morality," "ethics," and "law." *Morality* may be defined as those attitudes, actions, or behaviors of an individual or of a group which reflect that individual's or group's vision of the highest good. *Ethics* is a discipline one of whose functions is to study moral attitudes, actions, and behaviors analytically or descriptively, looking for consistency and coherency between them and the highest good they purport to reflect. The other function of ethics is prescriptive, or normative. It is to move from a description of what *is* happening in a situation fraught with moral ambiguity to suggest what *ought* to be going on if the vision of the highest good is to be translated accurately into what is said and done. This is the more difficult task of ethics, and it invites analytical criticism from others (which is one of the ways the cause of truth is furthered). The *law* may be considered to be the societal requirement, allowance, or prohibition of attitudes, actions, and behaviors which, in a given culture and at a certain time in history, are thought of as either moral or immoral. Obviously, just as morality changes from one cultural milieu to another and from one generation to the next, so the law reflects these differing perceptions. Fifty years ago racial discrimination was well entrenched in the United States. Not only was its immorality unquestioned, it was legally sanctioned and enforced in countless ways. The civil rights' movement began to challenge racism as immoral. As the movement gathered momentum, racist laws came under attack as being unconstitutional. Eventually, the moral perception of Americans and the discriminatory laws were changed. Ethics functions with respect to the law much in the same way as it does in regard to morality. It analyzes what is going on in particular laws, attempting to assess whether these laws accurately express a society's moral consensus. And it makes normative proposals which, if adopted, would render the law less immoral or more moral than before.

Medical ethics, therefore, is that discipline concerned with moral issues arising in the contemporary practice of medicine. With respect to these proliferating problems, various positions begin to be formulated and adopted—either in practice or theoretically. Some of these positions become entrenched in the law, either legislatively or through case precedents. In its analytical or descriptive mode, medical ethics will be interested in the facts adduced in support of a particular position—how accurate, extensive, or pertinent they are; in the implicit or explicit values of the various parties involved—how well or how poorly they are being respected and upheld, and whether consciously or unconsciously; and in the logical and rational consistency (or otherwise) of the arguments brought forward to bolster claims or to undergird conclusions. In its normative or prescriptive mode, medical ethics will attempt to go beyond analysis to suggest what ought to be happening, with reference either to particular cases or laws.

DEONTOLOGY AND UTILITARIANISM

At the rational level, medicine has traditionally responded to moral quandaries by appealing to basic principles, rather than in *ad hoc* fashion. That is to say, medical ethics, to use the language of philosophers, has functioned either deontologically or in terms of rule-utilitarianism. It may be useful to explain these terms. The world "deontological" derives from the Greek "deon," meaning "it is necessary" or "it is required." A deontological ethics is one in which certain things are required on principle, *ab initio,* at the outset, no matter what the circumstances or the consequences may be. It is morally necessary that we be truthful, that we maintain confidentiality, that we seek to benefit patients rather than ourselves, that we engage not to harm those in our care. The consequences of truth-telling, or preserving confidentiality, or acting beneficently or nonmaleficently, are not accorded primary significance in the process of deciding what to do in a given situation. Utilitarianism weighs the imagined results of various possible courses of action and decides which to follow on the basis of the set of consequences thought to be most beneficial (or least detrimental) to the largest number of relevant parties. Thus, rule-utilitarianism seeks to apply those rules, principles, or guidelines that experience has taught will produce the maximum amount of good (or the minimum amount of harm) for the greatest possible number. Tom L. Beauchamp and James F. Childress effectively demonstrate how medical ethicists with a deontological approach and a rule-utilitarian orientation, starting from different premises, can agree on concluding principles.[1] (Act-utilitarianism, the other major form of consequentialist ethics, enjoins those actions that will maximize the good or minimize the harm for the greatest number.)

MEDICOMORAL PRINCIPLES

Two primary medicomoral principles traditionally have informed the practice of medicine: preserving life and alleviating suffering. For the most part, these two principles can be applied concurrently, without conflict, to guide the physician's decisions and actions. However, in circumstances of critical or terminal illness, they sometimes come into conflict. Then it becomes possible to apply one principle only at the expense of the other. To continue, willy-nilly, to attempt to preserve life may, in fact, inflict rather than alleviate suffering. And to consciously strive to alleviate suffering may require abandoning the intention to continue to preserve life. In situations in which principles are in opposition to one another, the questions arise, Which principle ought to take precedence over the other, and when, and why? To these questions, we now must turn.

Some resolve a potential conflict between these two traditional medicomoral principles by insisting that, always and in all circumstances, preservation of life ought to take precedence over the concern to alleviate suffering. In terms of the diagram below, if X = birth, Y = death, and the curve = the human life span, they insist that CARE ought to take the unyielding and unremitting attempt to CURE, from X through Y; that is to say, the sanctity of the patient's life is valued above considerations of its quality, and death is perceived as an enemy to be warded off by any and all means, for as long as possible.

There are both patients and physicians who espouse this philosophy of care. Their putative motives warrant consideration. Some patients have urgent, unfinished business to attend to before they die: a book to complete, a project to finalize, a legacy of one kind or another to wrap up. Understandably, they are willing to purchase as much time as they possibly can, without regard for the quality of their lives, by insisting that everything feasible be done to maintain their physical existence. Others simply cannot come to terms with their own mortality and finitude. The threat of non-being is so intense that they are willing to endure all kinds of harms—iatrogenic or disease-related—in order to hold off the inevitable, to remain in being, for as long as possible. I suspect that many in this category support the cryonics industry (the claims of which are likely to be proved spurious).

With respect to physicians, various motives prompt the adoption of a CARE = CURE philosophy from X-Y. One has to do with research. If a breakthrough can occur in treating a patient with what is generally thought to be an incurable and terminal condition, this may benefit a whole population. Another motive is to be discerned when children are involved. In the case of children afflicted with terminal illnesses, research will often be an important consideration. Additionally, there is a further justification for a

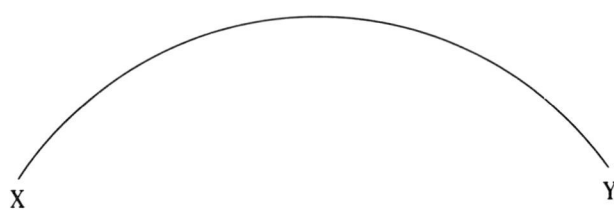

CARE = CURE philosophy: If unremitting, aggressive treatment can purchase for this child an extra year or two of life (at no matter what cost), that cost is worth paying because a year or two in the life of a 5- or 7-year-old represents a considerable proportion of the total life span. And, finally, just as there are patients temperamentally unable to come to terms with their inevitable mortality, so there are physicians incapable of accepting "defeat." And to stop treating a terminal disease aggressively is unfortunately equated with defeat by such physicians.

There is, however, another way of looking at this whole conundrum. It revolves around point Z (in the diagram below). Point Z may be defined as the moment when the difference between attempting to extend life (with meaning, as defined by the patient himself) and prolong death (in mindless and meaningless fashion) is discerned. Recognizing point Z, admittedly, is difficult. Three factors, at least, enter into its determination. One is the accumulation of *objective* clinical data: x-rays or CT-scan evidence that the disease is gaining the upper hand, further findings of untreatable metastases, disastrous blood counts, and so forth. A second is the *subjective* assessment of the patient himself that, having fought the good fight, the battle is no longer worth the prize: The deleterious effects of fighting on outweigh the benefits of sheer survival, without discernible quality. Last, there is *intuition:* the intuition of either the clinician or the patient, or both, that the time has come to switch from a mode in which attempting to extend life ought to be the primary concern to a philosophy in which the quality of life is seen as more important; where death may be regarded no longer as an enemy to be resisted, but rather as a friend to be afforded hospitality.

If the possibility is allowed of discerning point Z (and doing this requires more in terms of the art of medicine, perhaps, than its science), then another philosophy of care emerges. From X through Z, the principle of preserving life ought to take precedence over that of alleviating suffering; the value of the sanctity of life ought to predominate over quality of life valuations; death ought to be seen more as a foe to be attacked and defended against than as a colleague to be embraced; and CARE should take the form of a resolute attempt to CURE. But from Z through Y, these principles and values are reversed. Now, alleviating suffering ought to take precedence over the principle of attempting to preserve life. Now, the quality of life requires more

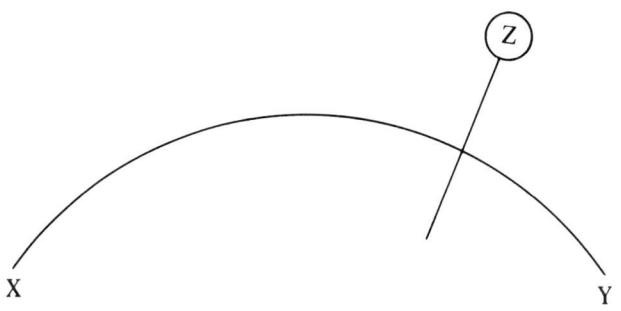

attention than the mere prolongation of physical existence. Now, death may appropriately be recognized and embraced as a welcome visitor. And now, CARE will take the form of ensuring comfort in the face of pain, being company with the dying person (rather than abandoning or segregating him), and facilitating a creative completion of the patient's inner journey (which will move spiritual counselors and companions from the sidelines to center of the playing field). Now, it will also be possible to view the withdrawal or withholding of aggressive life-sustaining technologies *as an appropriate expression of the concern to care.*

Accordingly, this chapter will be devoted to describing some principles that I have found helpful in the ICU in facilitating ethical decision-making about the withdrawal or withholding of aggressive, "heroic," life-sustaining technologies, and to identifying those who might be party to the decision-making process, along with their appropriate roles. At relevant points, reference will be made to major court decisions on withdrawing or withholding life-sustaining interventions. Recent legislation and policy statements having a bearing on the topic will also be considered.

Whether what follows is termed deontological or rule-utilitarian does not matter. What matters is that there *are* some guiding principles to help the intensivist make difficult ethical decisions. Five may be delineated. From my perspective, they serve as broad guidelines, rather than as rigid and inflexible context-invariant rules.

POTENTIAL FOR SALVAGEABILITY

The first is a common-sense principle first enunciated (to my knowledge) by Cynthia B. Cohen. It is that the criterion for admission to and continuance in an ICU is *the potential for salvageability*. As Cohen expresses it,

> All who are critically ill should not automatically be admitted to the ICU. A necessary condition for admission is that the patient be potentially salvageable, by which it is meant that the patient has a chance for returning to a state in which his or her life is not threatened. Patients who are immediately and irreversibly dying, and for whom it has been carefully determined that there is no known therapy, are not salvageable. They deserve comfort and support within the hospital but cannot benefit from intensive care.[2]

With respect to this first guideline, two qualifying comments are in order. One is that it is easier to apply at the time of admission to an ICU than when the discontinuance of intensive care is being contemplated because a patient is no longer deemed to be "salvageable." When admission to an ICU is being considered, it is usually sufficient that the patient be thought to have a 50/50 chance of recovery for the attempt to be made aggressively to preserve his life. But when it is becoming apparent that the patient is no longer salvageable and that, therefore, comfort and support rather than intensive care is more appropriate, a far higher level of certainty is mandated. Before agreeing to the discontinuance of life-sustaining therapies (because point Z is thought to have been reached), the intensivist wishes for a degree of certainty approaching 100%, rather than the 50% that sufficed at the outset.

A second qualifying remark is that the definition of salvageability is very much determined by the resources available. A simple analogy may serve to make this clear. If one were fortunate enough to inherit a Model T Ford (which had been locked in a garage for the last half century) and wanted it restored to its original, pristine, showroom condition, one could find craftspeople available to accomplish such feats. Their work is beautiful to behold. As long as there were no limit to the funds one was willing to expend on such a project, it is entirely possible that the Ford could be totally restored, with genuine parts, or with parts handmade to the original specifications. However, if one had to work within a restricted budget of, say, $5000, it is highly unlikely that the same goal could be reached. For $5000 it might be possible to restore the upholstery, the chassis, the motor, or even the body, to mint condition. But it is too much to expect that the whole car could be renovated. Labor and parts together would cost more than the $5000 available.

In the same way, as long as resources are infinite (or are thought to be infinite, as was the case when intensive care had its genesis in the 1960s), the definition of salvageability can be loose, and the threshhold for admittance to and continuance in an ICU can be low. But once resources are recognized as finite and limits on expenditures have to be set (as is now the case within cost containment systems), the definition of salvageability needs to be tightened and the threshhold of eligibility for initial and continued intensive care must be raised commensurately.

These two disclaimers notwithstanding, Cohen's principle is helpful. It reminds us that caring can encompass several different activities. At times, caring means furnishing a patient with a respirator or with renal dialysis. At other times, it requires no more than palliation for pain and the discomfort, for example, of constipation. It is to be hoped that caring never ceases. However, the *form* caring takes will be determined by medical and other factors, presently to be considered.

Further, Cohen's principle accords well with the findings of a Consensus Development Conference held at the National Institutes of Health on March 7–9, 1983, to discuss issues related to the practice of critical care medicine. The conference identified three categories of patients: [1] the patient "with acute reversible disease for whom the probability of survival without ICU intervention is low, but the survival probability with such intervention is high"; [2] the patient "with a low probability of survival without intensive care whose probability of survival with intensive care may be higher—but the potential benefit is not as clear"; and [3] patients "admitted to the ICU, not because they are critically ill, but because they are at *risk* of becoming critically ill. The purposes of intensive care in these instances are to prevent a serious complication or to allow a prompt response to any complication that may occur." The conference went on to state that

It is not medically appropriate to devote limited ICU resources to patients without reasonable prospect of significant recovery when patients who need those services, and who have a significant prospect of recovery from acutely life-threatening disease or injury are being turned away due to a lack of capacity. It is inappropriate to maintain ICU management of a patient whose prognosis has resolved to one of persistent vegetative state, and it is similarly inappropriate to employ ICU resources where no purpose will be served but a prolongation of the natural processes of death.[3]

PRESERVING LIFE

A second principle, mentioned earlier, is that of *preserving life*. This principle goes back to the Judaistic element in our Judeo–Christian heritage. The governing principle in Jewish medical ethics is the preservation of life. So fundamental in the tradition is this principle that things otherwise prohibited by Jewish law must be set aside to preserve life. "Thus even though it is forbidden to mutilate a corpse, heart and kidney transplants as well as corneal grafting are permitted, provided of course that the utmost care is taken to be sure that the person whose body is being used for the purpose is really dead."[4]

NONMALEFICENCE

A third principle is that of *nonmaleficence.* A duty not to harm is recognized in most deontological and rule-utilitarian ethical theories. According to Beauchamp and Childress,

> the concept of nonmaleficence is associated with the maxim *primum non nocere*—"above all, or first, do no harm"—which has wide currency in discussions of the responsibilities of health care professionals, particularly physicians. The origins of this maxim, however, are obscure. Scholars have been unable to locate it in the Hippocratic corpus . . . .[4]

Of course, harm can be variously defined: in terms of death, disability, distress, or deprivation of freedom and pleasure. Further, harms—however defined—have to be weighed against hoped-for, compensatory benefits: All medical interventions inflict *some* harm. Usually, the harm inflicted is minimal and the ensuring benefits are many. In the ICU, however, this may not always be the case. When someone has been determined to be no longer salvageable, there will be no hoped-for, compensatory benefit to offset the iatrogenic harms being inflicted by aggressive life-sustaining measures. Applying this principle, in such situations, then becomes fairly straightforward.

Allied closely to the negative principle of nonmaleficence is the positive concept of *alleviating suffering,* which goes back to the Hippocratic corpus. We have already alluded to this principle. Not to harm entails, as a corollary, a concern to alleviate suffering—whether physical or psychological. For the most part, in medicine, it is possible to apply the second principle (that of attempting to preserve life) and this third principle (doing no harm or alleviating suffering) simultaneously and without conflict. As has been remarked, however, in circumstances of terminal illness, the one principle can usually be upheld only at the expense of the other. Then a decision has to be made about which principle should predominate over the other, and when, and why. We have suggested how this ranking of principles might take place, and we shall return to this point later.

AUTONOMY

Fourth is the principle of *autonomy*. The origins of this norm can be traced back to the emphasis in the Judeo-Christian tradition on respect for persons. Respecting the personhood of others requires of us that we allow and enable them, as far as possible, to be self-determining agents. Immanuel Kant, in insisting that every human being always be treated as an end and never as a means to an end, embedded this principle more deeply in our Western tradition. (The tradition of Marxist countries, for example, points in another direction: that of elevating the common good above the autonomy of the individual. In our own country, the recent ruling by Charles J. Cooper, head of the Justice Department's Office of Legal Counsel, allowed employers to dismiss employees who have AIDS or who carry the AIDS virus; this represents a movement away from an emphasis on the autonomy of the individual to a concern, in this case clearly neurotic, for the common good). In recent decades, Ralph Nader and the consumer movement have applied the principle of autonomy effectively to relations between patients and their physicians. This movement has made us all aware that, in the language of transactional analysis, each person who becomes a patient ought to be treated not as a "child" by the physician–parent but as an "adult" in an adult–adult transaction. This militates against paternalistic decision-making on the part of medical caregivers, and requires that patients—as far as possible—be respected as equal partners in making decisions about their own destinies, and be encouraged to assume the responsibility this entails.

JUSTICE

Last is the principle of *justice*. Understood in its most basic terms, justice may be thought of as fairness. Fairness, when it comes to distributing scarce resources equitably, requires that we do not do for some what we are unwilling or unable to do for all. To expend three quarters of a million dollars on a single patient, who in the end dies in the ICU 14 months and 16 surgical procedures after admission, is one thing. To expend such colossal amounts of money on *all* potential ICU patients is another. Manifestly, it is impossible. The principle of justice, much to the fore these days in an era of cost-containment systems, poses the question, How can we fairly allocate ICU resources? How can we equitably distribute among the many claimants for our services those limited benefits we have to offer?

Let one thing be stated now, most emphatically: Decisions *within the ICU* ought not be made on economic, rather than on medical, grounds. It is simply not acceptable, from an ethical point of view, once having begun to offer a patient intensive care, to decide to discontinue aggressive therapy because it is now thought to be costing too much. Doing this would violate the moral contract entered into with the patient at the time of admission. This point of view is endorsed by the National Institutes of Health Consensus Development Conference on Critical Care Medicine, to which reference was made earlier.

Nevertheless, it is morally licit for considerations of distributive justice to enter into the decision-making process *before the patient is admitted to the ICU,* in terms of a raised threshhold of eligibility for costly, technological life-sustaining services. Given the finitude of our present-day resources, it is morally acceptable for a hospital to decide not to afford intensive care, for example, to any patient with a metastatic, terminal disease process. As long as this policy is publicly stated, beforehand, to everyone concerned—staff members as well as patients and their family members alike—there can be no objection to this attempt to raise the threshhold of eligibility for what the ICU is able to provide.

Application of Medicomoral Principles

Having enunciated five basic ethical principles pertinent to decision-making in the ICU, we must now attempt to rank them in order of priority and identify their points of applicability. As far as the first three are concerned, the following can be said. As long as the patient is still considered to be "salvageable" (as defined both medically and by the resources available), and is therefore on the X-Z segment of the curve, the attempt to preserve life ought to take precedence over the principle of doing no harm or alleviating suffering. However, once it is decided that a patient is no longer "salvageable," that is, is on the Z-Y segment of the curve, intensive care is no longer the most appropriate form of care, and the principle of nonmaleficence or alleviating suffering assumes priority over the attempt to preserve life. Defining "salvageability," both medically and in terms of the resources available (and thus deciding that the Z-point has been reached), is the key to reranking principles and accordingly reordering priorities from attempting to cure to comforting.

The fourth principle, autonomy, ought to have its place throughout the decision-making process. Insofar as possible, medical decisions ought not to be made by physicians acting unilaterally. (The emergency room setting provides one obvious exception to this general norm.) Usually, this is unproblematic if the patient remains conscious and competent. Difficulties in the continued exercise of patient autonomy arise when he becomes unconscious or incompetent. Various measures have been devised to meet these difficulties and will be discussed later.

As has already been suggested, the fifth principle, distributive justice, ought to have its place outside the ICU, in the arena of institutional and public policy, rather than within the ICU itself. Once treatment for medical reasons has been initiated, it is simply unacceptable to terminate treatment for economic reasons. Economic considerations should have their place in deciding which patients not to treat intensively in the first place.

As was indicated earlier, in situations in which aggressive therapy has been initiated but it has become apparent that the patient is no longer "salvageable," doing no harm (or alleviating suffering) now becomes more important than continuing with the (futile and potentially harmful) attempt to preserve life. If intensive care is no longer the most appropriate form of care and palliative or supportive care is indicated, who can and who ought to decide to limit treatment? A summary answer to this question is provided in Table 3-1. The summary points made in Table 3-1 are further explicated below, with reference to pertinent court decisions, legislation, and policy statements.

The principle of autonomy requires that patients assume the primary role in all decisions to limit therapy, whenever this is possible. Usually, the interest patients have in deciding to limit therapy is that of not wanting the process of dying meaninglessly and painfully prolonged when life can no longer be extended with "quality"—according to patients' own definitions. I say "usually," because occasionally there are patients who are so afraid of death that they will do anything and endure all manner of hardship to prolong the inevitable. Patients in this category present a different ethical problem: To what extent does an "unsalvageable" patient have the right to demand costly and possibly scarce ICU resources in a futile attempt to keep death at a distance? In this case, the principles of autonomy and justice are in conflict. Since autonomy is never an absolute, even in societies like ours (none of us is free not to pay taxes, or not to obey the highway code, or not to have our children immunized, or not to send our children to school), this may well be an area in which concern for the common good (represented by the principle of justice) ought to take precedence over the principle of autonomy (inadequately construed as unbridled freedom).

LIMITATION OR REFUSAL OF TREATMENT

If the patient is conscious and competent, there are no insurmountable obstacles in the way of his exercising the right to refuse treatment. This right has been recognized both by the American Medical Association and the American Hospital Association and is included in the commonly accepted "Patient's Bill of Rights." However, the case of *Bartling v. Superior Court*[5] is a reminder that this "right" cannot be taken for granted and of the fact that it has now been upheld by court action in a single jurisdiction. Mr. Bartling, 70 years old, had multiple medical problems. His condition had become compromised after a pneumothorax sustained during a biopsy of a lung mass. He had a chest tube inserted, was given a tracheostomy, and was placed on a ventilator. Throughout, Mr. Bartling remained conscious and competent and on several occasions attempted to remove the ventilator tubes. Mr. Bartling repeatedly requested that ventilatory support be discontinued.

TABLE 3-1. *Ethical and Legal Considerations in Critical Care Medicine: Who Can, and Who Ought, to Limit Therapy?*

	INTEREST IN LIMITING THERAPY	OBSTACLES IN THE WAY OF DOING THIS	HOW THESE OBSTACLES MAY BE OVERCOME	REMAINING PROBLEMS
THE PATIENT Should, ideally, play the *primary* and *central* role in limiting therapy	Not wanting death prolonged when life cannot be further extended with meaning and quality according to the patient's own definition. *Principle:* Autonomy	None, as long as the patient is conscious and competent *and* "unsalvageable" (irreversibly terminal)	Appeal to the "right to refuse treatment," recognized by the AMA and the AHA. The case of Mr. Bartling	
		Unconsciousness or incompetence	Natural Death Act (or its equivalent), Durable Power of Attorney for Health Care	Ignorance or neglect of these measures. Patient not legally "qualified." Patient not identified as having executed such a document
		The patient not yet seen as "unsalvageable," the disease process not yet seen as irreversible and terminal	Either: the Bartling precedent Or: The team continuing to treat. For how long?	Risk of litigation for assault and battery

THE FAMILY Should, ideally, play a role *secondary* to the patient and *advisory* to the team in decisions to limit therapy	(i) Same as the patient's, expressed above *Principle*: As above	The family's guilt over "ending the patient's life" by their decision. Defining "quality" of life for someone else	Prior unambiguous, regularly updated written statements of patient's wishes. Verbal testimony	Absence of any such statement, written or verbal. The family divided in its opinions
	(ii) Wanting to end their own suffering, rather than the patient's	The team's contract is always with the patient first and foremost: the family is secondary	The team continuing to act in accordance with the *patient's* express wishes (if known), or according to the *patient's* best interest, medically perceived	The possibility of legal repercussions from disgruntled family members. Documenting all decisions and collaborative decision making important
	(iii) Ulterior motivation: wanting to save further expense, or the desire to inherit	Again, the patient's interests take precedence over those of the family. Decisions must be made on medical, not economic, grounds		

TABLE 3-1. Ethical and Legal Considerations in Critical Care Medicine: Who Can, and Who Ought, to Limit Therapy? (Continued)

	INTEREST IN LIMITING THERAPY	OBSTACLES IN THE WAY OF DOING THIS	HOW THESE OBSTACLES MAY BE OVERCOME	REMAINING PROBLEMS
THE CRITICAL CARE TEAM Should, ideally, play a role *secondary* to the patient, but more *assertive* than the family in limiting therapy	Medical judgment about "unsalvageability" with the patient now perceived as terminal	Unrealistic attitudes in the family. Family members with unfinished business to complete. Legal hazards of withdrawing ventilatory, then intravenous, support. The case of *Clarence Herbert*	Continuing treatment *and* initiating emotional and spiritual support of family until family ready to let go. AMA guidelines following the *Barber* case	The possibility of civil, but not criminal, legal repercussions
	Medical judgment about the irreversibility of the patient's condition (vegetative state)			
SOCIETY: *Economically:* Society should *not* make decisions within the ICU itself *Legally:* Court decisions affect what happens in the ICU	*Principles:* Nonmaleficence, alleviating suffering Conservation of scarce resources *Principle:* Distributive justice	Policy decisions are typically made in *ad hoc* fashion, not in a rational, principled manner	Institutional guidelines for eligibility for ICU services, publicly proclaimed Societal involvement in policy decisions	The increased bureaucratization of medicine. Policies applicable across the board do not sufficiently allow for the uniqueness of individuals
	Autonomy of the patient. Privacy	Concern of institution and physicians that they will be sued by family members	Court decisions. Legislation policy statements discussed above	Still areas of ambiguity: Elizabeth Bouvia

The treating physicians and the hospital refused to withdraw ventilatory support and continued to restrain Mr. Bartling so that he could not do this himself. Richard S. Scott, a doctor and lawyer active in the right-to-die movement, took up this case on Mr. Bartling's behalf. The lower court denied the request for an injunction, restraining the hospital and the physicians from administering medical care to which the patient had not given consent. The case was appealed. Before the appeal court could rule, Mr. Bartling died, still connected to his ventilator. So important was this case deemed to be, however, that the Court of Appeal ruled posthumously, holding that " . . . competent adult patients, with serious illnesses which are probably incurable, but have not been diagnosed as terminal, have the right, over the objection of their physicians and the hospital, to have life-support equipment disconnected despite the fact that withdrawal of such devices will surely hasten death."

Typically, obstacles in the way of the patient being able to limit intensive care therapy have arisen only when he has become either unconscious or incompetent. From the patient's point of view, the prior concern was, How can I continue to exercise my autonomy beyond the point of unconsciousness and incompetence? From the physician's perspective, the consideration was, How does one do what the patient seemingly would have wanted, without becoming overly vulnerable to malpractice litigation? Early attempts to surmount these obstacles included the so-called Living Will (not yet recognized in all jurisdictions as a legally valid document) and the California Natural Death Act, or its equivalent. The Natural Death Act had several deficiencies. One major problem was that, according to the provisions of the Act, the Directive to Physicians could be executed only by persons who were at the time, and had been for at least 14 days previously, terminally ill—as defined in the Act. (Mr. Bartling was not terminally ill, as defined in the Act, when he asked to be allowed to exercise his right to refuse treatment.) This prevented the Natural Death Act from being of assistance to persons who, not being terminally ill beforehand, had later sustained massive, irreversible neurologic or physiologic insults, or both—whether iatrogenically or through accidents.

Because of these difficulties, California legislated its "proxy directive," commonly know as the "Durable Power of Attorney for Health Care," in January 1985. This document empowers any other person, selected by the patient, to make decisions regarding health care on the patient's behalf and in accordance with his expressed wishes, if he should later become unconscious or incompetent. Ordinary powers of attorney do not survive the makers' incompetence. This one remains in effect; hence its appellation, "durable." Several other states have since emulated California in this respect. All follow the recommendation of a presidential commission that durable powers of attorney are preferable to living wills "since they are more generally applicable and provide a better vehicle for patients to exercise self-determination."[6]

Typically, one obstacle in the way of attending physicians simply acceding to a patient's request to terminate life-sustaining treatment is that the patient may not be considered "unsalvageable" or terminal, on medical grounds. For a "salvageable" or "nonterminal" patient to decline treatment that could possibly restore him to functionality—at least for the foreseeable future—seems tantamount to a suicidal death wish or evidence of insanity. The (benignly paternalistic) instinct in such cases is to continue treating, hoping that either the suicidal impulse or the insanity will prove temporary and will later give way to retroactive consent. Yet there are people like Mr. Bartling in ICUs who are not terminal, crazy, or irrationally suicidal. Entirely rationally, they wish to exercise their right to refuse further aggressive treatment. The treating physician is then faced with a dilemma: either to presume that the patient being treated is in the category Mr. Bartling has compelled the court to recognize, or that the patient is somehow "incompetent" and that, therefore, his expressed wishes must be disregarded until such time as competency can be established. Either way, there are risks. Clearly, this could be a no-win situation for intensivists. From a moral standpoint, when in doubt it is better to treat than not to treat, since life is the precondition for all else of value. To deprive someone of life by not treating would therefore seem to constitute a more serious harm than abrogating patient autonomy and preserving life by treating intensively.

THE FAMILY'S ROLE

The role of the family in decisions to limit therapy should be secondary to the patient (on the strength of the principle of autonomy) and advisory to the critical care team rather than assertive. The distinction between advisory and "assertive" is important. To allow the initiative for decision-making to pass from the critical care team to the family (where the patient is no longer available as an active party to the decision-making process—either directly, or indirectly via a Durable Power of Attorney for Health Affairs) is, at the same time, to assign responsibility for the decision arrived at to the family. This means that later the family could come to feel guilty for decisions made that resulted in the death of the patient. Because it is the underlying disease process that usually causes patients to die, not the withdrawal or withholding of life-sustaining measures, it seems unnecessarily cruel to saddle the family with an additional burden of guilt for the decision to limit (futile) aggressive therapy. The critical care team should consult closely with the family in order to act in accordance with their interpretation of the patient's wishes, yet should themselves assume responsibility for the decision eventually made.

Ideally, the family's interest in limiting therapy would be identical to that of the patient: to not want dying to be protracted when life cannot be extended any longer with qualities consistent with the patient's own self-understanding. This presupposes that the family knows what capacities the patient would have considered indispensable for a meaningful life. When there is good evidence that the family does represent the patient's wishes and interests (either because of a prior written statement by the patient or reiterated verbal statements to which all members of the family could attest), there are no foreseeable problems. But when there is no prior written or verbal statement by the patient, and the family is divided in its opinions about what the patient would have wanted were he able to verbalize this, it would seem that the critical care team has no alternative but to "play it safe," that is, to be conservative and to continue to treat.

Occasionally, the critical care team may have reason to suspect that the family members are not representing the patient's best interests, but rather their own: either in seeking to alleviate their own suffering or, worse, in wanting to hasten the patient's demise in order to inherit an estate. Whenever such suspicions surface, the team has no alternative, morally speaking, but to remind itself that its primary obligation is to the patient, not to the family, even though the family may be the legal surrogate decision-maker. The burden of proof is on the medical caregiver. In such circumstances, the team will continue to act either in accordance with the patient's expressed wishes or in what is thought to be the patient's best interests, medically perceived. The reasons for so doing should be carefully documented in the patient's chart. For in such situations there is always the possibility that disgruntled family members will later sue the treating team for malpractice.

Occasionally it will be necessary to seek a court-appointed guardian to resolve the problem.

THE CRITICAL CARE TEAM

The term "critical care team" has been used in this discussion. Perhaps the reasons for a team approach in critical care and the dynamics within the team need to be addressed, however briefly. Apart from the technology, what makes modern intensive care possible is the sophistication and concentration of intensive care nurses in such units. Because of their extensive technical, pharmacologic, psychological, and nursing competence, registered nurses have developed and are steadily asserting their own distinct professional identity. No longer are they willing to be subservient to physicians; they are acknowledged caregivers in their own right, and seek to be recognized as such. Moreover, because of the nature of their training and the strategic position they occupy within ICUs (registered nurses are the one group of professionals in ICUs who are with the patient 24 hours a day), nurses have a pivotal role to play in the communication process: between other members of the team, between the team and the patient or family, and between various family members. For these reasons, it is important that nurses in intensive care units be regarded as the partners of physicians, not as their "handmaidens," and be accorded their due place in the team, especially with respect to the process of making decisions about the withholding or withdrawal of intensive care therapies. (Incidentally, the *Barber* case, to be discussed presently, illustrates the potentially devastating consequences of not according intensive care nurses an equal place as partners in the team. It was the supervisory ICU nurse, who for long had been disgruntled with what she considered to be unilateral decision-making by the intensive care physicians, who initiated a report to the district attorney whose assistant later charged Drs. Leonard Barber and Robert Nejdl with murder.)

Other members of the "team" may include community physicians, who often admit patients to ICUs, house officers (in teaching hospitals), respiratory therapists, social workers, chaplains, and, more and more, an ethics consultant or hospital ethics committee representative. A recent article in the *Journal of the American Medical Association* draws attention to the way residents at the bedside frequently think that their attendings are out of touch with current problems and ethical approaches. They experience considerable stress when attendings make decisions without discussing them beforehand, yet expect the residents to comply with these decisions, unquestioningly, after the fact. As the author points out,

> Little attention has been paid to the issue of whether residents are always bound to the decisions of their attending physicians, and whether it may ever be appropriate for residents to decline to participate in the life-sustaining care of patients on the basis of ethical grounds.[7]

Although the attending ICU physicians will ultimately have to take responsibility for decisions made in the ICU, difficult or complex decisions should always be arrived at in collaborative, rather than in unilateral, fashion. This makes good sense in terms of human interactions and relationships within the unit. It also makes good sense from a legal perspective. A decision, however controversial, that has been thoroughly discussed among the members of the team, carefully arrived at, and meticulously documented is the best defense against litigation.

LIMITATION OF THERAPY

The team's role in limiting therapy should be secondary to that of the patient (on the basis of the principle of autonomy) but assertive, not merely advisory, vis-à-vis the family. It is physicians who are licensed to practice medicine, not family members *per se*. As has been said, assertiveness on the part of the team (after careful consultation with the family) can alleviate substantially the family's guilt over "deciding to end the patient's life." After all, it is the disease process with which he is afflicted or the accident he sustained that, ultimately, will end his life, not any decision not to prolong meaningless suffering. The interest of the team in deciding to limit therapy ought to be primarily medical. On *medical* grounds, judgments ought to be made about a patient's "unsalvageability" or the irreversible chronicity of the patient's condition (*e.g.*, a persistent vegetative state). Such determinations trigger the reranking of principles discussed earlier, the switching from one form of care (intensive) to another (palliative), with the attempt to cure replaced by the concern to assure the patient's comfort. Such determinations will cause death no longer to be resisted but to be hailed as a welcome guest. The principle of alleviating suffering and nonmaleficence will now predominate over the principle of preserving life.

Humanitarian Reasons

The team may hesitate to implement decisions arrived at in this way both for humanitarian reasons and for fear of legal repercussions. The humanitarian concerns could include allowing a family with an unrealistic view of the patient's condition the time necessary to adjust to the reality of the situation, or allowing members of the family time to complete any unfinished business with the patient. An anecdote may illustrate this last point. After a 51-year-old patient in our ICU had been determined to be legally dead by the brain death criterion, she was ventilated for another week to allow her 18-year-old son time to complete his own unfinished business with her. He had left home in anger a year earlier and had not seen his mother after that. His siblings were present with her before her surgery (from which she never recovered), but he was not. When he finally arrived at the hospital, his mother was unresponsive. Nevertheless, he was encouraged to talk to her *as if she could hear and understand what he was saying to her.* During the week before ventilatory support was discontinued, he told her that he was sorry about his earlier behavior and that he loved her. Finally, when he had expressed what he had not previously verbalized and had begun to forgive himself for what had been amiss in his relationship with his mother, the respirator was disconnected. The patient died immediately.

Legal Repercussions

Fear of legal repercussions has been the major reason for the team's hesitation in implementing a decision based on good medical grounds. Initially, this fear was exacerbated by the case of *Barber v. People*,[8] in which two physicians, Leonard Barber and Robert Nejdl, were charged with murder and conspiracy to commit murder after life-support measures were withdrawn from Clarence Herbert, a patient in a deeply comatose state, in accordance with the wishes of the family. However, the court's eventual ruling and subsequent developments have relieved these anxieties considerably. Physicians are now *more* secure than they were before as they proceed to implement decisions about the withdrawal of life-sustaining procedures on medical grounds in accordance with family desires. The facts of the case are as follows.

Clarence Herbert, a 55-year-old security guard, had come into the hospital for an ileostomy closure. The operation had been completed successfully. While in the recovery room, Mr. Herbert went into cardiopulmonary arrest. He was resuscitated, intubated, and transported to the ICU, where he was placed on a respirator. He would never again regain consciousness. He went into what the physicians described as an irreversible coma, secondary to extensive brain damage. The EEG showed minimal brain activity. Mrs. Herbert and her eight children unanimously asked that ventilatory support be withdrawn from Clarence Herbert and that he be allowed to die naturally. They went so far as to express this in writing: "We, the immediate family of Clarence LeRoy Herbert, would like all machines taken off that are sustaining life. We release all liability to Hosp. Dr. & Staff." Three days after his cardiopulmonary arrest, Mr. Herbert was taken off the respirator. To the dismay of all concerned, Mr. Herbert did not die; he began breathing spontaneously. Two days later, at the family's insistence that intravenous feeding lines be withdrawn and that the nasogastric feeding tube be removed in compliance with their written request that *"all machines [be] taken off that are sustaining life,"* Mr. Herbert ceased to receive hydration and nourishment. Six days later, he died. Sandra Bardenilla, an ICU nurse, called the county health services department to file a formal complaint; the department referred the case to the district attorney. Deputy district attorney, Nikola M. Mikulicich, initiated the prosecution of Drs. Barber and Nejdl for murder. The physicians petitioned the Court of Appeal to issue a writ of prohibition against the trial court, restraining it from taking further action against them. The Court of Appeal did so, with Justice Fleming observing that "a murder prosecution is a poor way to design an ethical and moral code for doctors who are faced with decisions concerning the use of costly and extraordinary 'life support' equipment."[9]

Based on the decision in *Barber v. Superior Court*, the Board of the Los Angeles County Bar Association approved, on December 11, 1985, and the Board of the Los Angeles County Medical Association ratified, on January 6, 1986, a document entitled "Principles and Guidelines Concerning the Foregoing of Life-Sustaining Treatment for Adult Patients." In this document, it is expressly stated that *"all life-sustaining interventions, including nutrition and hydration, are legally equivalent. It is legally acceptable for the caregiver to withhold or withdraw any or all of them. It is recognized, however, that nutrition and hydration have a powerful symbolic significance to both the members of the general public and to many caregivers."* That is to say, the insertion of intravenous lines and nasogastric feeding tubes are regarded as *medical interventions* (which, like all medical interventions, may be withheld or withdrawn in appropriate circumstances), not "basic requirements" like food and drink.

In March 1986, the American Medical Association's judicial council approved a new policy on withdrawing medical treatment. In this far-reaching policy statement, the AMA proclaims that it would be ethical for doctors to withhold "all means of life prolonging medical treatment, including food and water, from patients in irreversible comas." The court decision in *Barber v. People*, these two policy statements by the joint LACBA–LACMA committee on biomedical ethics, and the position now taken by the AMA should go a long way toward alleviating intensivists' fears that the withdrawal or withholding of life-sustaining interventions, *including hydration and nutrition by means of IV and nasogastric feeding tubes,* could result in criminal action against them. However, the possibility of *civil* action remains.

Society's Impact

The last column in Table 3-1 has to do with society. Society impinges in many ways upon those involved in decisions to limit therapy in the ICU; however, society's primary impact is in terms of economic and legal constraints. From the economic perspective, society's interest in limiting therapy is based on the principle of distributive justice: the need to allocate fairly among the many claimants for them the limited resources available for intensive care. At present, public policy decisions in the United States are made in *ad hoc* fashion, rather than in a principled way, for example, according to the proposals of John Rawls.[10] As has already been asserted, I am convinced that if economic considerations are to enter into decisions about intensive care (as inevitably they must), they need to take effect at the policy level, *beforehand,* rather than in the clinical situation, *after the fact.* This is true both in terms of institutional and societal budgetary constraints. Inevitably, this will lead to increased bureaucratization in the practice of medicine, with the concomitant danger that policies applicable across the board will not prove flexible enough to meet the unique needs of individuals. Only those with strong convictions about the respect that is due to persons will be able to temper justice with mercy, and thus make "the system" work in a more, rather than less, humane fashion.

Society will have an increasing impact on decisions to limit therapy in the ICU in terms of court decisions and legislation. At this level, it is to be hoped that the guiding principle will be that of patient autonomy. At the same time, physicians acting out of respect for patient autonomy must be exonerated from all possible later legal repercussions. If this does not happen, self-interest on the part of the caregivers is bound to outweigh concerns about upholding the right of individual patients to be self-determining, as far as possible, in matters related to their medical care. Further court precedents are to be expected. One recently handed down is the verdict in the case of Elizabeth Bouvia, the quadriplegic who, in 1983, unsuccessfully sought court permission to starve herself to death at Riverside (CA) General Hospital–University Medical Center. Subsequently, she was again admitted to a southern California hospital. Again, the physicians treating her refused her request to remove a life-sustaining feeding tube. Again, she petitioned the court to order it removed. Her motive in now wanting the feeding tube removed, she claimed, was not to starve herself to death; rather, it was to be able to choose her own treatment. She believed that her caloric intake was sufficient, without IV hydration or nasogastric nutrition, to sustain life. Her physicians disagreed. Her "continued refusal to eat adequate food was viewed by the staff as an attempt at suicide starvation," county attorneys for the hospital stated in their court papers. This time, the court ruled in Ms. Bouvia's favor, and the nasogastric tube was withdrawn. Subsequently, when her physicians sought to deny her intravenous morphine for control of her constant pain, Ms. Bouvia again petitioned the court. The court ruled in her favor. She now receives food by mouth and morphine intravenously and appears not to be in imminent danger of dying.

CONCLUSION

At least five driving forces, together, continually create fresh ethical quandaries in the contemporary practice of medicine: the discovery of new diseases (such as AIDS); the advent of new technologies (such as the Jarvik VII implantable heart); fresh legal judgments and legislative measures; emerging economic constraints (DRGs and PPOs among them); and sociological phenomena such as nurses developing and asserting their own distinctive professional identities. Interestingly, all five factors conjoin and are focused in the modern ICU. Here the ethical issues are presented most acutely and with the utmost poignancy. It is possible, however, to approach these problems in a principled way, such as has been outlined in this chapter. It is also possible to identify those who, potentially, can participate in decisions to limit therapy, and to suggest what weight their respective contributions ought to have, and why. This, too, has been attempted in the preceding pages. It is to be hoped that what has here been presented at the reflective level will be helpful to those existentially bound up in the decision-making process in the clinical situation.

REFERENCES

1. Beauchamp TL, Childress JF: *Principles of Biomedical Ethics,* 2nd ed. New York, Oxford University Press, 1983
2. Cohen CB: Ethical problems of intensive care. *Anesthesiology* 1977; 17:217
3. *Critical Care Medicine:* National Institutes of Health Consensus Development Conference Summary, vol 4, no 6. Washington, DC, Department of Health and Human Services, 1983
4. *Dictionary of Medical Ethics,* p 263. Crossroad, New York, 1981
5. 163 Cal. App. 3d 190, 209 Cal. Rptr. 220
6. Deciding to forego life-sustaining treatment: Ethical, medical and legal issues in treatment decisions. In *The President's Commission for the Study of Ethical Problems in Medicine and Biomedical and Behaviorial Research.* Washington, DC, 1983
7. Winkenwerder W Jr: Ethical dilemmas for house staff physicians. *JAMA* 1985; 254:3454. Cf. the editorials in the same issue of *JAMA,* Moral disagreements during residency training and doctors' orders, pp 3467–3468
8. 147 Cal. App. 3d 1006, 195 Cal. Reptr. 484
9. *Barber and Nejdl v. Superior Court,* 147 Cal. App. 3d 1006 at 1011
10. Rawls J: *A Theory of Justice.* Cambridge, Massachusetts, Harvard University Press, 1971

Informed Consent   4
Laurence B. McCullough

KEY CONSIDERATIONS TO PRACTICE INFORMED CONSENT

There are five key considerations in applying a practice of informed consent in critical care medicine: (1) the elements of informed consent: (2) degrees of disclosure; (3) four strategies for obtaining informed consent; (4) informed consent in the care of incompetent patients; and (5) preventive ethics.

ELEMENTS OF INFORMED CONSENT

There is consensus in the literature on two main features of informed consent. First, it is a *process* involving the physician and the patient; it is not simply the signature of the patient on a hospital form or a nod of the patient's head. These are only indications that the process has taken place and should not be regarded as informed consent. Second, as a process, informed consent has three elements:

> The patient must be provided with an adequate amount of information about his or her condition, the ways in which it might be treated (including diagnostic interventions, not just therapies), the risks and benefits of alternative treatments, the prognoses of various treatments, and the risks, benefits, and prognosis of nontreatment.
>
> The patient must understand this information. He or she must interpret this information in terms of his or her values and beliefs, in an attempt to determine what, in his or her own view, is the best course of intervention.
>
> The patient must choose a course of intervention or nonintervention free of controlling constraints.

DEGREES OF DISCLOSURE

One central problematic feature of informed consent is the degree of disclosure required of the physician to satisfy the first condition of informed consent. The key word in the above formulation is "adequate." What is an adequate amount of information? Three standards have emerged, and all are relevant to critical care medicine. Each requires progressively more disclosure.

The first standard is the *professional community standard*, in which adequate disclosure is defined by the customary rules or traditional practices of the professional community of physicians. Increasingly, in a specialty like critical care medicine, the benchmark will be a national standard, not simply a regional or local one (*e.g.*, the risks of complications of arterial catheterization to monitor arterial blood pressure and gases). This is obviously a physician-centered standard; the other two are patient-centered.

The second standard of disclosure is the *reasonable person standard*, in which the physician discloses what a hypothetical reasonable person would want to know. "Reasonable" means that the patient is free of unreasoning fears and the like, can think clearly, and should participate in the decision. A helpful benchmark for disclosure under this standard is that the physician should share with the patient any information that has entered into his or her clinical judgment about diagnosis and about diagnostic and therapeutic interventions. The patient can then assess the risks and benefits of available alternatives and, indeed, whether to accept the physician's determination that a particular procedure be initiated.

The third standard of disclosure is the *subjective standard*. This is the most demanding standard. It requires that the physician aim for the ideal of providing for the patient all of the information that this patient, here and now, needs to know. Obviously, this standard makes the physician vulnerable to being second-guessed. Nonetheless, in some circumstances in critical care medicine, it is the appropriate standard.

STRATEGIES FOR OBTAINING INFORMED CONSENT

There are four ethically distinct situations in critical care, although they do not always occur in a temporal sequence. Obviously a patient can begin in situation one, proceed to situations two and three, and ultimately be in situation four. But a patient can also be admitted to the critical care unit in situation three and remain in that situation for some time, even indefinitely. Others can be admitted in situation two and change to situation one, because they experience a crisis of some sort. It is probably the case that only some patients proceed neatly through all four situations in a temporal order. These four situations, regardless of the temporal sequence, are ethically different, with different requirements for disclosure and communication. This heterogeneity requires a heterogenous approach to informed consent.

SITUATION ONE. The patient is in crisis, and he or she is at grave risk of loss of life or of serious disease, injury, or handicapping condition. There is usually little time to act, if action is to benefit the patient. In these circumstances the appropriate standard of disclosure is the professional community standard. The patient should be told of his or her condition, how it can be most effectively addressed, the most common risks and benefits of treatment, and the risks of nontreatment. The second and third elements will sometimes, perhaps frequently, be not fully satisfied. The operating assumption is that most reasonable persons would want to avoid unnecessary death, disease, injury, or handicap if reasonably safe and effective treatment is available. This assumption might be invalid in cases where the patient has made a prior determination of what he or she would want (*e.g.*, a living will or some other form of advanced directive) as might occur in a patient admitted in situation three who suffers a cardiac arrest and has a living will that explicitly rules out cardiopulmonary resuscitation as against his or her wishes.

SITUATION TWO. The patient has been stabilized, and further diagnosis and treatment remain to be done. In cases where situation one temporarily precedes situation two, it is not justified to assume that the patient's initial consent to intervention amounts to consent for continuing intervention. This is because the patient's condition must now be addressed in the long term. The kind of information the patient must consider in the first situation—what intervention will prove to be of *immediate* benefit—is different from the kind of information that must be considered and evaluated in the second situation—what diagnostic and therapeutic interventions will be of *continuing* benefit, and of how great a benefit. The reasonable person standard emerges in situation two as the appropriate standard of treatment, because the patient now has the time to assess his or her condition and its prognosis under alternative interventions. The critical care patient's needs in situation two can rarely best be met through a single course of therapy. In addition, some diagnostic and therapeutic interventions may carry considerable risk of failure and be accompanied by what most reasonable persons would regard as significant, long-term pain and suffering. These are important matters in the life of any person and are best decided by that person. For example, in situation two, code status should be discussed with the patient, and the patient's autonomous decision (*i.e.*, one that satisfies the three elements of informed consent) should be implemented.

SITUATION THREE. The patient's prognosis appears to be turning poor and it is not clear whether he or she will recover. Conversely, it is not clear whether he or she will not recover. This situation in critical care is distinctly different from the first two. In the first and second situations the physician has reason to believe that the patient will directly benefit from intervention; the patient is expected to recover and leave the hospital to resume his or her life. Interventions are undertaken with this goal as justification. In the third situation the physician cannot proceed with such confidence toward a beneficial outcome. The justification for continuing becomes that of going on to find out whether it is fully justified to continue, that is, to determine whether recovery to some reasonable degree is possible.

A major factor in meeting the first requirement of informed consent, adequate disclosure, is whether to share uncertainties with the patient. The physician's clinical judgment has shifted to the subjective mood and so should disclosure. The alternative is usually nondisclosure of information that shapes clinical judgment regarding further diagnostic or therapeutic interventions. Yet these usually involve significant levels of pain and suffering, as well as iatrogenic risks from invasive or painful monitoring techniques. Respect for the patient's autonomy requires that the patient know why his or her physician believes that such risks be considered, so that he or she can decide whether it is worth going on, that is, whether the patient can possibly change to situation two of critical care or whether he or she will change to situation four. The standard for disclosure in this situation should be a blend of the reasonable person and subjective standards.

SITUATION FOUR. The patient's prognosis turns grim, and reasonable and well-founded clinical judgment indicates that the patient is not expected to recover. He or she is judged either to be dying in a way that further intervention can no longer prevent or to be in a permanent "vegetative" state from which recovery is not expected. The decisions to be made in these kinds of critical care cases reach to the heart of the human experience: whether someone will be allowed to die, how someone will die, and how someone will be remembered by loved ones, friends, and those who cared for him or her. The subjective standard should therefore guide disclosure. Given the deep human significance of the issues to be decided, primary—indeed overriding—consideration should be given to the patient's decisions.

INFORMED CONSENT IN THE CARE OF INCOMPETENT PATIENTS

The above guidelines apply, obviously, to competent patients, those who are able to think and communicate (by speaking, writing, nodding) for themselves. Informed consent in the care of incompetent patients poses special challenges. Traditionally, physicians turned to family members for guidance. Physicians still do so, but now there are other factors to consider, including living wills and other advance directives, durable power of attorney, hospital ethics committees, and court review.

The main accent of informed consent is on the *patient's* values and beliefs and respect for them in the patient's life and decisions about medical treatment and care. Can this accent be sustained in caring for incompetent patients? The answer is a qualified "yes."

Adult critical care patients have already lived their lives according to values and beliefs that they have found significant and meaningful. Many of these values and beliefs have to do with medical care and being treated with dignity and respect by physicians, nurses, and hospitals. This is especially true of elderly patients, many of whom have given a good deal of thought to such matters as whether they want to be on a respirator or undergo resuscitation should they experience cardiac arrest. This dimension of aging in our society is too frequently overlooked in critical care.

When previously competent patients become incompetent, the following strategy seems sound. First, the physician should attempt to restore the patient to a condition of competence. This is sometimes the result of critical care interventions in situation one. When this result is achieved, the above four stategies can be followed. When the patient cannot recover to a condition of competence, previous values and beliefs—the patient's value history—should guide intervention. This value history may be given specific, even detailed, expression in a living will or other form of advance directive. The value history can also be reconstructed with the aid of family members, loved ones, and the patient's primary physician. Family members should not first be asked (as they often are), "What do you want us to do?" Rather, the questions are, "What was important to your spouse/parent/relative?" "On the basis of that, what do you think he or she would want us to do?" "Did your spouse/parent/relative say anything directly about the sorts of interventions we are considering, like resuscitation, respirators, and so on?"

Patients and families will most likely not have thought as much about specific diagnostic interventions when they are first proposed or if they have not been experienced earlier. But they will have values and beliefs about pain and suffering and how much pain and suffering are worth enduring to undergo medical interventions. This dimension of values and beliefs about medical care is especially important in developing a value history relevant to assessing the worth of diagnostic interventions that involve significant levels of risks of complications and of pain and suffering. These risks should be assessed in terms of the patient's values and beliefs about pain and suffering and how much should be endured to gain the expected benefits of the proposed diagnostic interventions.

Value histories are obviously relevant to all four situations in critical care. Hence, they should be obtained by critical care physicians routinely for incompetent patients. If a reliable value history cannot be determined, then the physician should be guided by his or her judgment of what is in the patient's best interests, taking into account the values and wishes of family members. In such circumstances, hospital ethics committees can play a useful role because they can provide a forum for careful and critical evaluation of the physician's judgment.

Some patients have never been competent, typically infants and young children, and perhaps adolescents. In these circumstances, the physician should be guided by his or her judgment of the patient's best interests, again in consultation with an ethics committee, if available. Judicial intervention may also be necessary in these cases.

The role of the family in cases of incompetent and never-competent patients has two parts. On the one hand, they are the moral fiduciaries of the patient. They are expected to authorize interventions that are in the patient's best interests, on the basis of respect for the patient's value history (in the case of formerly competent patients) and on the basis of values and beliefs that are important to them (in the case of never-competent patients). In this respect, the family's moral relationship with the patient parallels that of the physician, who is also expected to act in a way that protects and promotes the best interests of the patient. On the other hand, the results of medical interventions can sometimes have an adverse effect on the interests of family members. In this respect, the family is a third party to the physician–patient relationship, and their interests as third parties can be harmed by what the physician does. This is especially the case if critical care will result in long-term care for the patient, which in our society is usually provided by the family, for both children as well as elderly parents. Families should be assisted in distinguishing these two legitimate roles and in focusing first on what is best for the patient.

Increasingly, the critical care of no longer and never-competent patients is influenced by the law. Courts in a number of states have made landmark rulings that may influence the courts in other states. Legislatures have enacted statutes to sanction living wills and other forms of advance directives. Two responses to this potentially stressful situation seem appropriate. First, if the physician is uncertain about the legal dimensions of a case, he or she should consult with an attorney. Physicians are not trained to be experts in the law and are often erroneous in their legal judgments. Such consultations should be obtained and considered in clinical judgment. Beware the attorney who assures the physician that a particular intervention is always the safe course for the physician. It may not be in the patient's best interests. Rather, ask for an assessment of benefits and risks for the patient of appropriate alternatives. Second, court review of deeply conflictual cases is an option, but one that should be exercised after careful and thorough consideration. Courts in different, and even in the same, jurisdictions have handed down conflicting opinions regarding similar case situations. In addition, court hearings may introduce factors, such as an excessively strong desire on the part of the hospital to protect itself, that turn the primary focus away from the patient's best interests to those of third parties.

PREVENTIVE ETHICS

One unfortunate development in recent years has been to focus all of the attention on informed consent and decision-making on critical care itself. Should this patient be on full code status? Should we keep this patient on the respirator, or should we turn it off? Should we monitor blood gases on patients with increasingly poor prognoses or on patients who are dying? These are important questions, but they can be anticipated for many patients before they enter the critical care setting.

Many of the patients in critical care units in our hospitals suffer from chronic diseases and disabilities. The reason that they are in the critical care unit is that they have suffered an acute episode requiring hospitalization and intensive care. In many of these cases, such an event was predictable, given the patient's underlying chronic condition. This is especially the case with elderly patients whose chronic condition worsens, resulting in hospitalization.

There is a major role for primary care physicians, surgeons, and critical care physicians in what might be termed "preventive ethics." Recall the previous discussion of basing decisions regarding incompetent patients on the patient's value history. Probably the least advantageous time to obtain such a history is when the patient is in the critical care unit. Compared with the patient himself or herself, the family is the less advantageous source of such a history. Obviously, the best source is the patient. The primary care physician working with chronically ill patients can obtain a value history during regular visits with the patient. The future of the patient's chronic condition can be explained (it should have been already) and the possibility of hospitalization raised, including details about the sorts of interventions available. The surgeon can explain postoperative risks of various diagnostic or therapeutic interventions that might be indicated if the patient needs to be admitted to the critical care unit or if such admission is a standard postoperative strategy.

The patient should consider these matters and discuss his or her values and preferences with the physician. This information should be recorded in the patient's chart. If necessary and if the patient consents, the physician or surgeon should arrange sessions with the patient and the patient's family, so that they have the opportunity to learn what the patient wants for himself or herself if critical care hospitalization should occur, either as a part of the natural history of a chronic condition or as a result of complications of surgery.

The physician or surgeon should then ensure that the contents of the value history are communicated accurately to the patient's critical care physicians. The role for critical care physicians is twofold: first, to encourage their referring physicians to obtain value histories in advance; and, second, to act on those values histories when they provide adequate guidance about diagnostic and therapeutic interventions.

ETHICAL FOUNDATIONS OF INFORMED CONSENT

The concept and practice of informed consent entered the history of medicine in our century. The roots of this historical change were in the law at first, and later (in the last 20 years) in ethics. Informed consent cannot be found in the writings of medical ethics before the beginning of our century. As Beauchamp and Faden have recently shown, before our century, matters of disclosure or "truthtelling" were handled in one of two ways.[1] One view was that physician discretion should be the guiding principle, with patients being told little or nothing about their condition and treatment. Obviously, this approach would lead to minimal disclosure, even on a professional community standard. Patients were simply to accept what was offered to them, which was usually little more than comfort and support, given the extremely limited therapeutic power of medicine in previous centuries. A second view was that the physician should be forthcoming with the patient, including dying patients. The justification for this approach was twofold: first, such an approach benefits the patient by alleviating fears based on ignorance or uncertainty; and, second, this approach respects the dignity of patients.

The contemporary understanding of the ethics of informed consent derives from the second of these two approaches. The fundamental ethical principle on medical practice in the West, from its beginnings in Ancient Greece, has been that the physician should protect and promote the best interests of the patient. Until the beginning of our century, there was a single perspective on those best interests: that afforded by the knowledge, skills, and experience of physicians. Medicine, as a social practice and institution, took upon itself the task of defining for patients what was in their best interests. The phrase "do no harm" (of unknown historical origin and certainly not contained in the Hippocratic writings) captures the main thrust of this perspective by presupposing that physicians can and do know what harms to avoid for their patients and what benefits to seek for them. The overall goal, of course, is to undertake diagnostic and therapeutic interventions whose net effect is to increase the balance of good over harm for the patient and, when at the limits of knowledge and skill, at least to "do no harm."

In ethical theory the principle of beneficence directs us to seek for others in our dealings with them the greater balance of good over harm. Obviously, to apply this principle, one must have some sense of the goods to be sought and the harms to be avoided. Western medicine, drawing on pervasive values in our culture, claims to have such a sense when it comes to medical care. It seeks for its patients the goods of avoiding premature or unnecessary death and preventing, curing, or at least ameliorating disease, injury, handicap, and unnecessary pain and suffering (pain and suffering that are not achieving the other goods). Given this understanding of beneficence in medicine, we can say that there is a beneficence model of moral responsibility in medicine that directs the physician to those interventions that are beneficial to patients from medicine's perspective.[1]

The hallmark of the beneficence model is that its balancing of goods and harms is objective in character. By this I simply mean that the model requires the physician to avoid as much as possible idiosyncratic balancing among the goods and harms of the model. Thus, a worry that sharing uncertainties with situation-three critical care patients would be harmful must be based on more than one's own intuitions or experience. Rather, such judgments should have a firm empirical foundation in the experience of critical care physicians and patients. Objectivity in the application of the beneficence model, speaking more generally, thus means that the physician can give reasons and provide a justification for a clinical judgment about what is and is not the best interests of the patient.

As a result of the influence of law (with its principle of respect for the self-determination of individuals) and of ethics (with its principle of respect for the autonomy of individuals), another perspective on the best interests of the patient must now be acknowledged, that of the patient himself or herself. Human beings have values and beliefs by which they live their lives and which do not desert them when they become ill and find themselves in a critical care unit under a physician's care. Because these values and beliefs shape individuals and their lives, they are to be accorded respect. Otherwise, we treat each other as things, as "means merely" to our own ends, as the 18th century philosopher Immanuel Kant would put it. The ethical principle of respect for autonomy directs us to acknowledge and implement the autonomous decisions of others, those decisions that reflect or express their values and beliefs—even if, and especially if, those values and beliefs happen to differ from our own. This ethical principle is at the heart of the autonomy model of moral responsibility in medicine.[1]

The distinctive feature of medical ethics is that both of these models must be taken into account by physicians. Each directs the physician to important but incomplete views on what counts as the best interests of the patient. No account of the ethics of medicine will be adequate unless reference is made to both models.

This is certainly the case for informed consent. The beneficence model justifies the practice of informed consent on the grounds that it promotes important goods in patient care, chiefly trust and cooperation. In the absence of these two attitudes on the part of the patient, it is usually difficult, if not impossible, to seek for him or her the goods of the beneficence model. The beneficence model is also the primary ethical foundation of the professional community standard of disclosure, presumably because professional practice is based on a shared judgment of what level of disclosure promotes trust and cooperation. This matter, however, is open to empirical investigation and dispute. This is the reason why the professional community standard, although the legal standard in the majority of states, is being criticized in the medical ethics literature.

The autonomy model plays an obvious role in justifying the practice of informed consent, since the entire thrust of this model is to make the patient's perspective on his or her best interest the primary consideration. The autonomy model justifies both the reasonable person and subjective standards of disclosure. The autonomy model is also the primary justification for both the second and third elements of informed consent. The second element emphasizes respect for and attention to the values and beliefs of the patient by the physician. The third element emphasizes the importance of voluntary decisions on the part of the patient. Most accounts of autonomy in the literature acknowledge that full autonomy, in the sense of making decisions that are *un*constrained, is an ideal not open to achievement by our species. Rather, it is acknowledged that we act under a variety of internal influences (physical and psychological factors) and external influences (other persons and institutions). The goal of an autonomous decision therefore is a decision that is not *controlled* by such influences and thus is to this extent one's own.[2]

There is a temptation with the autonomy model to shift all responsibility to the patient along with decisional authority. This practice would represent a misunderstanding of both informed consent and the ethical principle of respect for autonomy. With respect to the latter, it is important to emphasize that informed consent is a two-party process. And, in critical care, given its four ethically distinct situations, there is a constant give and take between the physician's and patient's perspectives on the patient's best interests. For example, situation one care relies more heavily on a beneficence model-based approach to informed consent, whereas situation four care relies more on an autonomy model-based approach. The clinical realities of critical care medicine make impossible and thus impractical a single-model approach to understanding the ethical dimensions and thus the practice of informed consent.

Shifting the full burden of decision-making to the patient, under the guise of respecting his or her autonomy, usually amounts to just the opposite. This move is often made in frustration or even anger with the decisions a patient makes or with his or her general personality type (*e.g.*, the "demanding" patient). What it amounts to is an attempt to isolate or even psychologically to abandon the patient. "Here, you decide!" is not an offer to help a patient think through an often very difficult and perhaps tragic situation—as it should be under any reasonable interpretation of respect for autonomy—but is a power play that results in alienating the patient even further. In short, the introduction of the ethical principle of respect for autonomy into medical ethics along with the changes that this brings for such matters as informed consent should be seen as enriching the moral life in medicine.

SPECIAL CONSIDERATIONS

Although a great deal has been written about the ethical and legal dimensions of informed consent, less work has been done on its psychological dimensions. Important questions remain to be investigated, if informed consent in its three elements as described above is to become a more common practice in critical care medicine and medical practice generally.

These concern the psychological "markers" for the three elements themselves. The first element is fairly easy to measure, to the extent that it depends on what the physician discloses. To the extent that achieving a standard of disclosure depends on the patient's cognitive and affective capacities to absorb the information that is being disclosed, the first element of informed consent is more difficult to measure. Mental status examinations may provide some indication of the level of such capacities, but not as much as we need. These examinations attempt to measure such capacities as short-term memory, logical functioning, and the like, but do so with varying degrees of reliability, especially in the critical care patient.

The second element requires that the patient evaluate the disclosed information on his or her own terms. This involves the patient considering the risks and benefits of alternative interventions and their prognoses and rank ordering them from most preferable (or best) to least preferable (or worst). We very much need further study of the psychological markers that will indicate with some reliability when this process is occurring, how it can be facilitated and strengthened, and when it is completed.

The third element poses similar difficulties. Critical care patients are under a great deal of stress, as in the situation one patient in the early hours of care. However, it is important to recognize that a patient's diminished ability to make his or her own choices in the first hours of care, or at any other time during the course of hospitalization, does not necessarily imply that he or she has lost that capacity altogether. The whole point of distinguishing situations in critical care is to call attention to the changing capacity of patients for autonomous decision-making and to encourage the assumption that patients in situations two, three, and four, especially, possess a greater capacity for autonomous decision-making than commonly assumed. The main goal here is for the physician to identify and alleviate internal influences that threaten to control a patient's decisional capacity. Psychiatric involvement with and support of critical care patients may be of considerable use in striving for this ethically significant goal.

"To what extent is the patient making a decision to satisfy someone else?" is a question that is appropriately raised regarding the third element of informed consent. Here the someone else may be a family member, as well as a member of the health care team, including the physician. Again, the goal should be to prevent such influences from becoming controlling factors, even if we still have difficulty in identifying when an external factor has indeed become controlling. This is an especially important consideration for elderly patients who have absorbed the ageism of our society and thus suffer from reduced self-esteem. Ageism can also be exhibited by members of the health care team, an attitude that is without justification.

CONCLUSION

Informed consent as a practice is founded in the two main models of moral responsibility in medicine generally and in critical care medicine particularly. It has three elements and involves three standards of disclosure, all of which are relevant to critical care medicine. I have proposed four strategies for informed consent in critical care medicine and have addressed matters of informed consent and incompetent patients, along with the important role of the physician in preventive ethics. More study and full appreciation of the psychological markers of informed consent remain. Medical ethics has created for clinical medicine an important new area for investigating and improving the quality of patient care.

REFERENCES

1. Faden RR, Beauchamp TL: *A History and Theory of Informed Consent*. New York, Oxford University Press, 1986
2. Beauchamp TL, McCullough LB: *Medical Ethics: The Moral Responsibilities of Physicians*. Englewood Cliffs, NJ, Prentice–Hall, 1984

Judicial Involvement in Treatment Decisions: The Emerging Consensus

Christopher J. Armstrong

A decade has passed since the decision of the New Jersey Supreme Court in the case of Karen Ann Quinlan.[1] During that time 30 or more cases of precedent-setting significance concerning lifesaving treatment have surfaced and been decided in appellate courts. Doctors, surveying the results, have been skeptical and critical of the involvement of courts and lawyers in what they regard as an area of medical expertise. They point, with much justification, to the delays endemic to the judicial process, illustrated by frequent instances in which the court proceedings to determine whether lifesaving treatment should be withheld or withdrawn remained pending, still not finally decided, after the death of the patient.[2] Far from providing useful guidance, the court decisions have often seemed to physicians to be confusing if not outright inconsistent. Abstractions like "substituted judgment" seem to have little relevance to the realities of the situation confronting the doctor; and distinctions on which courts sometimes place reliance ("ordinary" versus "extraordinary" measures, "life-saving" versus "life-prolonging" treatments) have no clear medical meaning in the physician's view. Courts seem naive when they describe as "awesome" or "profound" decisions of a type that doctors have to make each day. They see the procedural apparatus of the judicial process, with the involvement of hosts of doctors, lawyers (often as many as three for the patient alone—a counsel, a guardian, and a guardian *ad litem*), and multiple levels of courts as impossibly cumbersome and exquisitely insensitive to the hardship on the patients' families at a time of maximum stress. Thus, doctors inevitably ask, what useful purpose is served by court involvement?

My theme is that the involvement of courts has been essential, particularly for the medical profession, in working out societal guidelines that had

---

1. *Matter of Quinlan*, 70 N.J. 10 (1976)
2. Instances include *Superintendent of Belchertown State School v. Saikewicz*, 373 Mass. 728 (1977); *Matter of Spring*, 380 Mass. 629 (1980); *John F. Kennedy Hosp. v. Bludworth*, 452 So.2d 921 (Fla. 1984); *Matter of Hamlin*, 689 P.2d 1372 (Wash. 1984); *Matter of Storar*, 52 N.Y.2d 363 (1981); *Corbett v. D'Alessandro*, 487 So.2d 368 (Fla. App. 1986)

not previously been articulated; that courts have succeeded in the task of establishing workable guidelines to a greater degree than physicians often appreciate; and that in setting these guidelines, courts have been consciously working toward minimizing their role in the future.

THE PROBLEM

The *Quinlan* case was not the beginning of the problem, but it was the beginning of the public debate about the problem. Before the *Quinlan* case and the enormous publicity focused on it, the public generally assumed that medical practitioners would always do everything in their power to sustain the lives of critically ill patients. Doctors, of course, knew better. They knew of instances where, by written or verbal orders, available resuscitation was intentionally withheld in the aftermath of cardiac arrest,[3] where severely defective newborns were permitted to die from treatable conditions,[4] and where hospitalization and antibiotic therapy were withheld from severely debilitated patients in nursing homes,[5] pneumonia, for example, being treated (in Osler's phrase) as "the old man's friend."

Doctors as a group were not eager to discuss these matters openly. Destroying the public misconception might impair confidence in the profession. Knowledge of the fact of choice would trouble many families unnecessarily. The wise family physician was treating the family as well as the patient, a family whose concerns and troubles he understood. Where difficult decisions had to be made, he would not hesitate to spare the family and take the burden on himself.

Three factors conspired to destroy the myth. One was the gradual breakdown of the once-intimate relationship between the doctor and the family. In an age of group practices and hospital-based or clinic-based practices and ever more rarified specialization, treating physicians were often relative strangers to the patient and his family. The second factor, to a large extent related to the first, was the growth of malpractice litigation, which made the doctor, knowing little of the family he was dealing with, chary of potential legal liability, and ever more cognizant of the dangers of acting in the absence of documented informed consent. The third factor, certainly the most dramatic and pervasive, was the revolution in drugs and technology. No longer was medical care "both cheap and useless,"[6] new discoveries, at first gradually and then exponentially, increased the range of treatment options and their potential impact to a point where, by the 1970s, it had become possible to sustain life in some form almost indefinitely in some cases if the

---

3. Rabkin, Gillerman, Rice: Orders not to resuscitate. *N Engl J Med* 1976; 295:364
4. Duff, Campbell: Moral and ethical dilemmas in the special care nursery. *N Engl J Med* 1973; 289:90
5. Brown, Thompson: Nontreatment of fever in extended care facilities. *N Engl J Med* 1979; 300:1246
6. Avorn: Benefit and cost analysis in geriatric care: Turning age discrimination into health policy. *N Engl J Med* 1984; 310:1294

technology could be brought to bear while the patient was still alive or, indeed, within a few minutes after his death. No longer could the fact of *choice* be submerged. It had to come, in Fried's words, "out of the closet"[7] and enter the public domain.

THE PUBLIC DEBATE

The problem made its public debut in the *Quinlan* case, and at first the results seemed reassuring to doctors. The problem had been aired; the court had sanctioned a decision to withdraw life-sustaining treatment; and the contention that such a decision could be indictable as homicide was seemingly put to rest. The court had suggested a seemingly viable decision-making process, involving consultation and consensus among the treating physician, the patient (if competent) or family, and a hospital ethics committee. It had exonerated medical practitioners from civil liability, and it had rejected the idea, anathema to most physicians, that courts should normally have to become involved in such decisions. Comfortingly, it had characterized such involvement as "a gratuitous encroachment upon the medical profession's field of competence."[8]

The *Quinlan* decision was followed within a year, however, by the influential *Saikewicz* decision in Massachusetts,[9] which rejected the *Quinlan* view and called (as the *Saikewicz* case was understood at the time) for judicial resolution of decisions to terminate treatment.[9a] Within a short time thereafter the New York Court of Appeals, in *Matter of Storar*,[10] emphatically rejected the developing substituted judgment doctrine that had played a role in the *Quinlan* decision and had been the cornerstone of the analysis of the *Saikewicz* opinion. The celebrated *Earle Spring* case brought "right to life" groups into the debate, charging euthanasia,[11] and in New York and some other states district attorneys were threatening prosecution of doctors who terminated life-sustaining treatment. Frustrated groups advocating "natural death" options sought relief from state legislatures, some of which passed natural death acts over often vocal "right to life" opposition that treated the

---

7. Fried: Terminating life support: Out of the closet! *N Engl J Med* 1976; 295:390
8. 170 N.J. at 50
9. *Superintendent of Belchertown State School v. Saikewicz*, 373 Mass. 728 (1977)
9a. *Saikewicz*, 373 Mass. at 758–759: "We reject the approach adopted by the New Jersey Supreme Court in the *Quinlan* case of entrusting the decision whether to continue artificial life support to the patient's guardian, family, attending doctors, and hospital 'ethics committee' . . . [S]uch questions of life and death seem to us to require the process of detached but passionate investigation and decision that forms the ideal on which the judicial branch of government was created. Achieving this ideal is our responsibility and that of the lower court, and is not to be entrusted to any other group purporting to represent the 'morality and conscience of our society,' no matter how highly motivated or impressively constituted."
10. *Matter of Storar*, 52 N.Y.2d 363 (1981)
11. *Matter of Spring*, 380 Mass. 629 (1980). The story of the involvement of right to life groups is recounted in Paris', "Death, Dying, and the Courts: The Travesty and Tragedy of the Earle Spring Case," Linacre Quarterly, Feb 1972

question of natural death as indistinguishable from abortion. The resulting "living will" legislation was often so narrow in scope as to be almost useless in the view of the advocates and so couched with legal conditions as to be intimidating to medical practitioners. What doctors most feared seemed to be happening. Far from providing understanding and guidance, the legal community—courts, legislatures, lawyers—seemed hopelessly enmeshed in conflict and confusion.

What the dismayed physicians were witnessing, of course, was the somewhat disorderly process of hammering out significant policy in a democratic country. Democracy encourages dissent; the federal system encourages a diversity of approaches. The process looks chaotic; but, when it works well, it forges a societal consensus that derives its durability from the fact that alternatives have been examined, tried, and found wanting.

Doctors were unrealistic in thinking that courts could provide instant, clean answers. Courts are not wiser than the society they serve. They are profoundly human institutions, not detached citadels. They are dedicated to principled decision-making (*i.e.*, to the resolution of disputes by reference to articulated principles which are applied uniformly in all like cases); but in the absence of legislation they must forge the governing principles, and in doing so they proceed by trial and error, reflecting in the process, with unsurprising fidelity, the conflicts of opinion in the larger society. Where these conflicts are deeply rooted, courts may be unable to forge viable solutions, as the *Dred Scott* case[12] and *Roe v. Wade*[13] eloquently testify.

Physicians who were critical of the confusion in the aftermath of the *Quinlan* and *Saikewicz* cases would do well to reflect on the conflicts within their own profession in the early stages of the debate. Many of the major court cases were marked by sharp divisions of opinion among doctors concerning the dictates of medical ethics.[14] Articles surveying physicians' attitudes in these matters displayed similar, deep-seated divisions.[15] The natural death movement had its roots in a societal revulsion to the excessive use of technology by some practitioners, based on "a technological attitude that threatens to become an abuse."[16] Many saw "the ultimate horror [not as] death but the possibility of being maintained in limbo, in a sterile room, by machines controlled by strangers."[17] In the description of one ethicist,

> When was the last time you heard anyone say: "The patient had a wonderful life; he fought the good fight; he has finished the race. He

---

12. *Dred Scott v. Sandford*, 60 U.S. (19 Howe) 393 (1856)
13. *Roe v. Wade*, 410 U.S. 113 (1973)
14. The *Quinlan* case was an example. Another was *Brophy v. New Eng. Sinai Hosp.*, 398 Mass. 417 (1986)
15. See Shaw, Randolph, Maynard: Ethical issues in pediatric surgery: A natural survey of pediatricians and pediatric surgeons, *Pediatrics* 1977; 60:588; Todres, Krane, Howell: Pediatricians' attitudes affecting decision making in defective newborns. *Pediatrics* 1977; 60:197
16. Quoted in the Vatican Declaration on Euthanasia, May 5, 1980, appearing in Appendix C of the Report of the President's Commission for the Study of Ethical Problems in Medicine and Biomedical and Behavioral Research, Deciding to Forego Life Sustaining Treatment (1983)
17. Steel: "The right to die: New options in California," 93 *Christian Century* (July–Dec 1976)

kept the faith. Now it is time for him to go to his Maker." Rather, is not the call: "He is dying. Do something." The most glaring example of that reality is that nobody dies in the hospital, they arrest! For the individual whose journey has indeed come to its conclusion, the individual with end-stage liver disease whose heart stops, we do not say: "At last he is at peace." Instead, we shout: "Code Blue." That is the problem.[18]

Unquestionably, most physicians sympathized with the concept of death with dignity, but many, as the court cases made clear, were genuinely concerned that the omission of lifesaving treatment or the termination of life support was indefensible on moral or legal grounds. The medical profession seemed as much in need of standards as the larger society; more so, for it was faced daily with treatment decisions that could not be put off.

THE EMERGING LEGAL CONSENSUS

On matters so fraught with emotion as the withholding or withdrawing of life-sustaining treatment, there can never be perfect agreement. Although some serious problems remain, the recent court decisions from across the country seem to be falling into some definite patterns that, to me, presage substantial agreement among courts on several principles of importance to physicians and hospitals. If this reading is correct, these principles can be relied on to govern future court decisions. These principles will derive stability from the fact that they are in harmony with the traditional and accepted roles of physicians, patients, and families in determining courses of medical treatment.

The largely settled principles are presented below, together with a brief discussion of the application of each.

(1) *A competent adult has a legal right to refuse medical treatment, a right that may be qualified in particular cases by one of four countervailing state interests.* The right to refuse treatment has been declared in so many decisions, in so many jurisdictions, as to be now beyond any dispute. It represents a definitive rejection, by the law, of the vitalist principle that underlies the thinking of many in the "right to life" movement: that human life must be preserved at all costs. Cases applying the principle have often involved elderly patients refusing major surgery, such as leg amputations,[19] Jehovah's Witnesses refusing blood transfusions,[20] or lucid patients with devastating conditions—Lou Gehrig's disease or quadriplegia—seeking removal of life support.[21]

---

18. Paris: "Terminating treatment for newborns: A theological perspective." *Law, Med Health Care*, p 122, June 1982
19. Examples are *Lane v. Candura*, 6 Mass. App. Ct. 377 (1978), and *Matter of Quackenbush*, 156, N.J. Super. 282 (1978)
20. E.g., *Matter of Osborne*, 294 A.2d 372 (D.C. 1972); *Matter of Melideo*, 88 Misc.2d 974 (N.Y. Sup. Ct. 1976)
21. E.g., *Satz v. Perlmutter*, 362 So.2d 160 (Fla. App. 1978), aff'd. 379 So.2d 359 (Fla. 1980); *Matter of Farrell*, 212 N.J. Super. 294 (1986); *Bouvia v. Superior Court*, 225 Cal. Rptr. 297 (Ct. App. 1986)

These amputation and transfusion cases illustrate that the state does not always insist "that human life be saved where the affliction is curable."[22]

The state interests that sometimes justify overriding the wishes of the competent patient have been repeatedly stated to be "(1) the preservation of life, (2) the protection of the interests of innocent third parties, (3) the prevention of suicide, and (4) maintaining the ethical integrity of the medical profession."[23] The first of these is often said to be "the most significant"[24] of the four state interests. Taken literally, however, it could destroy the free choice principle.[25] Recent cases have tended to sidestep it as a factor in cases of terminal or incurable illness. "The general state interest in the preservation of life—most weighty where the patient, properly treated, can return to reasonable health, without great suffering, and a decision to avoid treatment would be aberrational—carries far less weight where the patient is approaching the end of a normal life span, where the afflictions are incapacitating, and where the best that medicine can offer is an extension of suffering."[26] Cases involving the second state interest—protection of the rights of innocent third parties—have usually involved refusals of needed blood transfusions by healthy pregnant women[27] or by basically healthy treatable adults with young children to support.[28] Prevention of suicide—the third countervailing state interest—has not led to overriding a competent patient's refusal of treatment in any reported appellate case. Courts have universally accepted a distinction between suicide and allowing a life-threatening condition to take its natural course, without treatment or artificial life support.[29]

The fourth state interest—maintaining the ethical integrity of the medical profession—has carried different connotations in different decisions. To the *Quinlan* and *Saikewicz* courts, it meant a consensus of medical practitioners, where one could be shown to exist, that withholding treatment would be ethically unjustified in particular circumstances. Other courts have used the concept in which a patient seeks institutional treatment but seeks also to limit the course of that treatment in a manner violative of sound medical practice, for example, consenting to surgery while denying consent for any

---

22. *Saikewicz*, 373 Mass. at 742
23. *Saikewicz*, 373 Mass. at 741
24. *Id.*
25. The state interest in the preservation of life may play a decisive role in states that do not utilize substituted judgment analysis in cases of incompetent patients, because it can be invoked as a reason for continuing life support to patients who derive no benefit from treatment, such as those in a permanent vegetative state.
26. *Brophy v. New Eng. Sinai Hosp.*, 398 Mass. 417, 433, fn. 8 (1986), quoting from *Matter of Spring*, 8 Mass. App. Ct. 831, 845–846 (1979), rev'd. in part 380 Mass. 629 (1980)
27. *Raleigh Fitkin–Paul Mem. Hosp. v. Anderson*, 42 N.J. 421 (1964); *Crouse–Irving Hosp. v. Paddock*, 127 Misc.2d 101 (N.Y. Sup. Ct. 1985); *Matter of Jamaica Hosp.*, 128 Misc.2d 1006 (1985); *Jefferson v. Griffin Spaulding County Hosp.*, 247 Ga. 86(1985)
28. *Holmes v. Silver Cross Hosp.*, 340 F. Supp. 125 (D. Ill. 1972); *Application of President & Directors of Georgetown College*, 331 F.2d 1000 (D.C. Cir.), cert. den. 377 U.S. 978 (1964); *Winthrop Univ. Hosp. v. Hess*, 128 Misc.2d 804 (N.Y. Sup. Ct. 1985)
29. *Saikewicz*, 373 Mass. at 743, fn. 11; *Matter of Conroy*, 98 N.J. 321, 350–351 (1985)

necessary blood transfusions.[30] To some courts the concept has meant that a physician or hospital may not be required to act in a way that the physician or hospital views as immoral, as long as the patient may be transferred to the care of others who do not share that view.[31] The last application, of course, does not significantly qualify the patient's right to refuse treatment.

The trend in recent cases has been to emphasize that patient autonomy governs except in those situations in which the countervailing state interest is for some reason "compelling."[32] As J. Letts stated in *Satz v. Perlmutter,*

> It is all very convenient to insist on continuing Mr. Perlmutter's life so that there can be no question of foul play, no resulting civil liability, and no possible trespass on medical ethics. However, it is quite another matter to do so at the patient's sole expense and against his competent will, thus inflicting never ending physical torture on his body until the inevitable, but artificially suspended, moment of death. Such a course of conduct invades the patient's constitutional right of privacy, removes his freedom of choice and invades his right to self-determination.[33]

(2) *An incompetent patient has the same right as a competent patient to avoid treatment, and the right may be exercised in his behalf by an appropriate surrogate.* All courts accept this general principle, but there is some underlying disagreement as to the basis of the right and as to the manner in which it may be asserted. The *Saikewicz* court, using the term "substituted judgment," conceptualized the right as precisely analogous to the right of a competent patient to withhold consent. It envisions the surrogate's role as one of determining as nearly as possible what the incompetent patient would choose if he were competent to make a choice. The standard is said to be subjective; the surrogate will give or withhold consent based on the incompetent's choice, whether wise or foolish. Other courts tend to rely on the more traditional, "best interests of the ward" approach, which is said to be an objective determination. They focus on whether treatment will cause or extend suffering and whether the likely benefits of that treatment justify that suffering.[34] The substituted judgment approach, most plausible where the views of the patient were expressed at some time before he/she lapsed into

---

30. *Application of President & Directors of Georgetown College,* 331 F.2d at 1009; *United States v. George,* 239 F. Supp. 752, 754 (D. Conn. 1965); *John F. Kennedy Mem. Hosp. v. Heston,* 58 N.J. 576, 582–583 (1971).
31. An example is the *Brophy* case, 398 Mass. at 440–441, where the court agreed that the patient (who was in a permanent vegetative state) was legally entitled to the removal of a gastrostomy, but declined to require that the removal take place at the chronic care hospital where he was a patient. The decision noted that other nearby hospitals are available and willing to assume care of the patient during the removal and thereafter. Contrast *Matter of Requena,* 213 N.J. Super. 475 (1986), where a hospital was ordered to continue treating a woman with Lou Gehrig's disease despite her refusal to accept insertion of a feeding tube.
32. See *In re Torres,* 357 N.W.2d 332, 339 (Minn. 1984).
33. *Satz v. Perlmutter,* 362 So.2d at 164.
34. See, *e.g., In re Torres,* 357 N.W.2d at 338–339; *Matter of Hamlin,* 689 P.2d 1372, 1375–1376 (Wash. 1984).

incompetency, has been criticized as meaningless when applied to infants or to mentally retarded patients who have never been competent to have or express a meaningful choice.[35] Its advantage may be that it tends to facilitate consideration of intangible factors—those related to personal dignity, concern for loved ones, concern even for cost—that the surrogate knows, but cannot demonstrate, would enter into the thinking of most competent persons similarly situated. The objective, "best interests" test, if narrowly applied, can become bureaucratic, resulting in mechanical decisions to continue life support in situations where it is of no benefit to the patient, and is both exorbitantly costly and a source of anguish to the patient's loved ones, simply because it cannot be shown by reference to objective criteria, such as pain, that it is better for the patient not to prolong the ordeal.[36]

Fortunately, most courts have resisted the temptation to approach these cases mechanically and have blurred the theoretical distinctions between the subjective and objective approaches. When the patient's actual views are not known but it is clear that continued treatment is of no benefit, most courts have not imposed technical legal barriers to humane decision-making. Courts have been influenced by the thought of religious leaders that a decision not to treat may sometimes be justified "as an acceptance of the human condition, or a wish to avoid the application of a medical procedure disproportionate to the results that can be expected, or a desire not to impose excessive expense on the family or the community."[37]

(3) *The family of an incompetent patient is presumptively an appropriate surrogate to act in his behalf.* Although there has been little discussion of the principle in court decisions until recently, it has long been taken for granted by physicians and hospitals that they may look to parents, spouses, and children to give valid consent to treatment when the patient is incompetent to make the choice. In deciding that the family is presumed also to be the appropriate surrogate to participate in decisions not to continue treatment,[38] courts have confirmed the traditional view of the family's role.

The presumption may be rebutted. Circumstances may come to the attention of physicians or hospital staff indicating that the family is not an appropriate participant in the treatment decision. Obviously the presumption is strongest when applied to the immediate family of the patient, who live

---

35. See *Matter of Storar,* 52 N.Y.2d at 380
36. In New Jersey, for example, the *Conroy* case seems to require (where the incompetent patient's actual views are not known) that life support must be continued except where "the recurring, unavoidable and severe pain of the patient's life with the treatment [is] such that the effect of administering life-sustaining treatment would be inhumane." 98 N.J. at 366. See the moving protest against this restrictive standard by J. Stanton in *Matter of Visbeck,* 510 A.2d 125, 130–133 (N.J. Super. Ct. 1986). The *Storar* case indicates that New York law is similarly restrictive. See discussion in *Matter of Hier,* 18 Mass. App. Ct. 200, 206–207 (1984)
37. Vatican Declaration on Euthanasia, May 5, 1980. See fn.16, supra
38. *John F. Kennedy Hosp. v. Bludworth,* 452 So.2d 921 (Fla. 1984); *Matter of Hamlin,* 689 P.2d 1372 (Wash. 1984); *Matter of J.N.,* 406 A.2d 1275 (D.C. Ct. App. 1979); *In re L.R.H.,* 253 Ga. 439 (1984); *Barber v. Superior Court,* 147 Cal. App.3d 1006 (Ct. App. 1983). See also *Matter of Spring,* 8 Mass. App. Ct. 831, 840 and fn. 9 (1979), rev'd in part, 380 Mass. 629, 638 (1980); *Custody of a Minor (No. 1),* 385 Mass. 697, 707–710 (1982)

with him, and weakest in the case of distant relatives, who have to be searched out; strong when their view seems like the normal view of a loving and emotionally involved family, weaker when their view seems unconcerned or aberrational. As one court has stated, "[i]n individual cases, health care providers and courts have to be wary about idiosyncratic decisions made by surrogates."[39] An important and long-standing example is that courts have regularly overridden idiosyncratic choices of parents to refuse needed medical treatment for children.[40] Here physicians and hospital staff must necessarily rely on experience and common sense, knowing that they will not be held accountable if they act in good faith. Serious doubts about the role of a family in treatment decisions may sometimes necessitate the assistance of a court.

(4) *Court proceedings are generally unnecessary to secure approval of a decision to withhold or withdraw life-sustaining medical treatment, except in cases of dispute or where the incompetent patient lacks an appropriate surrogate to act in his behalf.* The *Quinlan* decision in 1976 rejected the notion that courts should decide termination of treatment cases on a case-by-case basis. Later cases, including the *Saikewicz* case in Massachusetts and *Leach v. Akron General Medical Center*[41] in Ohio, cast doubt on the *Quinlan* view, but it is now clear that all courts that have addressed the point, with the possible exception of Ohio's, have adopted the view that prior court approval is not legally required.[42] This is true even in Massachusetts, where the Supreme Judicial Court has clarified or amended its statement in the *Saikewicz* case, so as to make it clear that

> our opinions should not be taken to establish any requirement of prior judicial approval that would not otherwise exist. . . . [T]he standard for determining whether the treatment was called for is the same after the event as before; negligence cannot be based solely on failure to obtain prior court approval, if the approval would have been given. . . . Thus absence of court approval does not result in automatic civil liability for withholding treatment; court approval may serve the useful purpose of resolving a doubtful or disputed question of law or fact. . . .[43]

---

39. *Matter of Visbeck*, 510 A.2d 125, 132 (N.J. Super. Ct. 1986)
40. *Custody of a Minor*, 375 Mass. 733 (1978) (parents choosing vitamin treatment over chemotherapy for child with leukemia). *Jehovah's Witnesses v. King's County Hosp.*, 390 U.S. 598 (1966), and *Matter of Sampson*, 29 N.Y.2d 900 (1972) (parents refusing blood transfusions for children)
41. 68 Ohio Misc. 1 (1980)
42. *John F. Kennedy Hosp. v. Bludworth*, 452 So.2d 921 (Fla. 1984); *Barber v. Superior Court*, 147 Cal. App.3d 1006 (1983); *Parker v. United States*, 406 A2d 1275 (D.C. Ct. App. 1979); *In re L.R.H.*, 253 Ga. 439 (1984); *In re Torres*, 357 N.W.2d 332 (Minn. 1984); *Matter of Hamlin*, 689 P.2d 1372 (Wash. 1984); *Matter of Spring*, 380 Mass. 629 (1980); *Matter of Storar*, 52 N.Y.2d 363 (1981)
43. *Matter of Spring*, 380 Mass. at 636, 639. The earlier statement in the *Saikewicz* case (see fn. 9a, supra) was explained to mean only that, "when a court is properly presented with the legal question, whether treatment may be withheld, it must decide that question and not delegate it to some private person or group." 380 Mass. at 639

Some courts require that the decision of a family (or guardian) and attending physicians to terminate life-sustaining treatment be reviewed and approved by a third party, such as a hospital ethics committee,[44] other physicians,[45] or a prognosis committee.[46] If the incompetent patient does not have a family or guardian, ordinarily resort must be had to a court to obtain either the appointment of a guardian with the authority to act for the patient or a substituted judgment decision by the court.[47] New Jersey has adopted a unique procedure, applicable to patients in nursing homes, that requires the appointment of a guardian (whether or not the patient has a family) and involvement of the State's ombudsman.[48] When there is irreconcilable disagreement between physicians and family members, resort should be had to a court.

Courts appreciate the logistical impossibility of deciding all termination-of-treatment questions on a case-by-case basis. In the *Torres* case, for example, the Minnesota Supreme Court noted that "an average of about ten life support systems are disconnected weekly in Minnesota."[49]

(5) *The entry of a no-code (or DNR) order on a patient's chart does not require prior judicial approval.* The principal case on this subject is *Matter of Dinnerstein*, which held prior judicial approval unnecessary.[50] Most deaths in our time occur in hospitals; most are signaled by cardiac arrest.

> As it cannot be assumed that legal proceedings ... will be initiated in respect of more than a small fraction of all terminally ill or dying elderly patients, [a requirement of prior judicial approval of no-code orders] would require attempts to resuscitate dying patients in most cases, without exercise of medical judgment, even when that course of action could aptly be characterized as a pointless, even cruel, prolongation of the act of dying.[51]

When cardiac arrest is anticipated immediately as part of the terminal stage of incurable illness, resuscitation is manifestly inappropriate,[51a] whether or not the patient's family has been consulted. In such cases there is no real treatment decision to be made; rather, the situation "presents a question

---

44. *Matter of Quinlan,* 70 N.J. at 54
45. *John F. Kennedy Hosp. v. Bludworth,* 452 So.2d at 926
46. *Matter of Hamlin,* 689 P.2d at 1377–1378
47. *Matter of Conroy,* 98 N.J. at 381–382 (guardian); *Matter of Hamlin,* 689 P.2d at 1378 (guardian); *Custody of a Minor (No.1),* 385 Mass. at 708–710 (substituted judgment determination)
48. *Matter of Conroy,* 98 N.J. at 381–385
49. 357 N.W.2d at 341, fn. 4
50. *Matter of Dinnerstein,* 6 Mass. App. Ct. 466 (1978) There seem to be no reported cases concerning DNR orders in other jurisdictions.
51. *Matter of Dinnerstein,* 6 Mass. App. Ct. at 471
51a. "The purpose of cardiopulmonary resuscitation is the prevention of sudden, unexpected death. Cardiopulmonary resuscitation is not indicated in certain situations, such as in cases of terminal irreversible illness where death is not unexpected or where prolonged cardiac arrest dictates the futility of resuscitation efforts. Resuscitation in these circumstances may represent a positive violation of an individual's right to die with dignity." AMA standards for cardiopulmonary resuscitation (CPR) and emergency cardiac care (EEC). *JAMA* 1974; 227:837, 864

peculiarly within the competence of the medical profession of what measures are appropriate to ease the imminent passing of an irreversibly, terminally ill patient in light of the patient's history and condition and the wishes of the family."[52] When the death is not expected immediately but the patient is suffering from an untreatable, debilitating illness or is greatly enfeebled by the afflictions of age, the entry of a no-code order should normally be discussed with the patient (if appropriate) or the family.

There may be cases in which a "family, through ignorance, misunderstanding, fear, or guilt," demands resuscitation of an irreversibly dying patient or, conversely, insists "on a DNR order for a patient the physician believes has a good chance of recovering."[53] In such cases, after education or persuasion fail, the physician or hospital may find it appropriate to seek the assistance of a court.

(6) *A decision to terminate medical treatment is subject to the same legal standards as a decision not to begin the treatment.* Each court that has considered the question has agreed that no distinction should be drawn between withdrawing and withholding treatment. Leading decisions have been the *Barber* case in California, the *Conroy* case in New Jersey, and the *Brophy* case in Massachusetts.[54] A person who "has a right to refuse treatment in the first instance has a concomitant right to discontinue it."[55] This position accords with that taken by the influential President's Commission for the Study of Ethical Problems in Medicine and Biomedical and Behavioral Research in 1983.[56]

A contrary view was, until recently, prevalent among physicians, who doubtless reasoned from the principle that a physician, having undertaken care of a patient, should not abandon him or her.[57] But terminating a treatment is not abandonment if the treatment turns out to be pointless. Respirator support may be required to give time for evaluation, but if the evaluation shows that nothing can be done to benefit the patient, the reason for respirator support is gone. "From a policy standpoint, it might well be unwise to forbid persons from discontinuing a treatment under circumstances in which the treatment could be permissibly withheld. Such a rule could discourage families and doctors from even attempting certain types of care and could thereby force them into hasty and premature decisions to allow a patient to die."[58] Thus in 1983, the National Institutes of Health Consensus Development Conference on Critical Care Medicine concluded that "[i]t is inappropriate to maintain ICU management of a patient whose prognosis has resolved to one of persistent vegetative state, and it is similarly inappro-

---

52. *Matter of Dinnerstein,* 6 Mass. App. Ct. at 475
53. Paris, Reardon: Dilemmas in intensive care medicine: An ethical and legal analysis. *J Intensive Care Med* 1986; 1:75, 79
54. Respectively, 147 Cal. App. 3d at 1016; 98 N.J. at 370; 398 Mass. at 438
55. *Satz v. Perlmutter,* 362 So.2d at 163
56. Deciding to Forego Life-Sustaining Treatment at 181–183
57. *Ascher v. Gutierrez,* 533 F.2d 1235 (D.C. Cir. 1976)
58. *Matter of Conroy,* 98 N.J. at 370

priate to employ ICU resources where no purpose will be served but a prolongation of the natural process of death." That view is fully consistent with the decisions of all courts that have spoken to the point.

(7) *Rules concerning withdrawal of treatment apply equally to withdrawal of nutrition and hydration by artificial means.* Artificial means include intravenous feeding, nasogastric tubes, gastrostomies, central hyperalimentation, and the like.[59] The first and leading case of withdrawal of feeding was the *Barber* case in California, in which physicians, at the family's request, withdrew a nasogastric tube from a patient in permanent vegetative state.[60] The physicians were charged with murder. The court quashed the charges, holding that withdrawal of artificial feeding was no different from withdrawing any other medical treatment not benefiting the patient. "Medical procedures to provide nutrition and hydration are more similar to other medical procedures than to typical human ways of providing nutrition and hydration. Their benefits and burdens ought to be evaluated in the same manner as any other medical procedure."[61] The court adopted, in effect, the conclusion by the President's Commission Report the same year,[62] and since that time the position taken in *Barber* has in turn been adopted by every court that has spoken on the point.[63]

(8) *A physician or hospital acting in good faith will not be held civilly or criminally liable for acquiescing in the wish of the patient's family that artificial life-support measures be terminated.* This is a corollary of the principle that a court decision is normally not required or desirable except in cases of dispute or cases without an appropriate surrogate. Because decision-making within the physician–patient–family triad is authorized by the law, such a decision cannot in itself be a source of liability. Here the courts recognize that determinations when to continue and when to terminate treatment require a sophisticated exercise of judgment, and the law will not inhibit the physician's exercise of his best judgment by second-guessing it at a later date. Rather, the courts have indicated that the highest standard to which a physician will be held is that he must act without negligence and in good faith.[64]

The unusual action of the California courts in quashing the criminal prosecution in the *Barber* case should serve as an example to physicians that,

---

59. "Life-prolonging medical treatment includes medication and artificially or technologically supplied respiration, nutrition or hydration." Statement of American Medical Assn. Council on Ethical and Judicial Affairs (1986), also stating: "Even if death is not imminent but a patient's care is beyond doubt irreversible and there are adequate safeguards to confirm the diagnosis and with the concurrence of those who have the responsibility for the care of the patient, it is not unethical to discontinue all means of life-prolonging medical treatment."
60. *Barber v. California,* 147 Cal. App.3d 1006 (1983)
61. *Id.,* at 1016–1017. The language was adapted from *Lynn, Childress:* Must patients always be given food and water? *Hastings Ctr Rep* 1983; 13:17,20
62. Deciding to Forego Life-Sustaining Treatment, at 90, 288
63. *Matter of Conroy,* 98 N.J. at 372–374; *Brophy v. New Eng. Sinai Hosp.,* 398 Mass. at 435–440; *Bouvia v. Superior Court,* 179, Cal. App.3d at 1141; *Corbett v. D'Alessandro,* 487 So.2d 368, 371 (Fla. Dist. Ct. App. 1986); *Matter of Hier,* 18 Mass. App. Ct. 207–208
64. *Matter of Spring,* 380 Mass. at 639

in this sensitive area, the courts will not countenance the misuse of the criminal process for political reasons. Massachusetts' highest court has stated, "Little need be said about criminal liability: there is precious little precedent, and what there is suggests that the doctor will be protected if he acts on a good faith judgment that is not grievously unreasonable by medical standards."[65] The Florida Supreme Court has stated, "To be relieved of the potential civil and criminal liability, guardians, consenting family members, physicians, hospitals, or their administrators need only act in good faith. For them to be held civilly or criminally liable, there must be a showing that their actions were not in good faith but intended to harm the patient."[66] There is no reason to think that other courts, should the question come before them, will not act similarly to protect physicians and hospital staff who honestly exercise their best professional judgment in this complex and sensitive area.

CONCLUSION

It is difficult to appreciate how far the debate has moved in 10 years without surveying the contentions made to courts in *Quinlan* and other cases and comparing those contentions with where we are today. In the early stages of the debate, the focus was the applicability of criminal concepts, like murder and abetting suicide, and on the need to establish legal mechanisms, the most comprehensive being full court review in every case, to protect patients from possibly unscrupulous or uncaring decisions by doctors and families. The very language of the debate seemed to promise an unavoidable involvement of lawyers and courts in every case in which doctors and patients or their families decided to withhold or withdraw an available life-sustaining treatment. The norm implicit in the debate seemed to be that all available technologies should be applied and that any derivation from that norm was fraught with serious legal consequences.

By the end of the decade, in contrast, those fears have been very largely put to rest. Courts across the country have reached something approaching consensus on principles that comprehensively protect private decision-making within the traditional physician–patient–family triad and insulate the decision-makers from criminal and civil liability for decisions, not manifestly unreasonable, made in good faith.[67]

At the beginning of the decade, medical providers lay vulnerable to criticism because the public had little understanding of the life-and-death

---

65. *Id.* at 637
66. *John F. Kennedy Hosp. v. Bludworth,* 452 So.2d at 926
67. An excellent (although controversial) illustration of the protective attitude of courts toward private decision-making was the response of both the New York and Federal courts to attempts by outside agencies (both private and governmental) to intrude into the physician–family decision-making process in the much publicized Baby Jane Doe case. See *Weber v. Stony Brook Hosp.,* 95 App. Div. 2d 587 (1983), aff'd. 60 N.Y.2d 208 (1983); *United States v. Univ. Hosp. of State Univ. of New York,* 575 F. Supp. 607 (E.D. N.Y. 1983), aff'd. 729 F.2d 144 (2nd Cir. 1984)

decisions being made daily in health care institutions. The glare of publicity was inevitable. It was also uncomfortable. The debate was at times intemperate and vehement, but today medical providers are in a safer position because a significant part of the public has come to understand, if only in a general way, a truth long hidden within the medical profession: that an important part of the physician's role is knowing when the time has come to terminate medical intervention and to permit the passage to death.

Important Legal Decisions in Critical Care   6
S. David Register

IRREVERSIBLE CENTRAL NERVOUS SYSTEM INJURY/BRAIN DEATH

In 1956, Zoll published a description of the termination of ventricular fibrillation in humans by externally applied countershock.[1] Within the next 4 years, Safar described mouth-to-mouth ventilation[2] and Kouwenhoven described closed-chest cardiac massage.[3] Widespread clinical application of these techniques, now referred to as cardiopulmonary resuscitation (CPR), resulted in a significant number of patients in whom cardiac function had been restored following irreversible ischemic injury to the central nervous system (CNS).[4]

Before this time, there had been relatively little legal debate over the definition of death. Both federal and state courts approached the issue of death as a question of fact to be decided in every case by the expert testimony of physicians. The courts also made the assumption that the medical criteria for defining death were well established and not a source of controversy. Death was the cessation of life, and was defined by physicians as a total stoppage of blood circulation of the animal and vital functions consequent thereupon, such as respiration and pulsation.[5]

HARVARD BRAIN DEATH CRITERIA

In 1968, the Ad Hoc Committee of the Harvard Medical School published their landmark report "A Definition of Irreversible Coma."[5] The stated purpose of the committee was "to define irreversible coma as a new criterion for death." This new definition was needed for two reasons: improvements in resuscitative and supportive therapy had yielded a substantial number of patients who were comatose with no discernible CNS activity, and an increasing number of organs were needed for transplantation.

The committee began with the basic premise that "an organ, brain or other, that no longer functions and has no possibility of functioning again is for all practical purposes dead." They then defined the characteristics of a

TABLE 6-1. Harvard Criteria for Brain Death

(1) *Unreceptivity and Unresponsitivity*—A patient in this state appears to be in a deep coma with total unawareness of externally applied stimuli and inner need and complete unresponsiveness.

(2) *No Movements or Breathing*—A 1-hour period of observation by a physician is required to verify absence of spontaneous muscular movements, spontaneous respiration, or response to stimulation. The total absence of spontaneous ventilation is to be verified by turning off the ventilator in accordance with specific criteria.

(3) *No Reflexes*—There should be a total absence of elicitable reflexes. Pupils should be fixed and dilated. Ocular movement and blinking should be absent. There should be no evidence of postural activity (decerebrate or other). Other cranial nerve reflexes should also be absent. "As a rule the stretch of tendon reflexes cannot be elicited."

(4) *The Flat, or Isoelectric, Electroencephalogram (EEG)* —Although not required, is of great confirmatory value and should be used when available. Guidelines for EEG evaluation were specified.

permanently nonfunctioning brain in the Harvard criteria for brain death (Table 6-1).

The Harvard Ad Hoc Committee realized that this issue was more than just a medical problem: it was a "moral, ethical and religious" dilemma as well. The group also recognized that adoption of this position by the medical community would form the basis for change in the legal concept of death. However, the committee's report stated plainly that no statutory change in the law should be necessary, since the law treated this question essentially as one of fact to be determined by physicians.[5]

STATUTORY DEFINITION OF BRAIN DEATH

In 1970, Kansas became the first state to enact a statutory definition of death, allowing the application of the brain-death concept as an alternative means of declaring death. This legislation was quickly challenged in *State of Kansas v. Shaffer* following a homicide conviction using the brain-death concept. The court ruled that the statute applied "for all purposes in this state, including trials of civil and criminal cases."

In the decade that followed, a few other states adopted a statutory definition of brain death. The concept was challenged legally a number of times in appeals to homicide convictions. Most, but not all, of these cases involved removal of organs from the brain-dead person for transplantation. In each and every case, the courts upheld the brain-death concept as defined by the Harvard Ad Hoc Committee. However, most states still did not have a statutory definition of brain death. In the landmark case, *Commonwealth v. Golston*, the Massachusetts Court accepted the Harvard Ad Hoc Committee's definition of death for a homicide victim despite the lack of a statutory definition of death in Massachusetts.[4]

In 1978, the Kansas Supreme Court reviewed the Kansas Brain Death Statute. Not only did the court uphold the statute, but also it expressly recognized the need to maintain cardiopulmonary support following the pronouncement of brain death and to prepare the body for harvest and transplant of organs.[6]

ALTERNATE CRITERIA

Subsequently, a series of studies attempted to establish certain criteria for predicting failure of survival, that is, to establish criteria that predict "inevitable somatic or bodily death." Ouaknine reported that cardiac arrest generally occurred within 1 to 7 days, despite resuscitative measures, in patients with "absolutely nonreacting coma with bilateral, fixed, nonreactive mydriasis and absence of spontaneous breathing."[7] In 1971, Korein and Maccario prospectively studied 20 patients unresponsive to painful and auditory stimuli, without spontaneous movement, without spontaneous respiration, with fixed, dilated, and equal pupils, with no response to ice water calorics, intravenous administration of CNS stimulants, or to photic stimulation, and with an isoelectric electroencephalogram (EEG).[8] All 20 patients had "bodily death" within 48 hours. Ibe reported that all 72 patients who fulfilled unspecified brain-death criteria had cardiac standstill within 1 week.[9] In 15 patients with complete unresponsiveness, lack of spontaneous respiration, and absence of all cephalic reflexes, Becker reported a maximum survival time of 50 hours.[10] Plum and Posner also described a 50-hour maximum survival time in all 9 patients with unresponsitivity, lack of spontaneous respiration, flaccidity, absence of mesencephalic reflexes, progressive circulatory collapse, and loss of thermoregulation.[11] In Sweden, Ingvar added the technique of intracranial arteriography and reported that all 26 patients had somatic death within 14 days of the diagnosis of brain death.[12] In 1971 to 1972, the National Institute of Neurological Disease and Stroke conducted a nine-hospital cooperative study assessing brain-death criteria. The directors applied four sets of existent criteria retrospectively and demonstrated somatic death in all 503 patients.[13]

Acceptance by the public, the courts, and the medical profession of brain death as an alternate means of diagnosing death was greatly hastened by the realization that somatic death inevitably follows brain death. The rapid growth of organ transplantation programs across the country also hastened the acceptance of this new definition of death. However, there remained a large number of patients with irreversible CNS injury who did not meet brain-death protocols. These cases were dealt with quietly by the physician, family, or prognosis committee, but rarely by the courts, prior to 1975.[4]

IRREVERSIBLE CNS INJURY WITHOUT BRAIN DEATH

KAREN ANN QUINLAN AND THE DOCTRINE OF SUBSTITUTED JUDGMENT

Karen Ann Quinlan was the 22-year-old adopted daughter of Mr. and Mrs. Joseph Quinlan. Following the alleged ingestion of both tranquilizers and ethanol, she became comatose on April 15, 1975. In September 1975, Mr. Quinlan requested that Karen's ventilator be discontinued and that she be allowed to die. When the hospital and physicians refused to comply with this request, he filed a court suit seeking authority as legal guardian to discontinue ventilator support. Both Mr. Quinlan and Karen's physicians believed she would die if she were removed from the ventilator. The story was widely publicized by *Time* magazine and demonstrated to the entire world that the "right to die" had become a legal, as well as a moral and ethical, dilemma.

On November 10, 1975, Superior Court Judge Robert Muir, Jr., refused Mr. Quinlan's request to discontinue mechanical ventilation and allow Karen to die.[14] For his decision, Judge Muir was criticized by some members of the medical profession, the public, and the media. However, several important facts were not widely publicized by the media. First, Karen clearly did not meet brain-death criteria as established by the Harvard Ad Hoc Committee or by anyone else. She responded to pain with weak movement and her EEG was not isoelectric. Therefore, it was irrelevant that New Jersey at that time was not one of the eight states with a statutory definition of brain death since Karen Ann Quinlan was not brain dead. For the court and for the physicians involved in her care, discontinuance of mechanical ventilation would have been an active act intended to produce somatic death, that is, homicide. Second, Karen already was receiving mechanical ventilatory support. For many in the medical and legal professions, discontinuance of therapy was (and is) more difficult than withholding available therapy before it is initiated.[15] However, this distinction is no longer considered either legally or ethically valid (see Chaps. 3 and 5).

The lawyers presenting the case for Mr. Quinlan did not claim that Karen was brain dead, but nevertheless that she should be allowed to die. Their stated justification for this action included the following:

1. "Medical science holds no hope for Miss Quinlan's recovery." By this, they meant that she was not expected to regain normal cerebral function, not that somatic death was imminent.
2. "Miss Quinlan would want the respirator turned off." This concept was to be the source of considerable legal debate in future cases under the legal term of "substituted judgment."
3. "Doctors have no legal obligation to keep Miss Quinlan alive." However, "Judge Muir stated that a patient placed in the care of a

doctor expects that the doctor 'will do all within his human power to favor life against death.' " (This, too, was to become a point of controversy in numerous other court cases.)
4. "The wishes of the parents of an incompetent patient should be paramount in a doctor's life or death decision." Judge Muir disagreed. (This issue was later to become the central theme in legal debate over infanticide.)
5. "The constitutional right of privacy should allow parents or guardians to make the decision that an incompetent child's life should no longer be prolonged." Judge Muir, however, believed that previous legal right-to-privacy cases concerned the right to maintain a particular life-style, not the right to die.
6. "Freedom of religion should allow Miss Quinlan, a Roman Catholic, to die."
7. "The beauty and meaning of Karen's life was over and she should be allowed to die." In essence, Mr. Quinlan's attorneys argued that a quality-of-life decision should override the sanctity-of-life obligation. (This issue, too, was to become the center of legal debate which still rages in our courts today.)

Judge Muir's 44-page ruling stated that "judicial conscience and morality" indicated that Karen's case was being properly handled by "the treating physician." He held that despite the fact that the "victim is on the threshold of death, no 'humanitarian motives' can justify," under common law, "taking life." The debate regarding whether discontinuance of mechanical ventilation was an act of commission or omission, he felt, was "semantics," since either would result in death, and hence represent legal homicide. Importantly, Judge Muir stated that "there is no constitutional right to die that can be asserted by a parent for his incompetent adult child."

Because Karen Ann Quinlan was not brain dead, the public and the medical community as a whole understood and supported Judge Muir's decision. However, Mr. Quinlan's lawyers appealed the decision to the New Jersey Supreme Court, which reversed the lower court's decision and gave Karen's father, as legal guardian, authority to remove the "ventilatory support." Like the lower court, the New Jersey Supreme Court agreed that Karen was not brain dead and was not imminently terminal unless life support was withdrawn. However, in contradistinction to Judge Muir, the New Jersey Supreme Court assigned the right to make what now is commonly called a "quality of life" judgment.

A three-tier procedure was specified:

> Upon the concurrence of the guardian and family of Karen, should the responsible attending physicians conclude that there is no reasonable possibility of Karen's ever emerging from her present comatose condition to a *cognitive, sapient state* and that the life-support apparatus now being administered to Karen should be discontinued, they shall consult with

the hospital 'Ethics Committee' or like body of the institution in which Karen is then hospitalized. If that consultative body agrees that there is no reasonable possibility of Karen's ever emerging from her comatose condition to a *cognitive, sapient state,* the present life-support system may be withdrawn and said action shall be without any civil or criminal liability therefore on the part of any participant, whether guardian, physician, hospital or others.

The New Jersey Supreme Court ruled that "the state's interest contra weakens and the individual's right to privacy grows as the degree of bodily invasion increases and the prognosis dims." Thus, the court justified a quality-of-life decision by using a "substituted judgment" test, declaring that Karen's right to refuse treatment required that her guardian "render their best judgment . . . as to whether she would exercise it in these circumstances." Before assuming her vegetative state, Karen had verbally indicated on at least one occasion that she would choose not to live if confined to a ventilator.[16]

Eventually, Karen was removed from mechanical ventilatory support. To the surprise of her family and physicians, she breathed spontaneously and remained in her baseline vegetative state for several years until she finally died in 1986. Clearly she was not brain dead; the attempts to let her die were based on ethical decisions separate and distinct from those discussed by the Harvard Ad Hoc Committee.

Dr. C. Everett Koop, Surgeon General of the United States, has spoken and written extensively on the subjects of euthanasia and abortion. Following the 1973 United States Supreme Court decision *Roe v. Wade*[17] allowing abortion on demand, Dr. Koop predicted ten "natural consequences" of this landmark decision.[18] Several are relevant to the *Quinlan* case and to the issue of discontinuance of life support in general. Dr. Koop stated that "liberty leads to license." He pointed out that the New York Medical Society, less than a week after the Supreme Court's *Roe v. Wade* decision, took a stand in reference to a patient's right to die at the discretion of the patient's family, rather than the patient. He also stated that "the right to die leads to the right to kill in mercy." Two months after the Supreme Court decision, a Dutch jury found a physician guilty of murder after actively killing her mother who had terminal cancer but was pain free. A 1-week suspended prison sentence resulted.

Koop also predicted that the action of the Supreme Court in *Roe v. Wade* would contribute, first, to the process of depersonalization and, second, to the process of dehumanization. In his view, the Supreme Court declared unborn babies to be "non-persons." He pointed out that Lt. William Calley had expressed the opinion that the Vietnamese were not human beings when he was accused of unjustified killing of civilians. Both American Indians and blacks were once considered nonpersons in the United States as were Jews in Nazi Germany.

Leo Alexander, a Boston psychiatrist, was consultant to the Secretary of War on duty with the Office of Chief Counsel for War Crimes in Nüremberg. He pointed out that the Nazi dictatorship, like other recent dictatorships, was Hegelian in that moral, ethical, and religious values had been replaced by "rational utility."[19] What is most shocking is the degree to which organized medicine in Nazi Germany collaborated in the mass extermination of the chronically ill (to avoid "useless" expenses to the society), the mass extermination of racially, socially, or ideologically unwanted persons, and ruthless medical military research using "human experimental material."

These atrocities were not forced on an unprepared people. Years of mass propaganda gradually had altered the thought processes and values of the people. School textbooks included mathematics problems "stated in distorted terms of the cost of caring for and rehabilitating the chronically sick and crippled." For example, one problem asked how many new housing units could be built, and how many marriage-allowance loans could be given to newlyweds, for the amount of money it cost the state to care for "the crippled, the criminal and the insane."[19]

As a result of his experiences, Dr. Alexander stated,

> The case therefore that I should like to make is that American medicine must realize where it stands in its fundamental premises. There can be no doubt that in a subtle way the Hegelian premise of 'what is useful is right' has infected society including the medical portion of society. Physicians must return to their older premises, which were the emotional foundation and driving force of an amazingly successful quest to increase powers of healing and which are bound to carry them still farther if they are not held down to earth by the pernicious attitudes of an overdone practical realism.[19]

DECISION-MAKING FOR INCOMPETENT PATIENTS

Following the *Quinlan* court's lead, other courts allowed the "substituted judgment standard" to be used in cases where previously competent persons have no reasonable possibility of returning to a "cognitive, sapient state." The ruling has been applied to allow both withdrawal of life-support therapy and orders not to resuscitate in the event of a cardiac or respiratory arrest.

JOSEPH SAIKEWICZ

Ironically, the substituted judgment ruling has been applied in cases involving patients who were never competent and therefore had no possible opportunity to express their beliefs and desires with regard to matters such as these. The best known example is *Superintendent of Belchertown State School v. Saikewicz*.[20] Joseph Saikewicz was a profoundly retarded 67-year-old man with leukemia. Although chemotherapy offered a 30% to 50% chance of 2 to 13 months' remission, the court waived the relatively objective "best interest" standard in favor of the "substituted judgment" test. Therapy, accordingly, was withheld.

JOHN STORAR

Debate has also arisen as to what alternatives exist. Some believe that the *Storar* case in New York suggests that rejection of the substituted judgment standard would always "require treatment if a life of any semblance can be even briefly prolonged." This interpretation, however, appears to be a bit extreme.

John Storar had terminal bladder cancer. His mother requested that repeated blood transfusions be discontinued. The New York court rejected the substituted judgment test since Mr. Storar had been profoundly retarded throughout life, ruling that the substituted judgment standard in a case such as this was equivalent to asking "if it snowed all summer, would it then be winter?" The court, however, refused to terminate the blood transfusions since they did not cause "excessive pain" (as claimed by Mr. Storar's mother), and they improved his level of function.[21] Not surprisingly, Mr. Storar died before the legal controversy could be resolved.

Courts can reject substitutive judgment and yet authorize termination of treatment in appropriate circumstances. In the *Saikewicz* and *Storar* cases, the patients were incompetent but were conscious and active, and the proposed therapy could prolong their lives for at least a few months. I believe most competent patients would desire treatment under these circumstances. However, physicians, patients, and families often differ in their perceptions of the value of treatments. This has been observed when each group has been asked retrospectively about the value of treatment[22] and prospectively to see if another similar course of ICU treatment would be considered.[23] Therefore, withholding therapy from incompetent patients treats them differently from competent patients. Surgeon General Koop suggested that such quality-of-life judgments are analogous to those made in Nazi Germany and that America is on "the slide to Auschwitz."[24]

CLAIRE CONROY

A recent New Jersey case defined an even more elaborate method of decision-making for incompetent patients. Claire Conroy was an 83-year-old nursing home patient with severe organic brain syndrome who was unable to speak, eat, or move from a semifetal position. The trial court granted her guardian's request for permission to remove her nasogastric feeding tube, but the decision was reversed by the appellate court.[25] The New Jersey Supreme Court then reversed the appellate court's decision.[26] Although it acknowledged that the subjective substituted judgment test was meaningless for a patient who had not expressed a desire regarding life and death when competent, the Court authorized termination of treatment under either of two "best interest" tests: the "limited objective" test, in which there is some trustworthy indication of what the patient would have wanted, and the burdens of life with treatment outweigh its benefits; and the "pure objective" test, in which there is no such indication, but the burdens markedly outweigh the benefits.[19]

Although overruled by the New Jersey Supreme Court in *In re Conroy*, the ruling by the appellate court judge is notable:

> The trial judge . . . authorized euthanasia . . . If the trial judge's order had been enforced, Conroy would not have died as the result of an existing medical condition, but rather she would have died, and painfully so, as the result of a new and independent condition: dehydration and starvation. Thus she would have been actively killed by independent means . . .[25]

In re Conroy is not the only court case involving withholding of nutritional support as a means of hastening or causing death. Two California physicians were prosecuted criminally for terminating the intravenous feeding of a patient who was brain damaged but not brain dead. However, the prosecution was dismissed because the court held that cessation of life-support measures (feeding) "is not an affirmative act but rather a withdrawal or omission of further treatment." The court justified its decision by ruling that "medical procedures to provide nutrition and hydration are more similar to other medical procedures than to typical human ways of providing nutrition and hydration. Their benefits and burdens ought to be evaluated in the same manner as any other medical procedure." Similarly, *Severns v. Wilmington Medical Center* authorized a "no-code" order, no antibiotics for infection, and no reimplantation of a feeding tube for a comatose patient.[27]

Decision-making for incompetent patients is made even more difficult by the courts' inability to agree amongst themselves which cases need judicial involvement. The *Quinlan* New Jersey Supreme Court ruled as follows:

> We consider that a practice of applying to a court to confirm such decisions would generally be inappropriate, not only because that would be a gratuitous encroachment on the medical profession's field of competence, but because it would be impossibly cumbersome."

Instead the *Quinlan* court recommended oversight by hospital ethics committees with judicial review in unusual or exceptionally complicated cases.[14]

The *Saikewicz* court, however, strongly disagreed:

> We take a dim view of any attempt to shift ultimate decision-making responsibility away from a duly established court of proper jurisdiction to any committee, panel or group, ad hoc or permanent. Thus, we reject the approach adopted by the New Jersey Supreme Court in the Quinlan case of entrusting the decision whether to continue artificial life support to the patient's guardian, family, attending doctors and hospital 'ethics committee' . . . We do not view the judicial resolution of this most difficult and awesome question—whether potentially life-prolonging treatment should be withheld from a person incapable of making his own decision—as constituting a 'gratuitous encroachment' on the domain of medical expertise.[20]

SHIRLEY DINNERSTEIN

The *Saikewicz* ruling has been criticized for being unclear. Did the decision mean that a court presented with such a case should not delegate the resolution to others, or that all nontreatment decisions involving incompetent patients should be made by the courts? Most people interpreted the decision as requiring routine adjudication.

Matter of Dinnerstein is now cited as clarification of the *Saikewicz* ruling.[28] Shirley Dinnerstein was a 67-year-old woman in a vegetative state with no reasonable probability of recovery. Her family and physician sought court approval to enter a "no-code" order into her chart. The court ruled that such an order could be entered into the chart without judicial approval. The court also specifically referred to the questions raised by the *Saikewicz* ruling. The *Saikewicz* case was interpreted as applying only to treatments that could be "administered for the purpose and with some reasonable expectation of effecting a permanent or temporary cure of or relief from the illness or condition being treated." The *Dinnerstein* court ruled as follows:

> 'Prolongation of life,' as used in the Saikewicz case, does not mean a mere suspension of the act of dying, but contemplates, at the very least, a remission of symptoms enabling a return towards a normal, functioning, integrated existence.[28]

In *Matter of Spring*, the Massachusetts Supreme Court stated approval of the Dinnerstein decision but overruled the Appellate Court's ruling that judicial approval was likewise unnecessary before discontinuing dialysis treatments for a 78-year-old incompetent patient.[29] The Massachusetts Supreme Court agreed with the termination of dialysis in the *Spring* case (although by this time the patient had already died of other causes) but disapproved of delegating decision-making power to the family and physician. Thus, the Massachusetts Supreme Court declared "when a court is properly presented with the legal question whether treatment may be withheld, it must decide that question and not delegate it to some private person or group."[29]

Although the Massachusetts Supreme Court provided a long list of factors for physicians to consider, it failed to specify which set of factors would be sufficient to make prior judicial approval unnecessary. Thus, Massachusetts physicians still had to guess whether prior court approval was required, unless the situation clearly was governed by the Dinnerstein ruling.

Courts in other states also have made it difficult to determine when prior judicial approval is needed before termination of a particular therapy. For example, a New York intermediate court authorized discontinuation of mechanical ventilation of an 83-year-old patient who was comatose but not brain dead. The procedures set forth by the court for determining future need of judicial review in similar cases were so elaborate that they would require a minimum of four to six physicians, five attorneys, and one judge. New York's Court of Appeals upheld the decision to allow the discontinuation of mechanical ventilation (after the patient was already dead) but rejected the intermediate court's proposed procedures.[30] Instead, this Court stated the following:

> Neither the common law nor existing statutes require persons generally to seek prior Court assessment of conduct which may subject them to civil and criminal liability. If it is desirable to enlarge the role of the courts in cases involving discontinuance of life-sustaining treatment for incompetents by establishing a mandatory procedure of successive approval by physicians, hospital personnel, relatives and the Courts, the change should come from the legislature.[30]

Thus, it remains unclear in some states if physician and family can decide to terminate therapy without fearing civil or criminal liability for failing to obtain prior judicial approval. This uncertainty is exacerbated by the fact that in *Matter of Storar*, the New York Court of Appeals reversed the lower court's ruling that John Storar's blood transfusion could be discontinued.[21,31]

THE PRESIDENT'S COMMISSION

Because of the disagreement in the state court opinions (most of which were rendered long after the patient was dead), the President's Commission for the Study of Ethical Problems in Medicine recommended the approach suggested in *Quinlan*, that is, decisions made by the physicians and families with review by hospital ethics committees.[32] According to Rhoden, the commission noted that litigation is costly, creates long delays, and can seriously strain the relationships between the parties by forcing them into adversarial roles. Moreover, it exposes these private matters to the scrutiny of the courtroom and often to the glare of the public media.[16] It remains to be seen whether state courts and legislatures will adopt the Commission's recommendations.

ADVANCE DIRECTIVES FOR PATIENT CARE

NATURAL DEATH ACTS/LIVING WILLS

In 1976, California enacted the California Natural Death Act, the first statute to explicitly authorize a person to direct, in advance, that lifesaving treatment be withdrawn when death is imminent.[33] The act specifically required that a person must wait at least 14 days from the date that the terminal illness is made known before signing the document. However, approximately half of the patients to whom the act was potentially applicable in 1978 were comatose before the 14-day waiting period had elapsed and therefore did not benefit from it.

Since that time, a majority of state legislatures have passed similar Natural Death Acts designed to give legal validation to "living wills." Florida's "Right to Decline Life-Prolonging Procedures"[34] has been praised as particularly enlightened.[35] In brief, it holds that any competent adult can, at any time, direct in a written statement the withdrawal or withholding of life-prolonging procedures. The declaration may be given orally if the person is physically unable to sign a written statement. The declarant is responsible for notifying his/her physician of the declaration. However, in the event this notification is not possible, any person may do so. The declaration, written or oral, must be made a part of the patient's medical record. The attending physician must comply with the patient's directive or transfer the patient to another physician who will.

Living wills originally were not intended as legally binding documents. Instead, they were statements about a person's beliefs and desires should he/she become incompetent at a time when death was imminent.[36] However, the legal relevance of living wills was demonstrated recently by the Supreme Court of Florida in *John F. Kennedy Memorial Hospital v. Bludworth*. A lower court had ruled that the living will formulated by a competent person who had now become permanently vegetative could be implemented only by a court order authorizing a court-appointed guardian to consent to nontreatment. The Florida Supreme Court, recognizing that avoidance of litigation was a major purpose of living wills, ruled that family and physician can agree to withdraw life-sustaining treatments from a permanently vegetative patient without judicial review. The Court recommended that the patient's living will be strongly considered when making such a decision.

The Natural Death Acts of most states do not authorize withdrawal of life-sustaining therapy in patients with poor quality of life who are not imminently terminal; that is, in most states, directives to withdraw or withhold life-sustaining treatment come into effect only when the patient's death is imminent, such that treatment would merely prolong or interrupt the process of dying. According to the President's Commission, "The class of persons thus defined by many of the statutes, if it indeed contains any members, at most constitutes a small percentage of those incapacitated individuals for whom decisions about life-sustaining treatment must be made."[31] Most patients and many physicians, however, do not understand this important point. A patient who is not terminal may be asking the physician to go beyond the Natural Death Act's boundaries and withdraw or withhold life-support therapy because of "physical or mental disability."

Some living wills, such as the one first published by the Euthanasia Education Council, even request that "medication be mercifully administered to me to alleviate suffering even though this may hasten the moment of death."[36] Recalling two of Dr. Koop's ten predicted "natural consequences" of the *Roe v. Wade* decision ("liberty leads to license" and "the right to die leads to the right to kill in mercy"), we might anticipate further legislative and judicial attempts to broaden the scope of the Natural Death Acts to allow quality of life to be an increasingly important factor in the execution of the living wills.

As might be expected, Natural Death Acts have raised more questions than they have answered. For example, are physicians who refuse to follow the advance directives of a living will subject to civil or criminal penalty?

Are they obligated to execute the directives of a living will even if so doing violates their own personal moral, ethical, and religious convictions? In other words, what are the "rights" of the physicians? Finally, if a patient does not have a living will, can therapy still be terminated when appropriate?

DURABLE POWER OF ATTORNEY

Natural Death Acts, with the exception of that in Delaware, do not provide for appointment of a proxy decision-maker if the patient becomes incompetent. However, at least 42 states have statutes authorizing "durable power of attorney," that is, powers of attorney that remain in effect even if the person becomes incompetent.[32] More and more people are using these durable power of attorney statutes to appoint relatives or friends to make proxy health care decisions should they become incompetent.[16] Since these statutes were not originally intended for this purpose, further judicial and legislative clarification can be anticipated.

DO NOT RESUSCITATE

There is significant overlap between the issue of withdrawal of life support and the issue of withholding CPR in selected cases. Because CPR is a form of therapy, it is indicated in some situations but not in others. This conviction was clearly enunciated at the National Conference on Cardiopulmonary Resuscitation and Emergency Cardiac Care in 1974. The same year, the Standards for Cardiopulmonary Resuscitation and Emergency Cardiac Care published in the *Journal of the American Medical Association* contained the proposal that decisions not to resuscitate be formally documented in the patient's medical records and communicated to all staff involved in the patient's care. It was recognized by many physicians that CPR was intended to prevent sudden, unexpected death and is not indicated in certain situations such as terminal illness in which death is not unexpected. However, fear of liability often caused "do not resuscitate" (DNR) orders to be verbally communicated but not included in the medical record.[37]

In 1976, Rabkin published a report intended as a proposed policy statement for hospitals concerned with regulating the process whereby orders not to resuscitate may be implemented.[38] In discussing the problem, Rabkin referred to an "irreversibly, irreparably ill patient whose death was imminent." The report suggested that the initial medical judgment on the appropriateness of an order not to resuscitate should be made by the primary physician after discussion with an ad hoc committee composed of physicians, nurses, and others. It also recommended obtaining consent for the order from the patient (if competent) or family (if the patient is incompetent). Documentation of the patient's condition, the recommendation of the ad hoc committee, the patient's (or family's) consent, and a formal order not to resuscitate should then be clearly recorded in the patient's medical record.

As stated previously, the family and physician of Shirley Dinnerstein asked the courts for a declaratory judgment that a doctor can enter a "no-code" order for this type of patient without prior judicial authorization. The court agreed that prior approval was not necessary; concurrence of family and physician was all that was required for a "no-code" for this incompetent patient.[28]

PATIENTS OF QUESTIONABLE COMPETENCY

Thus far, I have discussed patients who were clearly not competent to make decisions about their own medical therapy. Even more problematic, though, are patients who are neither clearly competent nor incompetent. Frequently, questions on competence are not raised until a patient's expressed choice is not in agreement with the physician's recommendation.

Assessment of a patient's competence is complicated by the lack of a uniform, widely accepted definition. The legal presumption, however, is that a patient is competent to make treatment decisions until proven to be otherwise. Mental illness or the inability to perform certain functions does not necessarily prove incompetence.

Once again, though, the inconsistency of our legal system is apparent. In *In re Quackenbush*, the refusal of a 72-year-old man to allow lifesaving amputation of his gangrenous feet was upheld by the court.[39] The *Quackenbush* court cited an excerpt from the *Quinlan* ruling: "The State's interest 'contra' weakens and the individual's right of privacy grows as the degree of bodily invasion increases and the prognosis dims. Ultimately, there comes a point at which the individual's rights overcome the State interest."[14] Because Mr. Quackenbush was elderly and because his quality of life after amputation was predicted to be poor, the court upheld his refusal of lifesaving surgery. The court explicitly noted the contrast between Mr. Quackenbush's case and that of a young patient who could be returned to excellent health by a minimally invasive procedure such as a blood transfusion.[16]

The President's Commission[32] suggested that the determination of competence is best made by the physician, family, and hospital ethics committee without routine recourse to the courts. Accordingly, the Commission offered a list of considerations for determining competency (Table 6-2).

The ruling in *State Department of Human Services v. Northern*[40] suggests that an otherwise competent patient who refuses lifesaving medical therapy may be declared incompetent so that the treatment can be given.[40] And yet,

> inherent in the requirement of informed consent for treatment is the recognition that a competent patient has a right to choose to forego treatment. Legal recognition of this right to refuse is based on the common law right to bodily integrity, which underlies the informed consent doctrine. It may also be based on the constitutional right to privacy, which protects an individual's right to make his or her own decisions about fundamental personal matters. This right to privacy has been held to extend to a person's decisions about medical treatment.[16]

TABLE 6-2. President's Commission Criteria for Determining Competency

(1) Does the patient possess the ability to understand the relevant facts and alternatives?

(2) Is the patient weighing the decision within a framework of values and goals?

(3) Is the patient able to reason and deliberate about this information?

(4) Can the patient give reasons for the decision in light of the facts, the alternatives, and the impact of the decision on the patient's own goals and values?

COMPETENT PATIENTS

INFORMED CONSENT AND REFUSAL

The requirement of patient consent for medical treatment is not a new concept in medicine or law. Early court cases involved failure of physicians to obtain consent (which constitutes the intentional tort of battery) or exceeding the scope of the given consent. More recently, the concept has shifted away from mere "consent" to "informed consent," that is, a physician who fails to provide the patient with information sufficient to allow him/her to make a free and fully informed choice may be found liable to negligence for falling below the professional standard of care.

The requirement for advance disclosure of risks of treatment is an area of considerable legal debate. Most courts require the plaintiff to prove that adequate disclosure of the risks of the treatment would have caused a "reasonable person" to refuse consent. However, some courts have ruled that this objective "reasonable person" standard is too rigid and does not allow a person's subjective values and beliefs to be considered.[16] In addition to "informed consent," a few courts have dealt with what has come to be called "informed refusal." For example, the California Supreme Court recently held that a physician may be found negligent for failing to inform a patient of the risks of not having a Pap smear to test for cervical cancer.[16]

The legal concepts of informed consent and informed refusal are of tremendous relevance and importance in the ICU. Patients must be thoroughly informed of the risks of accepting and refusing treatment. However, many times it is not possible to obtain informed consent from a critically ill patient. In general, proxy consent (usually from the family) is required for treatment of the ICU patient who is no longer competent to give informed consent. In a medical emergency, in which consent cannot be obtained but failure to treat will result in imminent harm, the law makes an exception to the informed consent doctrine and considers consent to be implied from the circumstances.

Two other legal concepts allow exception to the requirement for informed consent: "waiver," in which the patient states that he/she does not want to be fully informed about the treatment, and "therapeutic privilege," in which the physician withholds information which will be emotionally harmful to the patient. The concept of therapeutic privilege is not yet well defined legally.[16]

STATE'S INTERESTS

As referred to in *Quackenbush*, the State has "interests" that must be legally weighed against the patient's right to refuse lifesaving therapy.[39] "Courts have frequently listed the potential State interests involved as (1) the preservation of life, (2) the protection of dependent third parties, (3) the prevention of suicide, and (4) the preservation of the ethical integrity of the medical profession." The *Quackenbush* Court found none of these four state interests sufficiently strong to order lifesaving surgery.[16,39] With the continued weakening of Judeo–Christian influence, and the corresponding shift from a "sanctity of life" doctrine to a "quality of life" doctrine, I predict that future courts will increasingly follow the lead of the *Quackenbush* court.

Jehovah's Witnesses

One or more of the above state's interests have been applied in cases involving the religious objection of Jehovah's Witnesses to blood transfusions. Courts have ruled that it is unfair to force physicians to institute surgical therapy without the ability to provide medically indicated blood transfusions, and have ordered blood transfusion (*i.e.*, for a critically ill young mother who, as a Jehovah's Witness, refused blood transfusion). Because her 7-month-old child would be effectively abandoned, and because she was critically ill, the court ruled that the patient was "not in a mental condition to make a decision."[16]

In the 1970's, however, courts ruled differently, upholding many refusals for blood transfusion, even for Jehovah's Witness patients with dependent children. Thus, "there is a trend away from the approach taken in earlier cases, which analogized foregoing treatment to committing suicide, and toward respecting competent refusals of medical treatment."[16] The President's Commission stated that "A competent patient's self-determination is and usually should be given greater weight than other people's views on that individual's well being."[32]

WITHDRAWAL OF THERAPY FROM MINORS

ROE V. WADE

Without question, the 1973 United States Supreme Court *Roe v. Wade* decision was the most controversial court ruling of modern times.[16] With what Justice Byron White referred to as "raw judicial power," the Supreme Court struck down legislative restrictions on abortion in every state of the nation. As stated by President Ronald Reagan,

> Our nationwide policy of abortion-on-demand through all nine months of pregnancy was neither voted for by our people nor enacted by our legislators—not a single state had such unrestricted abortion before the Supreme Court decreed it to be national policy in 1973 . . . make no mistake, abortion-on-demand is not a right granted by the Constitution.[40]

President Reagan also noted that "We cannot diminish the value of one category of human life—the unborn—without diminishing the value of all human life." Another of Dr. Koop's predicted "natural consequences" of *Roe v. Wade* was that abortion would lead to infanticide.[18] His prediction was accurate. In November 1974, the International Correspondence Society of Obstetricians and Gynecologists asked obstetricians how they dealt with live births in abortions. A Philadelphia physician wrote the following:

> At the time of delivery it has been our policy to wrap the fetus in a towel. The fetus is then moved to another room, while our attention is turned to the care of the gravida. She is examined to determine whether placental explusion has occurred and the extent of vaginal bleeding. Once we are sure her condition is stable, the fetus is evaluated. Almost invariably all signs of life have ceased.

Ironically, some states have statutes on their books requiring an abortionist to make every effort to resuscitate the baby he has just aborted. Dr. Mary Ellen Avery, professor of pediatrics at Harvard University and physician-in-chief of Boston Children's Hospital, suggested that if on abortion the infant is large enough to survive in the neonatal ICU, the physician should make the decision about caring or not caring for the child.[41]

Much more common than infants who survive abortions, though, are infants with congenital birth defects. These, too, have become a target for some in our society, raising important legal questions. Immediately following *Roe v. Wade*, *Time* magazine reported a quotation by Nobel Prize winner Dr. James D. Watson, codiscoverer of the structure of DNA. Dr. Watson's statement had originally had been published in *Prism* magazine, a publication of the American Medical Association.

> "If a child were not declared alive until three days after birth, then all parents could be allowed the choice only a few are given under the present system. The doctor could allow the child to die if the parents so choose and save a lot of misery and suffering. I believe this view is the only rational, compassionate attitude to have."

These words really are not surprising. Although *Roe v. Wade* legalized abortion throughout pregnancy, Justice Blackmun's decision included the statement that "we need not resolve the question of when life begins." Thus, from a legal standpoint, we do not know when life begins. Another of Dr. Koop's predicted "natural consequences" of the *Roe v. Wade* decision was creation of a "schizophrenic" medicolegal environment.[18]

The issue of withholding medical treatment from a child is, legally speaking, even more complicated than withholding medical treatment from an incompetent adult, because the rights of the child's parents are also involved. In general, parents have a legal right to make fundamental decisions regarding their children. The United States Supreme Court has ruled that "It is cardinal with us that the custody, care, and nurture of the child reside first with the parents, whose primary function and freedom include preparation for obligations that the state can neither supply nor hinder." And yet, the appropriate legal standard to be upheld is that of the child's best interests. One court ruled that "While . . . [the child] 'belongs' to his parents, he belongs also to his state . . . the fact that the child belongs to the state imposes upon the state many duties. Chief among them is the duty to protect his right to live and grow up with a sound mind in a sound body and to brook no interference with that right by any person or organization."[42]

PARENTAL REFUSAL OF TREATMENT

In the past, courts ordered needed medical treatment, such as blood transfusions for children of Jehovah's Witness parents, when the parents refused to provide it.[42,43] In *Custody of a Minor* a Massachusetts court ordered resumption of chemotherapy treatments for Chad Green's acute lymphocytic leukemia, after such treatments had been stopped by Chad's parents, and prohibited further treatments with laetrile, megadose vitamins A and C, folic acid, and enzyme enemas which already had caused chronic cyanide poisoning, hypervitaminosis, and possible colon injury.[44] In other cases, the courts overruled a father's refusal to permit tonsillectomies and adenoidectomies for his children and a mother's refusal to permit medical and dental care for her child with cavities, dental fractures, and an umbilical hernia.

Parents' refusals of medical treatments have not always been overruled by the courts. In *In re Seiferth*,[45] the court refused to overrule the parents and to order cleft lip repair for a 15-year-old because the condition was not emergent. In *In re Green*,[46] the court upheld the parents' refusal of splenectomy for their child with sickle-cell anemia since the underlying disease would still be fatal.

WITHHOLDING THERAPY FROM INFANTS

BABY DOE

In 1972, a Maryland infant with Down's syndrome and duodenal atresia was allowed to starve to death after his parents' refusal of corrective surgery. In 1982, in Bloomington, Indiana, the "Baby Doe case" made national headlines. Because he had Down's syndrome, Baby Doe's parents refused consent for surgical correction of his tracheoesophageal fistula. Their decision was upheld by the court. Neither the underlying syndrome (trisomy 21) nor the tracheoesophageal fistula would necessarily have been fatal during infancy with appropriate medical and surgical therapy. However, the family and physicians were given legal (judicial) permission to allow the infant to die by starvation. In the words of President Reagan,[40]

> The death of that tiny infant tore at the hearts of all Americans because the child was undeniably a live human being—one lying helpless before the eyes of the doctors and the eyes of the nation. The real issue for the courts was *not* whether Baby Doe was a human being. The real issue was whether to protect the life of a human being who had Down's syndrome, who would be mentally handicapped, but who needed a routine surgical procedure to unblock his esophagus and allow him to eat. A doctor testified to the presiding judge that, even with his physical problem corrected, Baby Doe would have a 'non-existent' possibility for 'a minimally adequate quality of life'—in other words, that retardation was the equivalent of a crime deserving the death penalty. The judge let Baby Doe starve and die, and the Indiana Supreme Court sanctioned his decision.

President Reagan also wrote that "the basic issue is whether to value and protect the lives of the handicapped, whether to recognize the sanctity of human life. This is the same basic issue that underlies the question of abortion."

Baby Doe I Rule

In response to the Bloomington Baby Doe case, President Reagan directed the Department of Justice and the Department of Health and Human Services (DHHS) to apply civil rights regulations to protect handicapped newborns. A memorandum to Richard Schweiker, then Secretary of the DHHS, instructed him to notify hospitals and health care providers that Section 504 of the 1973 Rehabilitation Act "forbids recipients of Federal funds from withholding from handicapped citizens, simply because they are handicapped, any benefits or services that would ordinarily be provided to persons without handicaps." In May 1982, the DHHS Office for Civil Rights issued a "Notice to Health Care Providers," informing hospital administrators that they risked losing federal funds if their hospital allowed nourishment or medical treatment to be withheld from handicapped infants.[47] The notice stated that "It is unlawful . . . to withhold from a handicapped infant nutritional sustenance or medical or surgical treatment required to correct a life-threatening condition if: (1) the withholding is based on the fact that the infant is handicapped; and (2) the handicap does not render the treatment or nutritional sustenance medically contraindicated."

Although well received and praised by many, the DHHS notice was considered unnecessary or offensive by some professional and medical organizations. The American Hospital Association formally denied that hospitals have in any way been guilty of discrimination and promised "to assure that such simplistic solutions to complex situations involving health care delivery are avoided." The American Academy of Pediatrics argued that

DHHS' effort "to solve this complex problem through strict interpretation and enforcement of the letter of Section 504 may have the unintended effect of requiring treatment that is not in the best interest of handicapped children."[48]

In March 1983, the DHHS issued a rule requiring hospitals receiving federal funds to post warning signs in pediatric wards, nurseries, neonatal ICUs, and delivery suites stating that "Discriminatory failure to feed and care for handicapped infants in this facility is prohibited by federal law. Failure to feed and care for infants may also violate the criminal and civil laws of your state." A toll-free 24-hour "hotline" was established to allow violations of the rule to be reported to DHHS. Calls to the DHHS hotline caused nonmedical DHHS investigative teams to be sent to a number of hospitals. Meanwhile, however, the American Academy of Pediatrics, the National Association of Children's Hospitals and Related Institutions, and Children's Hospital National Medical Center filed suit against DHHS challenging the rule. In April 1983, the United States District Court for the District of Columbia declared the rule invalid for several reasons, including failure of the DHHS to give advance notice of the rule. Judge Gesell declared that the rule was "arbitrary and capricious" and "virtually without meaning beyond its intrinsic *in terrorem* effect."

Baby Doe II Rule

In July 1983, the DHHS issued a revised set of regulations with the mandatory 60-day advance notice comment period. The required notices were smaller and only needed to be posted so as to be visible to medical and nursing staff. In response to the criticism by the American Academy of Pediatrics,[48] the new rule stressed that Section 504 applies only "when non-medical consideration, such as subjective judgments that an unrelated handicap makes a person's life not worth living, are interjected in the decision-making process." Care of infants for whom treatment would be futile was exempted from the regulations. The new rule also called for the establishment of Infant Care Review Committees (ICRC). Thus, violations of Section 504 would be reported first to the hospital ICRC (if one existed), followed by the state child protective agencies, and finally to the DHHS hotline, if necessary.

BABY JANE DOE

While the DHHS was preparing the Baby Doe II rule, Baby Jane Doe was born with multiple congenital anomalies, including microcephaly, hydrocephalus, and spina bifida. The baby was transferred to Stony Brook University Hospital for corrective surgery. When the parents refused to consent to surgery, an attorney filed suit in New York State Court seeking the appointment of a guardian *ad litem* and a court order for the corrective surgery. The court granted these requests, but the Appellate Court reversed both decisions, and the New York Supreme Court affirmed the Appellate Court's decisions.[41]

Meanwhile, DHHS received an anonymous complaint that Baby Jane Doe was discriminated against because of the denial of medical care, thus violating Section 504 of the Rehabilitation Act. The hospital refused requests by the United States Surgeon General and DHHS for access to Baby Jane Doe's medical records, causing the federal government to file suit in the Eastern District of New York. The District Court ruled that the hospital's treatment of Baby Jane Doe did not violate Section 504 of the Rehabilitation Act. The Court also ruled that the hospital was not required to disclose Baby Jane Doe's medical records. In February 1984, the Court of Appeals for the Second Circuit upheld the District Court's decision "in a broadly written opinion holding that Section 504 does not apply to treatment decisions involving critically ill newborns."

In March 1984, the American Medical Association and five other organizations filed suit in New York against the DHHS and Secretary Margaret Heckler, challenging the Baby Doe II Rule. In May 1984, the United States District Court for the Southern District of New York struck down the Baby Doe II rule, calling it "invalid, unlawful, and without statutory authority."

As a result of the national attention received by the Baby Doe and Baby Jane Doe cases, House and Senate bills seeking to protect handicapped children were introduced in the 98th Congress of the United States. In September 1984, a compromise was reached to amend the Child Abuse Prevention and Treatment Act of 1974. "The Child Abuse Amendments of 1984 (Public Law 98–457) created a new category of child abuse and neglect, that of medical neglect." The law requires state child protective agencies "to pursue any legal remedies," including court proceedings, "as may be necessary to prevent the withholding of medically indicated treatment from disabled infants with life-threatening conditions."

Shapiro and Frader[41] summarized the Act as follows:

> Withholding indicated treatment is defined by the Act as the failure to 'provide treatment (including appropriate nutrition, hydration, and medication) which, in the treating physician's or physicians' reasonable medical judgment, will most likely be effective in ameliorating or correcting all such [life threatening] conditions.' Physicians are exempt from this legal responsibility to treat when 1) 'the infant is chronically and irreversibly comatose'; 2) the 'treatment would (i) merely prolong dying, (ii) not be effective in ameliorating or correcting all the infant's life-threatening conditions, or (iii) otherwise be futile in terms of the survival of the infant'; or 3) the treatment would be 'virtually futile' and 'under the circumstances would be inhumane'.

The Act was signed into law by President Reagan in October 1984. The DHHS then issued final regulations to implement the Child Abuse Amendments and guidelines for the establishment of hospital ICRCs. The exemption for treatment that would "merely prolong dying" refers to cases in which death will occur "in the near future" and not to more lingering deaths, such as from Tay–Sachs disease. The exemption for treatment that would be "virtually futile" and "under the circumstances inhumane" refers to cases in which treatment involves significant suffering "for an infant highly unlikely to survive." Failure of a state to adhere to the regulations may result in loss of federal child abuse funds.

REFERENCES

1. Zoll P, Linenthal A, Gibson W, et al: Termination of ventricular fibrillation in man by externally applied electric countershock. *N Engl J Med* 1956; 254:727
2. Safar P: Mouth-to-mouth airway. *Anesthesiology* 1957; 18:904
3. Kouwenhoven W, Jude J, Knickerbocker G: Closed-chest cardiac massage. *JAMA* 1960; 173:1064
4. McIntyre KM: Medicolegal aspects of cardiopulmonary resuscitation and emergency cardiac care. In McIntyre KM, Lewis AJ (eds): *Textbook of Advanced Cardiac Life Support*, p 277. Dallas, American Heart Association, 1983
5. Beecher H, Adams R, Barger C, et al: A definition of irreversible coma. *JAMA* 1968; 205:85
6. Curran W, Hyg S: Settling the medicolegal issues concerning brain-death statutes: Matters of legal ethics and judicial precedent. *N Engl J Med* 1978; 299:32
7. Ouaknine G, Kosary IZ, Graham J, et al: Laboratory criteria of brain death. *J Neurosurg* 1973; 39:429
8. Korein J, Maccario M: On the diagnosis of cerebral death; a prospective study on 55 patients to define irreversible coma. *Clin Electroencephalogr* 1971; 2:178
9. Ibe K: Clinical and pathophysiological aspects of the intravital brain death. *Electroencephalogr Clin Neurophysiol* 1971; 30:272
10. Becker D, Robert C, Nelson J, et al: An evaluation of the definition of cerebral death. *Neurology* 1970; 20:459
11. Plum F, Posner T: *Diagnosis of Stupor and Coma*, 2nd ed. Philadelphia, FA Davis Company, 1972
12. Ingvar DM, Widen L: Mjärndöd—Samm anfattning av ett symposium. *Läkartidningen* 1972; 69:3804
13. Black P: Brain death. *N Engl J Med* 1978; 299:339
14. *In the matter of Karen Quinlan*. 70 NJ 10, 355 A2d 647, 1976
15. Cassem NH: Ethical considerations in critical care. *Refresher Courses in Anesthesiology*. American Society of Anesthesiologists 1977; 5:13
16. Rhoden NK: Deciding about treatment in the ICU. In Benesch K, Abramson NS, Grenvik A, et al (eds): *Medicolegal Aspects of Critical Care*. Rockville, Aspen, 1986
17. *Roe v. Wade* 410 US 113 (1973)
18. Koop CE: *The Right to Live; The Right to Die*. Wheaton, Tyndale House, 1976
19. Alexander L: Medical science under dictatorship. *N Engl J Med* 1949; 241:39
20. *Superintendent of Belchertown State School v. Saikewicz*, Massachusetts Supreme Judicial Court No. 5JC–711, 1977
21. *In re Storar*, 52 NY2d 363, 420, NE2d 64, 1981
22. Danis M, Gerrity MS, Southerland LI, et al: A comparison of patient, family and physician assessments of the value of medical intensive care. *Crit Care Med* 1986; 16:594
23. Charlson ME, Sax FL, McKenzie R, et al: Resuscitation: How do we decide? A prospective study of physicians' preferences and the clinical course of hospitalized patients. *JAMA* 1986; 255:1316
24. Koop CE: The slide to Auschwitz. In Reagan RW (ed): *Abortion and the Conscience of the Nation*. Nashville, Thomas Nelson, 1984

25. *Matter of Claire Conroy,* 464 A2d 303 NJ App, 1983
26. *Matter of Claire Conroy,* 486 A2d 1209, NJ, 1985
27. *Severns v. Wilmington Medical Center, Inc.* 421 A2d 1334, Del Superior, 1980
28. *In re Dinnerstein,* 380 NE 2d 134, Mass App Ct, 1978
29. *Matter of Spring,* 405 NE 2d 115, Mass, 1980
30. *In re Eichner,* A2d, 637E, March 28, 1980. NY Supreme Court, Appellate Div
31. Kapp MB: Decision-making in critical care: Is the law an impediment or scapegoat? *Crit Care Med* 1986; 14:247
32. *Decision to Forego Life-Sustaining Treatment: Ethical, Medical and Legal Issues in Treatment Decisions.* President's Commission for the Study of Ethical Problems in Medicine and Biomedical and Behavioral Research. Washington, DC, US Government Printing Office, 1983
33. 1976 Cal Stat, Chapter 1439 (Natural Death Act), Sept 30, 1976
34. Life-Prolonging Procedure Act of Florida, Ch 765 FS, 1985
35. Kirby RR, Civetta JM: Critical care outcome. In Brown DL (ed): *Risk and Outcome in Anesthesia,* pp 184–212. Philadelphia, JB Lippincott, 1988
36. Bok S: Personal directions for care at the end of life. *N Engl J Med* 1976; 295:367
37. McIntyre KM: Medicolegal aspects of cardiopulmonary resuscitation and emergency cardiac care. In McIntyre RM, Lewis AJ (eds): *Textbook of Advanced Cardiac Life Support.* Dallas, American Heart Association, 1983
38. Rabkin MT, Gillerman G, Rice NR: Orders not to resuscitate. *N Engl J Med* 1976; 295:364
39. *In re Quackenbush,* 156 NJ Super, 282, 283 A2d 785, 1978
40. Reagan RW: *Abortion and the Conscience of the Nation.* Nashville, Thomas Nelson, 1984
41. Shapiro RS, Frader JE: Critically ill infants. In Benesch K, Abramson NS, Grenvik A, et al (eds): *Medicolegal Aspects of Critical Care,* pp 65–67. Rockville, Aspen, 1986
42. *John F. Kennedy Memorial Hospital v. Heston,* 48 NJ 576, 279 A2d 670, 1971
43. *In re Pogue,* No. M-18-74 (Super Ct DC Nov 1, 1974)
44. *Custody of a Minor,* 393 NE 2d 836 (Mass 1979) and 434 NE2d 601, 607 (Mass 1982)
45. *In re Seiferth,* 309 NY 80, 127 NE 2d 820 (1955)
46. *In re Green,* 12 *Crime & Delinquency* 377 (Child Div, Milwaukee County Ct, Wis 1966)
47. Discrimination Against the Handicapped by Withholding Treatment or Nourishment: Notice to Health Care Providers (DHHS, 47 Fed Reg 26, 027, 16 June 1982)
48. Strain E: The American Academy of Pediatrics comments on the "Baby Doe II" regulations. *N Engl J Med* 1983; 309:443

Iatrogenesis 7
Joseph M. Civetta

*I*atrogenesis, or as Kane titled a 1980 paper, "Just What the Doctor Ordered,"[1] must have originated soon after one human being undertook to provide some form of medical care for another. Interestingly, however, its recognition in print awaited the evolution of high-technology medical care. In 1956, Barr titled an article "The Hazards of Modern Diagnosis and Therapy—The Price We Pay."[2] Moser, in the same year, described the phenomenon as "diseases of medical progress."[3] One commonly thinks of technical misadventures when considering the problem of iatrogenesis in the intensive care unit (ICU). A pneumothorax following an attempted subclavian venipuncture or the use of a mechanical ventilator certainly is a well-recognized complication. The magnitude of the problem on a general medical service at a university hospital became startingly clear in a report by Steel and his coworkers.[4] They defined iatrogenic illness as any illness that resulted from a diagnostic procedure or from any form of therapy. They also included harmful occurrences (*e.g.*, injuries from a fall or decubitus ulcers developing during hospitalization) that were not natural consequences of the patients' diseases. However, they wished to stress that the term "iatrogenic" should not be construed to mean that there was any culpability on the part of the physician or hospital or that the illness was necessarily preventable. They found that 36% of 815 patients had an iatrogenic illness. In 9% of all persons admitted, the illness was considered major in that it threatened life or produced considerable disability. In 2%, the iatrogenic illness contributed to the patient's death. In all, 497 iatrogenic occurrences were discovered in these 815 patients. Finally, the presence of any iatrogenic illness significantly increased the risk of death during that hospitalization.

In 1983, Eugene Robin admonished us to take "a critical look at Critical Care" in a very provocative editorial.[5] He described four types of harm that can occur to patients, expanding the concept of iatrogenesis. These included technical errors in the laboratory, which lead to erroneous results. If the technical error is not appreciated, any decision or intervention based on this result can have only potentially harmful effects. A second category that he named "iatrodemics" was defined as the epidemic of systematic misdiagnosis or mismanagement of patients caused by the poor application of science or technology to patient management or, more simply, interpretive errors leading to incorrect decisions. A third type included those harms most commonly considered iatrogenic problems—the physical injuries to patients that result from invasive procedures selected or performed inappropriately. Finally, he characterized a fourth category as informational overload or having such a plethora of data, measurements, and results that the correct identification and selection of proper priorities are impeded.

We will consider the entire problem of iatrogenesis from the broader perspective of the clinical care process previously described in Chapter 2, titled "The What and When of Clinical Decision-Making." To appreciate the actual impact of iatrogenic acts of omission as well as commission, it should be useful to examine each element of clinical care: (1) the existing status of the patient; (2) recognition of newly acquired diseases or complications; (3) the decision-making process; (4) diagnostic evaluation; (5) the interventions used; (6) definition of outcome; and (7) evaluation of clinical care.

EXISTING STATUS OF THE PATIENT

We will examine two different perspectives: first, the proper selection of the patient for intensive care and, second, the patient's own effect on the probability of an iatrogenic occurrence. Selection of inappropriate patients is considered in detail in Chapter 1, titled, "Setting Objectives: Perspectives for Care."

Steel notes that the prehospital status of the patient affects the likelihood of subsequent iatrogenic occurrences, reflecting the influence of the patient on the likelihood of iatrogenesis.[4] Patients who were sick before admission, transferred from a nursing home or other acute care hospital, or judged in critical to poor condition by a physician on admission all had a significantly increased incidence of complications. These patients were more likely to be elderly and to be treated in the ICU, but the impact of these factors on statistical analysis was contained in prior health status and location before admission.

Because medications produced the highest number of iatrogenic complications, not surprisingly a greater exposure produced a greater frequency of complications and a greater number of major complications. In the patients with no complications, 7 drugs, on average, were used, whereas those with major complications were subjected to 17 different medications. Since iatrogenic occurrences require the interaction of a patient and the medical care system, the length of stay predicted the likelihood of a complication and the likelihood of a major complication. Thus, patients who escaped complications stayed about 1 week, those with minor complications were under care for about 2 weeks, and those with severe complications were hospitalized for nearly 3 weeks. Although it is clear that these predisposing conditions and temporal relationships must increase the risk of iatrogenic complications, they are also determinants of the patients that are in most need of our care. We must remain especially sensitive to these associations as we continue to deal with the high-risk population.

RECOGNITION OF NEWLY ACQUIRED DISEASES OR COMPLICATIONS

Many specific diagnoses have similar clinical presentations, and individual cases rarely present in a "classical fashion." This, then, is a fertile field for another type of iatrogenic occurrence. Of course, we are always at risk for missing the subtle presentation of an uncommon problem, and indeed our delight in the clinical pathologic conference reflects our fascination with the obscure or unlikely diagnosis, which serves to further our exhaltation of the clinician–detective. Another obvious problem is incorrectly attaching a name to a particular clinical presentation. We might consider that a "differential diagnosis" is a cautious method of hedging one's bets.

There are other problems as well. As soon as an incorrect diagnostic "label" is attached to a specific patient, the thinking and investigating expended on uncovering unknown factors usually cease. Thus, the real illness eludes identification and continues to exert its effects unabated, undiagnosed, and untreated. This effect is further perpetrated when each succeeding group of practitioners accepts the erroneous label and fails to reevaluate the situation. One case history should suffice. A quasi-ritualistic work-up of a fever in a critically ill postoperative patient included the search for pulmonary complications such as atelectasis or pneumonia, urinary tract infection, wound infections, bacteremias secondary to invasive monitoring catheters, and so on. This patient had an increased white blood cell count, a positive tracheal culture, infiltrates visible on chest radiograph, and purulent tracheal secretions. The label of pneumonitis was affixed to this patient; however, the true source of the fever and signs of inflammation was a septic antecubital vein, which would have been amenable to simple excision. Unfortunately, this diagnosis was not made until one week later, thus delaying the procedure designed to rid the host of the septic source. Ultimately, 3 months later, the patient died of sepsis and multiple organ system failure. At postmortem examination, multiple abscesses throughout the kidneys and lungs were found; cultures contained the same organisms that were identified in the septic vein.

DECISION-MAKING PROCESS

Medicine has been described as both art and science. The frequency with which the imprecise term "art" is used reflects the clinician's inability to identify the necessary data base used to form decisions or to relate this decision to subsequent diagnostic evaluation, therapeutic interventions, or clinical expectations for survival. The result is that the clinical decision-making process rarely is documented in the medical record, which prevents subsequent analysis of the total process of care. The particular diagnosis does not uniformly result in specific diagnostic and therapeutic interventions, and we can consider this one of the most important iatrogenic aspects of our care. Without demonstrated efficacy, parochialism and biased opinions are exhalted as examples of the art of medicine. Let us return to Robin's definition of iatrodemic: the epidemic of systemic misdiagnosis or mismanagement of patients caused by the poor applications of science or technology to patient management. He selected the treatment of acute respiratory failure for analysis. Of 19 therapeutic modalities considered *a priori* to have therapeutic effect, he believed there was scientific evidence to support only two, and this evidence could be considered only as partial support.

Although this area must be considered an important priority for future investigation, we must continue to practice today at the bedside; thus, the art of medicine will continue. Our teaching and research must reflect a new perspective—gaining understanding of the decision-making process does not demean the role or ability of the experienced expert clinician. It emphasizes the necessity to identify the data collected and the reasoning used, which leads this singular clinician to conclusions missed by the rest of us.

DIAGNOSTIC EVALUATION

We are faced with a vast array of potentially useful diagnostic tests. Particularly in the ICU, many of these tests can be done repetitively. Often, the explosion of utilization has been glibly attributed to a better awareness on our part to perform these tests of proven superiority to the traditional methods of history taking and physical examination. However, the proper timing, sequence, and repetition of diagnostic testing have not been studied relative to outcome criteria such that we could consider that we understand how many and how often laboratory tests should be used. We recently examined ten ways (Table 7-1) to improve the efficiency of care by diminishing unnecessary laboratory testing. We believe that this approach might resolve the dilemma of controlling costs while maintaining the quality of care, and it could impact favorably on total patient care by diminishing the incidence of Robin's four harms, thus lessening iatrogenesis. Hospital laboratory charges and the frequency of 28 commonly used tests were abstracted from itemized patient bills of 50 patients treated in April 1983 and, 8 months after the interventions, in a second group of 50 patients treated in February 1984. The total number of tests (Table 7-2) decreased by 2803 (42%), or 56 per patient per admission. In 1983, 2254 blood gases were performed, or 45 per patient. In 1984, the number was 1313, or 26 per patient. We have been astounded at the average of 23 tests per patient per day. As a result of the interventions planned and implemented, this number was reduced to 13 in February 1984 and has continued to decrease to approximately 8 per patient per day at the present time. No change in the severity of illness, distribution of patients, duration of ICU stay, length of hospitalization, or hospital mortality was noted. For our 12-bed unit, this could be extrapolated to diminish the total number of tests by more than 40,000 per year.

Our changes in what Stern and Epstein identified as "physician practice style,"[7] the how and why tests were generated, reduced charges in the ICU

TABLE 7-1. Ten Ways to Diminish Laboratory Charges

(1) Principles of management
(2) Elimination of standing orders
(3) Classification of patients
(4) Written guidelines for laboratory testing
(5) Mandatory communication among care givers
(6) No repetitive orders
(7) A single order for a single test
(8) Removal of monitoring catheters
(9) Constant administrative attention
(10) Feedback

with the attendant necessary diminution of the possibilities for Robin's types of harm and, thus, had an impact on patient care. Insecurity, inexperience, habits, training patterns, traditions, and fatigue seem to be the factors responsible for the proliferation of testing. This model of decreasing laboratory testing demonstrated that the quality of care was not dependent on our practice style and that "costly" and "high quality" were not necessarily synonymous. We must learn to distinguish the necessary yet costly elements from those which are unnecessary and contain the potential only for harm.

INTERVENTIONS USED

We should learn to make a distinction between "therapeutic" interventions and "manipulations." Therapy implies a chance for cure, that is, scientific evidence links outcome to the application of a particular remedy. It is for this reason that prospective randomized trials are considered proper for evaluating new forms of therapy. We can consider "manipulations" as the minute-to-minute responses to abnormalities in physiologic variables based on a constant stated or unstated desire to return as many of these abnormalities to normal in as short a period as possible. Because these efforts do not seem to affect outcome, the only possible results are deleterious. The obvious

TABLE 7-2. Overall Utilization

	1983	1984	COMMENT
ICU Days (% hospitalization)	15%	19%	Not different
Total Tests	6703	3900	↓ 2803; $p<0.05$
Tests/Patient	134	78	↓ 56 (42%)
Total Blood Gases	2254	1313	↓ 941
Blood Gases/Patient	45	26	↓ 19; $p<0.025$
Total Tests/Patient/Day	23	13	↓ 10

Mean values per patient are reported.
T test for two means used for statistical comparisons.

iatrogenic result after a nonindicated subclavian venipuncture, the pneumothorax, represents, in fact, only a small subset of all iatrogenic aspects of inappropriate evaluation, diagnosis, testing, and interventions. However, let us focus on a unique perspective of pneumothorax. In 1978 Ludwig and Kienzle published a study of 77 cases of pneumothorax occurring in an autopsy population of 3500 patients.[8] Eight were discovered in adult patients who had been receiving mechanical ventilation. The unsuspected undiagnosed tension pneumothorax could be postulated as at least a contributory cause of death in 0.15% of the deaths analyzed in this series and 0.3% of the patients receiving mechanical ventilation in their hospital. This would project to a total of approximately 500 patients per year in the United States alone—twice the number of airline fatalities in 1987 and a risk of health care far greater than many other conditions that have captured media attention. It is important, therefore, to focus on the particular and restricted definition of iatrogenesis, too, since the prevalence worldwide of potentially treatable complications contributes to overall ICU mortality in an unknown but probably significant way.

In addition to iatrogenesis associated with physical measures, it is important to reemphasize that Steel noted that exposure to drugs was a particularly important factor in iatrogenic illness.[4] In fact, 42% of the total occurrences were drug related compared to 35% related to diagnostic and therapeutic procedures and 23% classified as miscellaneous, such as falls, dietary management, transportation, or nursing procedures. Of the drug-related complications, 19% were considered major. The list of the most commonly associated drugs included nitrates, digoxin, aminophylline, antidysrhythmics, anticoagulants, penicillins, antihypertensives, propranolol, and benzodiazepines. Major complications occurred in a third or more of patients who had complications due to digoxin, anticoagulants, antihypertensives, or propranolol. Drug-related iatrogenic occurrences must be extremely prevalent in our ICU patients, given the degree of illness and frequency of usage. If many drugs can be presumed to represent "manipulations," we may be able to decrease the major complication rate significantly. Steel concluded that although it may be logically sound to speculate that the benefit of hospitalization far exceeds the risk, because of the severity of illness of the population in hospitals, the natural progression of disease, and the value of alternative modes of therapy, mechanisms must be developed to assess the hazards of hospitalization in an ongoing manner. Technological, educational, and administrative means can then be sought to reduce the number and severity of untoward events, and the efficacy of such efforts can be ascertained.

DEFINITIONS OF OUTCOME

Definitions of outcome are considered in detail in Chapter 9, titled "Prediction and Definition of Outcome in a Cost-Sensitive Era." One of the most important issues we must face in critical care is the distinction between therapeutic efforts that may return a patient to a productive life and continued ineffective efforts that only prolong the patient's dying, extend the family's grief, and deplete society's resources. We must develop a proper evaluation of outcome, which must include the discrimination between potentially curable patients and those already dying or beyond therapy, the duration of therapy, and the resources used. These are obviously factors beyond the traditional statistical analysis of mortality. Without such data, the complex interrelationships among legal, ethical, and societal aspects cannot be resolved. Due to the continually rising costs for medical care, our leadership in promoting the understanding and delineation of these complex clinical care interrelationships must supplant solely economic motivations as the major driving force to determine the future of medical care. We must not forget Fein's important observation that we live in a society, not an economy.[9]

Medical knowledge and our professional skills may not be able to treat each devastating critical illness, but we must not view this with a sense of failure. Rather, it is an opportunity for the expression of those unique human resources that aid the family and patient in coping with the dying process. The opposite course, persisting in hopeless situations, completely blocks the achievement of these important objectives.

EVALUATION OF CLINICAL CARE

It is not surprising, given the limitations that have been discussed in the first six steps of the clinical care sequence, that iatrogenesis abounds and that its effects extend far beyond technical complications. The incidence of complications due to technical error is only the tip of the iceberg. We must continue to practice on a daily basis, but we must accept the responsibility to investigate, quantitate, and delineate the clinical care sequence so that the subtle effects introduced by bias and lack of understanding (*i.e.*, iatrogenesis in its broadest sense) can be minimized. Fuchs' exhortation that we "consider the possibility of contributing more by doing less" is important.[10] The immense amount of data usually collected in the ICU must be organized to determine its use and relevance. We must learn what is the necessary and sufficient data base. However, we must not forget that the societal, not merely the economic, impact of medical care must remain our principle consideration. We must first "contribute more" by achieving a greater understanding of the medical care process. Only then can we knowledgeably "do less" at the bedside. The ultimate effect in purifying, clarifying, distilling, and delineating bedside intensive care will be to eliminate misinterpretations, misdirections, and misadventures—iatrogenesis.

REFERENCES

1. Kane RL: Iatrogenesis: Just what the doctor ordered. *J Community Health* 1980; 5:149

2. Barr DP: Hazards of modern diagnosis and therapy—The price we pay. *JAMA* 1956; 159:1452
3. Moser RH: Diseases of medical progress. *N Engl J Med* 1956; 255:606
4. Steel K, Gertman PM, Crescenzi C, Anderson J: Iatrogenic illness on a general medical service at a university hospital. *N Engl J Med* 1981; 304:638
5. Robin ED: A critical look at critical care. *Crit Care Med* 1983; 11:144
6. Civetta JM, Hudson–Civetta JA: Maintaining quality of care while reducing charges in the ICU: 10 ways. *Ann Surg* 1985; 202:524
7. Stern RS, Epstein AM: Institutional responses to prospective payment based on diagnosis-related groups: Implications for cost, quality, and access. *N Engl J Med* 1985; 312:621
8. Ludwig J, Kienzle G: Pneumothorax in a large autopsy population: A study of 77 cases. *Am J Clin Pathol* 1978; 70:24
9. Fein R: On measuring economic benefits of health programmes. In McLachlan G, McKeown T (eds): *Medical History and Medical Care: A Symposium of Perspectives,* pp 179–220. London, Oxford University Press, 1971
10. Fuchs VR: A more effective, efficient and equitable system. *West J Med* 1976; 125:3

Avoiding Legal Problems 8
David B. Mishael

No simple theory can be offered to explain the proliferation of medical malpractice suits. Lawyers and physicians have tossed around their own explanations for years, without much success. Substandard medical care is the explanation given by many plaintiffs' lawyers. Yet, that explanation does not explain why the most seasoned physician is sued, despite having rendered medical care within the acceptable standards. Since no two medical conditions, or malpractice cases for that matter, are alike, it is difficult to determine why some situations lead to lawsuits. In analyzing several malpractice cases, certain trends begin to surface. These trends or similarities, when quantified, suggest the impetus for the filing of many cases.

One recurring similarity is the failure of the physician to appreciate the human emotions involved in medicine. Unfortunately, this may be the direct result of medical school training. Too many schools teach the philosophy "that a physician should not become personally involved with a patient's condition." Medical schools have suggested that a physician must remain objective and cannot do so if personal emotions are involved. But if this theory is taken too far, the physician becomes divorced from humanity. This results in the development of a poor bedside manner. The end result may be a malpractice suit.

Opening lines of communication is essential to creating a respectful and friendly rapport and is the means through which the physician senses some of the nonmedical needs of the patient or family. Several years ago the family doctor or general practitioner (GP) made house calls and developed a friendship with families. Ironically, the proliferation of lawsuits has increased as we see declining numbers of physicians desiring to become GPs. A direct corollary can be made, however, that the GP was and still is less likely to be sued because he/she is a friend of the family or patient, and no one desires to sue a friend.

Perhaps the second greatest pitfall is the failure of one medical provider to communicate findings or observations concerning a particular patient to another treating physician. Information that is lost in transition leaves the physician in an unfortunate situation, as medicine cannot be practiced appropriately when all the information is not available.

The initiating forces that lead to malpractice claims are often only the tip of the iceberg. They do not reveal some of the most damaging elements that make the case difficult to defend. Since most cases are filed months and even years after treatment, memories tend to dissipate, and the reasons for the application of certain treatments are forgotten. The patient's chart (*i.e.*, the written record) is often the only remaining source that might shed some light on why a particular treatment was given. The failure of physicians to appreciate the need for thorough and accurate charting creates innumerable problems in defending cases years later. Either the reasons for treatment are never documented, or the chart is so sparse that one wonders whether the physician was actually treating the patient. In the eyes of the jury, "if it was not written down, it was not done."

The intensivist is not immune from these suits and is likewise open to these potential errors in judgment. Unlike normal hospital medical floors, the intensive care unit (ICU) offers certain unique qualities, which, if not appreciated in a medical–legal sense, may lead to malpractice suits. With the requirement of closer observation, one-on-one care, and the use of sophisticated machines, the potential for errors increases.

This chapter's purpose is to highlight problem areas in the ICU and explain some of the common mistakes that lead to claims. In an effort to express realistically the errors that occur, case examples are used. Suggested techniques are offered in the hope that similar situations can be avoided or handled more appropriately. My first suggestion is to apply the knowledge you gain from reading Chapter 13, titled "Understanding Reactions of Patient and Family," in your everyday practice.

COMMUNICATION BREAKDOWNS: A PRECURSOR TO THE MALPRACTICE CLAIM

LACK OF RAPPORT

All human beings make mistakes, physicians included. The physician's error, however, can be devastating because the recipient of the error is a human body and mind. Death, physical pain, paralysis, brain damage, or deformities are often the ultimate result of physician-induced error. Sometimes these unfortunate outcomes are the result of medically accepted complications that occur in the absence of malpractice. Due to breakdowns in communication, physicians are sued not only in situations of medical error, but also as a result of the medically accepted complication.

Using the medical complication scenario, several reasons may lead to a suit under such circumstances. In some instances, physicians have failed to develop a rapport with the patient or family. This problem occurs with some frequency with the medical consultants who are called in only briefly to assist with one element of a given patient's condition and feel that they do not have time to develop a rapport. When a complication arises, the physician may see the need to speak to either the patient or family for the first time. Since usually the patient and family are now upset or scared, they may not be too receptive, and in some instances they may not wish to talk at all. The problem plaguing the physician is simply that no relationship or communication foundation preexisted the complication, which might have otherwise allowed the physician the ability to broach the subject more easily. In these situations, the family or patient may leave the hospital thinking that an error occurred, when indeed it was an acceptable complication. For the physician, it is too late. The family or patient may institute a lawsuit on the belief that what occurred was a medical *faux pas*.

Sometimes the patient or family will ask the physician to explain certain untoward events and the mechanism by which they occurred. It behooves the physician to take the time to explain what happened. If the physician fails to do so, the recipient may not know that what occurred was a complication as opposed to a mistake. Believing a mistake occurred, the patient may file suit. Unfortunately, once the suit is filed, the patient's lawyer, or a medical expert hired by the lawyer, may scrutinize the chart and find other peculiarities. Although these peculiarities may not necessarily constitute malpractice, when combined with the complication, they reflect poorly on the physician's care. Further, what was once suspected to be a complication may now become more believable, considering the appearances of poor overall treatment.

FALSE EXPECTATIONS

Probably the most frequent reason for lawsuits when complications arise is the creation of false expectations. A concern of all patients and families is the welfare of the patient. Whether due to curiosity, concern, or insecurity, patients and families perpetually inquire as to the severity of the condition and the prognosis. Too often the physician feels the need to instill a sense of optimism without painting the true picture. I have heard the following examples of physician-uttered optimism in many malpractice cases: "She should come out of this just fine"; "She'll be up and around in no time"; and "No one has ever died of this disease, so don't worry." Although the physician may feel this optimism will assist the patient in having a positive outlook, it will be an insignificant factor when adverse consequences occur.

If after hearing these statements the patient were to deteriorate or die, the family or patient (assuming the patient lived) will require a good explanation if the physician hopes to avoid being sued. The problem confronting the physician is the unrealistic or "false" expectations created in the patient or family. The physician has made the prognosis so positive that no one expects a negative outcome. The patients or their families may never have been advised of the potential complications. When they occur, suspicions arise, since only good results were expected. They begin to think that a mistake must have occurred; otherwise, the patient would have been "up and around by now." The stimulating force for a malpractice case has been set in motion.

The foregoing situations should not occur if the physician follows a few simple steps before the complications arise. Initially, the physician should institute an orientation session for both the patient and the family. In the ICU setting, I would suggest that the physician explain the "team approach to medical care," perhaps the type of monitoring equipment being used for that given patient, the potential need for consultations, the role the consultant may play, and who the patient or family should speak to for daily reports or to answer any questions they might have. The orientation should be ongoing, so that if new monitoring equipment or consultants are called in, the patient and family are kept abreast of the patient's medical state. This orientation will create lines of communication between the physician and patient and may also put the patient at ease. The rapport that develops gives the physician that little extra "in" which may be used when unfortunate medical problems occur.

With the lines of communication in place, the physician should always tell the truth, regardless of how unfortunate the news might be. If the physician explains that the medical condition sometimes results in certain complications or explains the downside risks of certain forms of treatment, the patient and family will be preconditioned and perhaps even anticipate the complication. If the complication were to arise, they would not be shocked or lose confidence in the physician; to the contrary, they may feel more confident in the medical care being provided since the physician foresaw the event before it ever occurred. In turn, the complication is not viewed as a physician error but as a medically accepted event.

INCONSISTENT STATEMENTS

A unique quality of the ICU is the number of staff necessary to monitor and treat patients on a one-on-one basis. With more health care providers treating a given patient, the potential for communication breakdowns is greatly increased. A problem that can occur, with increasing probability, is the passing of inconsistent information to the patient or family.

The communication pattern that leads to this error is similar to the way rumors begin. For example, the infectious disease consultant indicates to the chief resident that the patient has a lung infection or pneumonia. The resident in turn advises the nurse before going off shift to pass this information on to the oncoming staff. For reasons that may never be identified, by the time the information reaches the next shift, the patient is said to be suffering from a pneumothorax. If the family was advised initially that pneumonia might be present, and then are told it might be a pneumothorax, they may begin to wonder if anyone actually knows what is transpiring. If an untoward event were to occur, without the inconsistency having been cleared, the family might be curious as to whether anyone actually knew what was going on. They might perceive the situation as a failure to diagnose, or they may question why one physician knew what was happening, yet the others did not. The attitude expressed by many plaintiffs in these instances is that if they are going to be charged such high fees for health care, the health care providers should be competent. It is a combination of expense mentality and the appearance of ineptness in times of deteriorating medical conditions that lead people to sue.

Preventing inconsistent statements is sometimes difficult. I would recommend the most senior physician for each shift be designated as the source to provide information to the patient and family. Though families often prefer to speak with only one or especially one physician in particular, the necessity for 24-hour staffing patterns with time off to recuperate may make this desire impossible to meet. The senior physician should have more experience in the functioning of the ICU and more knowledge of the disease processes. Unlike the less experienced physician, the senior physician can express the situation or condition with less chance of committing errors or misstating a particular medical phenomenon. I believe it would be beneficial to designate a set time each day for the discussion, so the family or patient can anticipate receiving answers to the questions and can be assured that everything possible is being done.

The senior physician should strive to learn the most current condition of a patient before conferring with the family. The chart should be reviewed, and, if any test results have not reached the chart or consultants have failed to note their findings, telephone reports should be sought. If the test results are not available, the physician should so indicate during the discussion. The potential always exists that the test results will change the physician's opinion. Failure to so indicate may place the physician in an awkward position if the physician had said only minutes earlier that the patient was progressing, when indeed the test results reveal otherwise.

With one physician conducting the review, the likelihood of inconsistencies occurring is lessened. If the consultants' findings are too complex to explain, a joint report by the consultant and the intensivist should be used. A second benefit of this technique is the perception of being organized and well informed. Psychologically, the patient and family will feel more confidence in the physicians.

No technique is perfect, and inconsistencies will still occur. When they do, the intensivist should immediately approach the patient or family and explain in logical terms how the inconsistency arose and how it has been resolved. The more time that elapses before an explanation is given, the longer the patient or family may dwell on the inconsistency and begin to sense incompetency.

CONFLICTING OPINIONS; CRITICIZING OTHERS

Sometimes inconsistent statements are not the product of communication breakdowns. Instead, they result from purposeful statements or opinions. Time and again, physicians and nurses openly criticize treatment rendered by others. When the patient and family overhear these critical statements, they are more likely to pursue a malpractice suit, especially if they feel the problem is directly related to the criticized treatment. This stands to reason since a physician of the same hospital is criticizing one of his/her own staff members. One would not expect a fellow staff member to speak out unless it was a serious mistake.

It is important to understand why these critical statements are made, so that perhaps they can be avoided before they ever reach the stage of being expressed. The forces behind them are often a product of the environment. Hospitals, like all other large business firms, have hierarchies and internal politics. Not infrequently one service may find itself pitted against another concerning the other service's response time to calls, the other service's knowledge or lack thereof, or even the soon-to-be-available space on a given floor. Competition occurs daily. One physician or service may envy another service or might hold feelings of animosity toward them. As a result, critical opinions may be expressed as a vendetta or as a rationalization for one's own shortcomings.

At times this occurs on an even smaller scale. One particular physician may not get along with his peers in the ICU. Such a person is an easy focus for blame should a patient's condition become worse. For example, an intern or first-year resident may have treated a nurse as inferior, thereby upsetting the continuity of the team approach. The nurse, who may have years of experience beyond the resident or intern, may indeed be correct in his/her medical judgment. After years of receiving such ridicule, the nurse might seek revenge by exposing the physician to unnecessary criticism.

The least mentioned reason for "uncalled for" criticism, yet the most prevalent, is the ego. The competition among residents, the desire to be recognized, and the hope to be named chief resident are all matters that cause aggressiveness. Perhaps the need to criticize occurs because during the early stages, in undergraduate studies, premedical students learn that "survival of the fittest" is the only way to get ahead. The term "cutthroat" competition is often mentioned by premedical students. By carrying this philosophy into their residency, young physicians still feel the need to be "cutthroat." Older physicians also have tendencies to behave in this fashion. Sometimes their attitude is due to competition surrounding research projects. Institutions have even become jealous of others because one institution may compete against another for patients. The need to fill beds and conduct medicine as a business is part of the blame for this mentality.

Ego problems also occur with nurses. In the following example, the nurses' egos were hurt and rebounded only to the detriment of the patient. The case arose in the neurosurgery ICU, when a postcraniotomy patient did not receive adequate monitoring. The patient was placed on neurologic watch, and the nurses had to complete a neurologic watch sheet. The family requested a private duty nurse be retained to monitor the patient throughout the night. The full-time nurses were well trained to provide such care and were insulted that someone felt it necessary to hire a private duty nurse. As a result, the full-time nurses would not even enter the patient's room to monitor him. Unfortunately, the private duty nurse was not trained to understand neurologic signs and failed to appreciate the patient's rapid neurologic deterioration. By morning, when the new nursing staff arrived and entered the room to check on the patient, it was already too late. The night shift nurses were quick to criticize the private duty nurse in front of the family, saying, "This would not have happened if the private duty nurse knew what she was doing." As it turned out, the hospital nurses were said to have been negligent for failing to periodically monitor the patient. Thus the nurses' egos prevented them from providing appropriate care. Their need to seek revenge led them to openly criticize the private duty nurse, although admittedly the private duty nurse failed to provide adequate care.

Other cases have arisen in which the ICU physician, for some unknown reason, felt compelled to criticize the prior treating physicians. There is little doubt that ICU patients find their way into the ICU from other medical floors, and even other hospitals, due to complications or deteriorating conditions. The conditions may have been due to surgical complications, perhaps problems arising out of orthopedic injuries, or for numerous other reasons. Once the patient arrives, the role of the intensivist is to provide quality care. The intensivist was not present during the initial treatment and therefore has no place rendering comments even within his/her field of expertise. Yet it is amazing how many times physicians in the ICU, including consultants, will criticize the care rendered by preceding or current physicians. The majority of times, the comments have no foundation or basis in fact. Unfortunately, when the patient and family are advised that the care rendered was poor or resulted in the current state, they will pursue a malpractice claim. The physician who was so quick to criticize may retract prior statements after the suit has been filed.

To avoid animosity and the potential for revenge by other staff members or physicians in the community, you need to treat your peers with courtesy and respect. Keep in mind that after each patient is discharged, the staff you work with will remain. The team approach will fail if you cannot work together, and the only party who will suffer as a result will be the patient.

Your ego and competitive nature must remain in check. Commenting to the patient or family on treatment rendered by others is an absolute mistake, especially when no foundation exists to support the opinions. This does not mean that constructive criticism to another physician must be avoided. Certainly each of you should strive to better the care being provided to a given patient, and if such care calls for criticism, speak directly to the person of whom you are being critical. It may turn out that what you are criticizing is the state-of-the-art treatment under the circumstances.

Those who practice in teaching hospitals require additional commentary. The young residents should appreciate the wisdom of the ICU nurses and treat them equally. You will learn that the nurses may know more than you initially. Even after practicing for several years, you will be pleasantly surprised how often the ICU nurse will be of great assistance.

Teaching hospitals also structure their ICU with a different chain of command. A "fellow" or senior resident is usually in charge of the first- and second-year residents. At times, they may feel the need to remind others of their superiority. They may "dump" on the younger residents since this was the way the system treated them at their younger stage. Such actions will only increase the animosity between residents, which may lead to revenge tactics.

For example, in one particular case a first-year resident thought a computed tomography (CT) scan was necessary after evaluating a patient. The senior resident disagreed, and the physicians began to argue. The CT scan was not done for several hours, and as it turned out the patient was harboring a subdural hematoma. Perhaps for revenge purposes, the younger resident refused to sign his own note.

After the malpractice suit was filed, one of the questions posed to the resident in deposition was "whether some procedure existed whereby the first-year resident could have called the attending to advise of the conflicting opinions." The answer is simple. Every ICU should provide access to attending physicians so that an objective forum exists to resolve disputes. The chain of command should not be used as a "dumping ground" for senior physicians to unload matters they do not wish to handle. The ICU patient will benefit if the ICU team functions in concert, and therefore competition among residents should be restrained.

INFORMATION LOST IN TRANSITION

Another problem resulting from providing health care through the team approach is the potential for information to be lost or go unreported. Inherently, the team approach requires reliance on others to communicate pertinent test results, observations, and symptoms to the treating physician. Lifesaving medications and emergency consultations may or may not be ordered, depending on whether the information has been communicated. Failing to provide the information to the physician is like asking someone to complete a puzzle without having all the pieces.

The case example cited earlier of the deteriorating craniotomy patient illustrates the problem. Reliance was placed on the nursing staff to monitor the patient and communicate any untoward signs to the attending physician. The failure of the nurses to make periodic assessments prevented the physician from learning about the patient's deteriorating condition. The information that would have been gained had the nurses observed the patient was simply never made known.

Another case illustrating this point arose when an orthopedic patient was transferred to the ICU. The patient had been placed in a halo device to allow his cervical fracture to heal. While he was on the orthopedic floor, orders were written requiring the nursing staff to cleanse the pin sites. At the time of the transfer, the attending physician did not write new orders. The ICU nursing staff failed to cleanse the pin sites for several days after transfer. Unknown to all involved was the fact that the patient's seizure disorder, necessitating transfer, was directly related to a pin site infection which had spread to the brain. Had the attending physician communicated with the intensivist, in all likelihood new orders would have been written.

There is no easy solution to this problem. The foregoing are only a few little examples of the myriad of circumstances that can lead to uninformed care. One suggestion is to create a communication network that functions consistently on a daily basis. Patient rounds are one means to keep updated. Perhaps a central depository should exist next to the patient, where all recent test results should be maintained. Any changes in orders or treatments and the monitoring of certain vital signs can be included.

Nurses and other support staff should be able to contact the intensivist directly at any moment. If daily rounds are used, representatives of each service that make up the team should be present. Strategies and patient care plans can then be updated regularly. The intensivist should alert all team members during the meeting to be on the lookout for potential problems concerning each patient, so that they can focus their care on specific matters. By following this practice, each service should know what others are doing, and the chances for confusion or contraindicated treatments are decreased.

When patients are transferred to the ICU from other medical floors or hospitals, the prior attending physician should be consulted to review past orders and treatment. Not only is the attending physician an important source of information but also he/she can function as the initial conduit through which the intensivist can begin developing a rapport with the patient and family. The attending physician makes a serious error in thinking that he/she can wipe his/her hands clean now that the patient is in the hands of the intensivist. The failure of the attending to appreciate his/her role during the transfer may implicate him/her in a future malpractice claim.

DOCUMENTING THE MEDICAL CHART

From a pragmatic standpoint, time does not permit documentation of all care in a patient's medical chart. Medical emergencies, volume of patient load, short staffing, and business enterprise philosophy are some factors that may prevent the physician from recording all activities in the patient's chart. Regardless of time constraints, the patient's chart should support the medical care rendered.

REASONING PROCESS IN WRITING

Three years after the fact, when a physician takes the stand in a courtroom, the physician may not recall the infinite wisdom displayed when he/she felt it necessary to change the patient's medication. Hopefully, the medical record was well documented and can help refresh the physician's recollection. If not, the physician can only offer plausible reasons for his/her actions at the time. If the physician failed to record his/her reasoning, the plaintiff's lawyer might ask the following question: "If you felt it so important to change the medication at the time, why did you not indicate in the chart your reasons for doing so?"

Opportunities will no doubt arise when medications and forms of treatment will require changes. Laboratory results or trends in symptoms may necessitate the change. A patient's deterioration may prompt unusual interventions. A thought process should always exist which the physician follows before making the change. During the thought process, physicians draw from their education, experience, and case studies to formulate the basis for their decisions. Although it is not plausible to document all the factors leading to the change in treatment, the general indications or explanation for the change should be documented. By such conduct the physician will be able to show, through documentation on the chart, that he/she was not "picking at straws," but instead completed a rational thinking process before making such an important decision. Likewise, this will leave the impression that the decision was not made in haste but was well reasoned.

LEGIBILITY

Routinely physicians and nurses will review the chart before seeing the patient to orient themselves about the patient's condition. Those caring for the patient during the earlier shifts will have documented their observations and findings. The medical record may be the only source of communication at times between physicians and other health care providers who do not cross paths. A certain amount of reliance is therefore placed on the earlier notations in the chart. If the subsequent treating physician is unable to read the earlier notes, an important sign can be missed, and important decisions may not be made. The potential for misinterpretations can also lead to improper care. For the same reason, proper medical nomenclature and abbreviations should be used.

When a patient's case finds its way into the legal setting, the ability of the physician to read the chart may become a focal point. In many depositions physicians testify "that their normal routine encompasses reviewing the chart before seeing the patient." When asked to read the progress notes that preexisted the involvement of the physician, the physician stumbles through and often states that "he or she cannot interpret various notations." The plaintiff's lawyer may then ask the rhetorical question: "Well, if you cannot read the note before yours in the chart, you really did not know the full extent of the patient's condition, did you?" The jury may then question among themselves whether the physician actually knew what was transpiring with the patient before he/she instituted treatment.

Clearly, the communication process through charting functions at a better level when the handwriting of physicians and nurses is legible. Subsequently, the physician who routinely reviews the chart can spend more time treating the patient instead of attempting to decipher what a fellow associate has previously written, and errors due to misinterpretations will occur less frequently.

REPETITION

After years of training and schooling one would expect the physician to be more independent than what the medical records sometimes reveal. For reasons still unclear to me, physicians will write a note in the progress notes that repeats almost *verbatim* the progress note written by another physician 3 hours earlier. Over the course of several days or a period of several hours the chart that contains repetitious notes will begin to sound as though it were created in an echo chamber. The implications of a repetitious note include the thought that the physician who wrote the repetitious note never saw the patient, but simply wrote a note to cover himself/herself.

Assuming that the note writer did see the patient, one may question why the note is identical to an earlier note. Perhaps the subsequent physician is lazy or not competent to assess the patient on his/her own.

The full impact of repetitious note writing can best be appreciated under the following hypothetical situation:

> A patient is documented to be recovering well following surgery. At 12:00 noon, 2 hours after surgery, and at 3:00 in the afternoon, 5 hours after surgery, the subsequent treating physician essentially writes *verbatim* in the progress notes the exact postoperative findings that appeared earlier in the chart immediately following surgery. At 3:01 P.M. the patient suffers a respiratory arrest and dies.

In all likelihood the competency of the subsequent treating physician will be questioned. The plaintiff's lawyer may suggest that the subsequent treating physician never really evaluated the patient, otherwise the notes of 12:00 noon and 3:00 would have shown a deteriorating condition. The plaintiff's lawyer may also allege that the subsequent treating physician never saw the patient at 12:00 or 3:00, but, instead, several days after the patient's demise, the physician came into the hospital and created fraudulent notes to give the appearance that he/she saw the patient twice in the afternoon before the patient died.

The problems surrounding repetitious note taking can easily be overcome if the physician takes the time to evaluate the patient and document all observations and findings present at the time of each visit with the patient. The physician may want to make reference to laboratory studies or other documentations in the chart that may not have existed at the time of earlier visits. The timing of these studies will confirm that the note is not a duplicate of an earlier note. Also by including notes concerning current laboratory results, the physician shows that he/she is constantly keeping up with the patient's condition.

Another problem with repetitious note writing is the fact that there may exist certain diagnostic studies in the chart that will contradict the contents of the note. For instance, if the physician copies an earlier note where the hematocrit and hemoglobin were found normal, the repetitious note written hours later may be in error because more recent studies may indicate a severe drop in those values. The repetitious note would be highly suspect if the case were to result in litigation.

FRAUDULENT OR LOST RECORDS

A medical malpractice case may be won or lost depending on the status of the medical records. I recall in one particular case that the medical care was believed to be defensible in court until it was learned that the defendant physician had secretly created two charts for the same patient. The physician's credibility was destroyed, and the case was settled quickly.

In recent years states have developed various laws to protect the patients' rights in having an accurate and complete record of the care they received. In several states a physician can be found guilty of a second-degree misdemeanor or a criminal charge if he/she fraudulently alters, defaces, or falsifies any medical record or causes any of these offenses to be committed.[1] In the face of a malpractice case an allegation of criminal misconduct can only strengthen the case against the physician. Alteration of records may also lead to license suspensions or restrictions being imposed.[2] Recreating a progress note, substituting operative reports, changing the time on test results, backdating a note, and discarding a record or test result easily constitute fraudulent attempts to alter or deface the medical record. A physician is only cheating himself/herself if he/she believes such actions cannot be proven. Handwriting analysts are readily available and with new technology can "date" the ink and examine the pages to see whether imprints or depressions exist that would show whether the page was originally a part of the chart or a page slipped in at a later time.

Most hospitals are required by law and the standards of the Joint Commission on Accreditation of Hospitals to maintain medical records, which include treatment notes and reports.[3] If a medical malpractice suit is filed and important notes that are usually a part of the chart are not present, various problems will arise. If the absence of the note sufficiently hinders the patient's ability to proceed with the lawsuit, the burden of proof, which normally is held by the plaintiff, may shift to the doctor or hospital, requiring that they bring forth evidence to rebut a presumption that they were negligent.[4] The effect of a missing note may therefore require the physician to prove his/her innocence, or nonnegligence, first. Defending a malpractice case under such circumstances is similar to starting out "behind the eight ball." Before the lawyer can even defend the medical issues involved he/she must first overcome a burden of proving nonnegligence due to the missing record.

---

1. Cal Penal Code §471.5; Fla Stat §395.0165(1); and NY Penal Law §175.05
2. Fla Stat §395.0165(2); Ill Rev Stat Ch 111, §4433(21) and (22); Mass Gen Laws, Ch 112, §5(C); NJ Stat §45:9-16(H) and (I); and NC Gen Stat §90–14(6); see also *Matter of Jascalevich*, 442 A 2d 635, 182 NJ Super 455
3. Fla Admin Code §10D–28.059(3); and JCAH Chapter 9 (Medical Record Services §§9.1, 9.1.2, 9.1.3, 9.2.2.8, 9.2.2.9, 9.2.2.9.1, 9.2.2.12.
4. See *Public Health Trust of Dade County v Valcin*, 507 So 2d 596 (Fla 1987)

CHARTING UNTOWARD EVENTS

The inevitable is bound to happen. An endotracheal tube may be placed improperly or may come out, depriving the patient of oxygen. An unforeseen or unanticipated complication may also occur. The treating physician has a duty to document these occurrences in the patient's chart. Failing to do so can subject the physician to various penalties, some of which were enumerated in the preceding section. If a lawsuit were to arise, other health care providers may have witnessed the occurrence and will so testify. The physician who failed to document such events will undoubtedly lose credibility when asked, "Why did you not chart such an important occurrence?"

If the physician knows for a fact the cause of the untoward event, it should be documented along with a description of the untoward event. In the endotracheal tube example, the physician should simply indicate that "the endotracheal tube came out," and the time it was observed should be documented. If the physician or nurse does not know the cause of the untoward event, he/she should not document speculations or guesswork. Often health care providers will document their intuitions, yet they may have no expertise in that particular field. If the physician comments in the chart on a subject matter outside his/her specialty, it immediately becomes guesswork. Once charted, the guesswork is "engraved in stone," and many lawsuits are filed as a result of such speculative statements in the chart.

If a physician-induced error occurs, not only should it be charted, but also an incident report should be completed and furnished to risk management. Incident reports can be completed by anyone and, therefore, speculation or guesswork can be included. In most states a certain privilege is afforded to incident reports that will either prohibit their disclosure or limit their use as evidence.[5]

In the ICU, physicians and nurses will encounter cases in which death is inevitable. If such is known, they should chart the existence of such a fact and follow through their normal charting procedures. Anticipated deteriorating signs should be documented, perhaps with references as to how the patient's family is holding up emotionally and what is being done to assist them in their time of need.

In situations in which "no-code orders" are on the chart, the physician should document, when the appropriate instance arrives, that in the light of the "no-code order," cardiopulmonary resuscitation or other life-sustaining treatments were withheld. By doing so, the physician indicates the reasoning behind his/her actions or lack of actions.

INFORMED CONSENT

In matters concerning informed consent for a particular procedure or regimen of treatment, all discussions should be recorded. Those who are present at

---

5. Fla Stat §395.041(4); and NY Pub Health Law §§2805–J, 2805–L, 2805–M

the time the risks are explained to the patient or family should be identified in the note. Although numerous risks may be associated with the treatment, those that are explained orally should be documented in the chart. Most hospital charts also contain standard consent forms. It behooves the physician to make sure that all risks associated with the procedure are documented on the form before the patient reads and signs it. If the patient's condition increases the probability of one particular risk occurring, the consent form should so indicate, along with a notation to that effect being placed in the progress notes.

Another problem that can occur with the consent form is the failure of the physician to document completely the procedures or treatments for which consent was obtained. On many occasions a procedure or treatment may entail more than one step in the process before it is completed. If the consent form reflects only the first step, the physician is acting without the patient's consent if he/she were to apply the second and third steps of the treatment. Unfortunately, preprinted consent forms do not always provide sufficient space to document the extent of the treatment being consented to. If the consent form lacks available space, another document should be attached to the consent, providing a more detailed account of the procedure so that the patient is fully aware of what he/she is consenting to.

In some situations the patient may not speak English, and an interpreter will be needed to explain the treatment, its purpose, and the risks associated with the form of treatment. In these situations, the interpreter should cosign the form and document that the patient fully understood the interpretation. The patient's signature should follow the interpreter's. Having the interpreter sign first will prevent the patient or plaintiff's lawyer from later suggesting that the interpreter signed the document after the procedure.

CHARTING IN GENERAL

Notations made in the medical chart are often perceived as a reflection of the author's attitude or ability. If a physician writes jokes in the chart, he/she will be perceived as cavalier and unprofessional. For example, in one particular obstetric case a resident examining an obese patient in labor documented "fundal height forever." The term "forever" is improper since fundal height is measured by a ruler. After the hospital was sued for malpractice arising out of the delivery of a brain-damaged baby, the notation was no longer perceived as a joke by the defendant physician and, indeed, assisted the plaintiff in establishing a general cavalier attitude on the part of the hospital staff.

The medical record is not the place to resolve arguments or controversies between physicians. The risk management department of every hospital should be consulted if problems arise between physicians since such problems may prevent proper patient care from being rendered. Residents-in-training should consult with their superiors if problems arise.

If a physician or nurse forgets to document something and remembers the following day, he/she should not go back to the prior day's records and attempt to "squeeze in" the information on the chart. The health care provider should simply record the information in the chart the day it is recalled, indicate when the matter occurred, and the reason for its being charted a day late. If the physician were to attempt to squeeze the information in the notes for the prior day, he/she may become suspect. Plaintiff's lawyers sometimes will suggest that the physician wrote the note in at a later time for protection in a future lawsuit.

The preprinted hospital medical record forms have certain boxes and columns where information is to be placed. Some columns are labeled with the heading of "Time." Certain boxes may be labeled "diagnosis," "plan," or "medications," and most forms provide a place for the physician's signature. Inevitably, sometimes the columns and boxes are left blank. Rest assured that at some point if a lawsuit arises and these areas are blank, a lawyer will ask, "Why do you think the hospital has these forms made up?" Documenting the time of the note is essential. The physician who picks up where the prior physician left off will be able to properly determine whether another evaluation is necessary if the preceding note is timed hours earlier. Without the time being reflected in the earlier note, the oncoming physician may mistakenly assume that the last evaluation was recent.

A new focus in malpractice cases is the failure of the physician or nurse to document both positive and negative findings. The nurse or physician normally charts significant positive findings such as symptoms that evidence deterioration. Some importance, however, should be given to certain negative findings because they may evidence improvement or a change in a patient's condition. For example, if a patient presents with one pupil larger than the other, it may suggest some intracranial involvement. If the eyes were later to become symmetrical, it might be construed as a negative finding and not documented. There is obviously some importance in this negative finding since it indicates both a change in symptoms and possibly some improvement. Failing to document the presence of symmetry allows others to speculate that perhaps the patient's pupils remained asymmetrical for a longer period of time.

Prediction and Definition of Outcome in a Cost-Sensitive Era

9

Joseph M. Civetta

COST CONSIDERATIONS

When costs for medical care exceeded 10% of the Gross National Product (GNP) a few years ago, responses varied and included changes in medical care financing,[1] high visibility for costly technology,[2] and the introduction of cost effectiveness as a perspective for viewing medical care.[3] Intensive care deserves special scrutiny because it generates approximately 15% of total hospital costs,[4] and thus represents approximately 1% of the GNP. Recognizing the varying goals for intensive care and the current status of predictive indices, there are three potential methods for achieving control of costs: reevaluating criteria for admission, diminishing charges generated during the intensive care unit (ICU) admission, and attempting to hasten discharge. The "appropriate" patient must be considered one who could not survive without intensive care but who actually does survive given such care. This patient is difficult to define accurately, and patients admitted to most ICUs include those who might otherwise be considered too sick or too well. Patients who are "too well," that is, those who could survive without intensive care, often are given observation and intensive nursing care and consume a small portion of ICU bed days. If terminally ill patients are excluded, patients who are severely ill usually die rapidly and, again, use few bed days. Control can be achieved by evaluating—and diminishing—expenditures while patients are in the ICU. Restriction of unnecessary diagnostic testing preserves patients from harms associated with incorrect test results and interpretations, technical errors from inappropriate procedures, and the confusion resulting from too much data. Limitation of the ICU stay is, actually, most important for patients who ultimately die. We must recognize the distinction between living and dying. When our efforts cannot have a salutary outcome in terms of survival, we must change directions and accept the inevitability of death. This subject is covered in greater detail in Chapter 3. Suffice it to say that the average patient who dies spends twice as long in the ICU as those who live. Earlier recognition will alleviate suffering and stress for patient, family, and ICU staff and will conserve limited resources.

DEFINITION OF OUTCOME

Our generation seems increasingly fascinated by science and technology; in many ways, the spectacular accomplishments of science gain greater attention than artistic endeavors of similar singular brilliance. It is not surprising that the current emphasis in intensive care reflects this societal fascination. Prediction of outcome fits into the broad area of clinical judgment, clearly one of medicine's arts. Faced with the 20th century requirement for precision, clinical judgment has become devalued and is deemed of lesser value. Not surprisingly, intensive care physicians have attempted to analyze the tremendous mass of data pertaining to critically ill patients in order to quantitate illness and predict outcome. It was hoped that these data, when subjected to proper statistical techniques in sufficient quantities, would provide a more precise and accurate tool to replace the uncertainties of clinical judgment alone. The basis of all predictive systems can be viewed in Figure 9-1, relating the patient, the disease, the physician, and the nurse. With respect to the intensive care illness, the patient, having reached a certain age and accumulated certain named diagnoses, has an acute exacerbation of prior illness

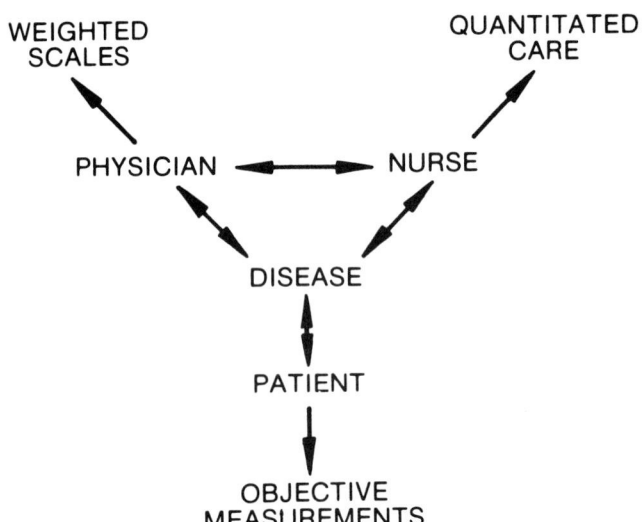

FIGURE 9-1. Prediction of outcome, based on relationship of the patient, the disease, the physician, and the nurse.

or contracts a new disease entity. The physician attempts to list the individual diseases, assess the severity, and select appropriate modalities of treatment. The nurse, reacting to the patient's physiologic condition and the physician's orders, forms an independent assessment, which translates into the bedside quantity of care given. Outcome must reflect more than survival from the disease that prompted ICU admission. An evaluation of a 6-month sample of 375 patients admitted to the surgical ICU (SICU) at the University of Miami/Jackson Memorial Medical Center showed that 22% of these patients died.[5] However, 20% of the patients who eventually died had at one point improved sufficiently to be discharged from the ICU with the expectation that they would survive hospitalization. Others were discharged to nursing homes and chronic care hospitals. Thus, mortality alone does not provide sufficient information to determine whether intensive care was successful, and prediction of success or failure based only on observed mortality will be problematic. Other goals include individual unit performance evaluations, interunit comparisons, and assurance of commensurate severity in patients entered in prospective studies. No index has yet achieved the goals set out by their developers. In the words of the National Institutes of Health (NIH) Consensus Development Conference on Critical Care Medicine,

> The combination of life-threatening diseases, finite resources, invasive therapeutic and monitoring techniques and high costs makes the need for adequate data on which to base decision a high priority. Such research is aimed at determining how ICUs can be used for the maximum benefit of the ICU population. This research should include procedures for "triaging" patients so that admission is not denied to patients who can most benefit from an ICU as well as excluding patients who have no reasonable chance to benefit. Research aimed at developing accurate outcome predictors as a function of initial presenting condition, diagnoses, and other on-going prognostic variables should be encouraged.[4]

This encouragement was offered after the panel had evaluated the various indices to be discussed in this chapter. The problem, simply stated, is that the data available at ICU admission may not be the data needed to determine outcome in the broad sense described above. We are well aware of the random appearance of late catastrophic events that uniquely determine outcome. These may be related to therapeutic interventions or an unpredictable clinical event such as a new myocardial infarction or cerebral vascular accident. These events often account for the deaths that occur after the patient has been discharged from the ICU. Expanding upon the NIH Conference statement, severity of illness is not the only determinant of the suitability of a patient for ICU admission. If this were true, we could safely exclude patients who were "too well" for ICU admission or deny admission to those who had no reasonable chance of survival. Yet, restrictive admission policies would have little effect on the utilization of limited ICU resources and the moral, ethical, and legal problems concerned with determining survivability in an individual patient.

COST AND COST EFFECTIVENESS

The element of resource allocation, though not fundamental to medical care, is now fundamental to reimbursement for that care. We must, therefore, examine some of the problems associated with this approach.

The relation between cost and charge is difficult to unravel for many reasons. Certain areas of the hospital, such as the laundry and utilities, create costs without generating any revenue. These costs may be apportioned in different ways to various charges, such as medications and laboratory tests. Furthermore, over the years, charges have been raised according to formulas applied under the auspices of government or third party payers. For instance, if a charge were "too high," the excess might be apportioned to another charge that was below the limit or ceiling (Fig. 9-2). Accordingly, to trace an individual charge backward to the fundamental costs is often impossible. "Best guess" estimates in our hospital range from a cost of 35% of charges for laboratory determinations to 70% for the daily bed charge. In 1985, the average charge for the total hospitalization of our SICU patients at the University of Miami/Jackson Memorial Medical Center was $31,000,[5] but this represented a 24% decrease from the $41,000 average bill in 1983.[6] For the sake of projecting the effect of a prospective payment system, a 6-month sample (375 patients) was used to calculate payments under the diagnosis related group (DRG) classification system, using the formula applied by the government's fiscal intermediary in Florida. Reimbursement for Medicare patients in 1985 was made according to the formula of basic payment for selected DRG plus 26.77% of the total hospital charges. The sum of these theoretical payments under the individual DRGs would have been $6,856,000 ($9113/patient), and the total reimbursement would have been $13,226,000 ($17,634/patient). If all patients had been reimbursed using

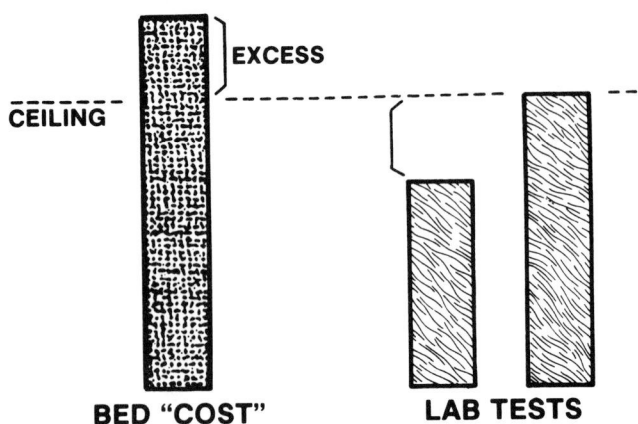

FIGURE 9-2. Apportionment of excess hospital charges from bed "cost" to laboratory tests.

these formulas, our medical center would have suffered a "loss" of $10,540,000 ($14,076/patient).

Whether prospective payments, indeed, will be applied to all admitted patients, resulting in these catastrophic losses, or whether across-the-board restrictive controls[7] or responses to perceived limitations in reimbursement[8] will be forthcoming, it seems sensible to examine the reasons for these costs to understand how we might approach the problem of control from within the medical profession.

From the perspective of the ICU, there are three potential methods for control: redefining criteria for admission, diminishing charges generated while the patient is in the ICU, and attempting to hasten discharge.

The number of patients admitted is not as indicative of resource utilization as are the patients days consumed (the product of the number of patients each day and the number of days considered). The 375 patients recently studied consumed 1664 days of intensive care. Of these 375, 110 patients were admitted for 1 day and ultimately survived. These patients were, for the most part, elderly patients undergoing major elective surgery with a known risk of postoperative complications. Additionally, 14 patients were admitted and died during the first 24 hours. Together, these 124 patients represented 34% of admissions yet used only 5% of the patient days and generated 8% of the total charges. Thus, elimination of these patients by developing restrictive admission policies would not result in a major reduction in charges.

SEVERITY OF ILLNESS

These two groups represent the opposite ends of the severity spectrum: the least severe ("too well") are discharged quickly because little care is needed, and the most severe die rapidly despite maximum therapeutic efforts. We can delineate a more important group as "critical" patients, those whose outcome is in doubt. This "critical" group constitutes the most important focus to understand the drain on resources. Twenty-eight patients (7%) used 583 (35%) of the ICU days and generated 36% of the total charges, yet 12 (44%) still survived. Thus, this "critical" group (*i.e.*, those who use the highest percentage of ICU resources) can never be excluded from ICU admission (Table 9-1).

PREDICTION AND RESOURCE UTILIZATION

Our inability to predict survival or death accurately on admission presents society with an unclear picture concerning the desirability of continuing therapeutic efforts. If we could define accurately that a patient had a 10%, 1%, or 0.1% chance of survival, society could decide if it wished to pay for treatment of 9, 99, or 999 patients with fatal illnesses in order for medical

TABLE 9-1. Spectrum of Severity of Illness

	LEAST					"CRITICAL"						MOST
	Living						Deaths					
	1	2	3–4	5–6	7–13	>13	>13	13–7	6–5	4–3	2	1
ICU STAY (DAYS)												
PATIENTS	110	71	52	27	21	12	16	20	9	10	13	14
ICU DAYS USED	110	142	170	146	184	258	325	182	49	35	26	14
CHARGE/PATIENT ($K)	20	20	28	30	60	113	71	55	36	23	18	23

Both rapid recovery (least severe = little care needed) and rapid death (most severe = little time for/success of intervention) are relatively low in charges. The "critical" patients (outcome in doubt = nearly equal chance of survival/death = midway along severity spectrum) require the most time and generate the highest charges.
ICU stay (days) = length of ICU admission until discharge as hospital survivor for living or in deaths, length of ICU admission for those who died in ICU or before hospital discharge.
Charge/patient ($K) in thousands of dollars.

care to achieve 1 survivor. Given our average charges, this would represent the investment of $300,000, $3,000,000, or $30,000,000 per survivor. One problem is that no current prognostic indicator can give us this level of precision, and a second is that there is no clear directive from society (the people, the government, and the insurance carriers) as to how much should be expended in a single case.

However, Oregon has recently taken a major step in deciding how resources would be spent. Organ transplantation was not funded by the state government so that the same amount could be allocated to a greater number of infants, presumably with a greater societal return.[9] The stance of course creates far more questions about allocations, the total allocated, the valuation of individual lives, and so on. This attitude is the reverse of usual societal practice according to Engelhardt,[10] whereby identifiable individuals are selected for care while failing to come to the aid of unidentified statistical lives that could have been saved with the same or fewer resources. Statistical lives is Schelling's term for unknown persons in possible future peril.[11]

It seems highly unlikely that the "critical patients," those who spend 3 weeks in the ICU before clear-cut separation or resolution is achieved, can ever be separated on the day that admission is requested. The identifiers, whether physiologic abnormalities or therapeutic interventions, are short-range predictors.

COST-CONTAINMENT EFFORTS

Since restrictive admission policies should not be used, and it probably will never be possible to differentiate the survivors from the dying patients on or before ICU admission in the "critical" high-utilization group, we must address our cost-containment efforts toward the other two areas of control: expenditures while patients are in the unit and the decision for discharge. In general, it is well recognized that ICU deaths are often associated with multiple organ system failure (MOSF) and sepsis.[12,13] It is important to note that our true therapeutic efforts, that is, interventions that cure disease, are limited in these patients. Multiple organ system failure is characterized by involvement of the central nervous system (CNS), the liver, immune system or host response, renal function, and coagulation, among others. We do not have effective therapeutic modalities in these states. Our two control measures, then, can be to restrict unnecessary diagnostic testing and the variations in treatment during this phase, recognizing that the desire to influence outcome often creates minute-to-minute manipulations and repetitive laboratory testing in the hopes that these will change outcome. In reality, the converse is true: excessive efforts carry no chance for improvement, thus, leaving only the possibility for errors, iatrodemics, and iatrogenic occurrences.[14,15]

Instead of devoting our energies to manipulations and useless testing, we should focus our attention on assessment and evaluation to determine when the patient has no chance for survival: living has ceased and dying has begun. This is important because it is an equally valid goal for medical care to alleviate suffering—and to avoid prolongation of dying when death is inevitable.

In our 375-patient sample, 82 (22%) patients died after being treated in the ICU for an average of 7.7 days per patient. These patients used 632 ICU days, which represents 38% of the total expended for all 375 patients. We might set a goal, therefore, to bring the percentage of days expended on dying patients into a reasonable proportion to the percentage of dying patients. If this were possible—by this I mean that we could identify more accurately the point at which living ceases and dying has begun—we could hope to equalize the duration of stay for survivors and patients who died. Since the average duration of those who survived was 3.5 days per patient, this would imply a "savings" of 3.2 days per dying patient, or 262 patient days. This would represent a savings of 16% of the total ICU days *without* restricting admissions and *without* changing outcome. The difficulty we now face in separating living from dying patients is the result of an unwanted and, perhaps, unexpected by-product of intensive care: creation of the prolonged dying state, which is unprecedented in human history. Current terms in common use reflect our discomfort in dealing with these concepts. Most often, we speak of termination of life support and discontinuation of life-sustaining treatment when, from another perspective, we could say termination of dying and accepting death, the natural end of human existence.

Clearly, it may be difficult to achieve clear distinction or resolution from the perspectives of the patient, the family, medical profession, and society in all cases, but that should not diminish the strong sense of need to make these decisions as early as possible in the truly "critical" patient.

GOALS FOR INTENSIVE CARE

All ICU patients are not similar in terms of the goals of ICU admission, the dimensions for care used, or the resources necessary. They can be separated by goals into three groups: patients admitted for intensive observation or "monitoring only," patients who are stable physiologically but need extensive nursing care, and patients given essentially full-time medical and nursing care. Intensive observation is a necessary goal for ICU care today because it represents a quantum of care impossible to achieve on a routine nursing unit. As an important corollary, however, we must be certain that observation is the only necessity: excessive ordering just because the patient is in the ICU must be avoided, and routine or "automatic" laboratory testing should be avoided. Approximately 20% of our patients are considered "monitoring only."

In the second group, nursing care in excess of that available on general nursing units is needed. Since the patients are, by definition, physiologically stable, there is little moment-to-moment medical need; the physician's role is primarily anticipatory. Unnecessary manipulations and tests should be avoided because these cannot improve outcome and can only increase costs.

These patients make up the bulk of our ICU population, 60% of total admissions.

The physiologically unstable patients make up 20% of our admissions. Physicians at the bedside generate a proliferation of orders, testing, and manipulations, which seem to be proportional to the perceived degree of the illness. However, even in these patients, utilization can be reviewed, perceptions changed, and use curtailed in many ways without compromising the "quality of care."

We must remember that the plethora of information generated by unrestrained laboratory testing and uncontrolled utilization of nursing time results in the creation of a vast array of data to be digested on a day-to-day basis. Robin termed this "informational overload."[14] It can be a cause of potential harm to the patient as a result of the inability of the physician or nurse to detect important abnormalities and to prioritize an approach because of the overwhelming amount of data to be evaluated. Curtailing unnecessary testing and unnecessary nursing activity will diminish the frenetic yet unproductive activity common to many ICUs. When the hubbub abates, the necessity for clear thinking and assessment on the part of the physician stands out: this is clearly the most important tool to achieve cost-effective use of the ICU.

Testing and technology may also be considered in three steps of increasing utilization. The "observation only" patients must have few, if any, tests ordered: by definition, repetitive testing is not the quantum of care necessary, rather it is the extensive observation not possible outside the ICU. Patients admitted for intensive nursing care often have associated physiologic derangements such as acute respiratory failure and cardiovascular dysfunction. They therefore tend to be fitted into parochial methods of treatment or clinical "protocols." Each unit usually defines the laboratory testing to be used. Routine or automatic ordering usually attempts to establish screening procedures so that fatigue or inexperience will not cause an important test to be overlooked. At other times, extensive testing is considered necessary to avoid risk exposure. Most often, however, it is not the absence of a test result in the chart that results in a malpractice suit. The real issue is the difficulty in clinical decision-making, committing a judgment to the medical record and communicating it to the patient and family.

We must remain committed to treatment of the patient with a poor but possible salutary outcome. Although we recognize that a 1% or 10% chance of survival clearly translates into a preponderance of similar patients who will die, we—both the medical profession and society—wish to achieve success when possible. This desire must recognize that over-utilization of resources, including materials, personnel, and time, does not help attain the successful outcome in the low-probability case.

We used laboratory testing as a model to determine whether modification in existing patterns of care could be accomplished without affecting the quality of care because the frequency of laboratory tests can be quantified;

thus, assessment before and after interventions was feasible.[6] Although increased efficiency was one goal, we hoped that the process would also lead to better teaching methods based on improved decision-making in the care of patients. These investigations could improve cost effectiveness and simultaneously contribute to our specific knowledge and understanding of bedside intensive care. In 1983, laboratory charges were $10,000, and the calculated ICU laboratory charges (calculated from the frequency of 28 identified tests abstracted from the patient's bills) were $6,160. The patients spent 15% of their total hospitalization in the ICU but generated 61% of their total laboratory charges during this period of time. We were astonished to find that we had ordered 134 tests per patient or 23 tests per patient per ICU day. In 1984, after the interventions had been made, laboratory charges were $6,300, and the calculated ICU laboratory charges were $2,894, representing a decrease of $3,226 or 53%. Total number of ICU tests per patient decreased by 56 (42%). Six months later, the frequency was again assessed and had diminished even further to approximately eight tests per patient per ICU day. This latter figure has remained stable for the past 2 years. We have diminished laboratory testing by 67%, or more than 60,000 tests per year, in our 12-bed unit. Total charges have diminished more than $3,000,000 and, using the 35% cost-basis, represents a $1,000,000 savings to the hospital. It is important to note that the mortality, distribution of patients by Therapeutic Intervention Scoring System (TISS) class, and average TISS score have remained the same throughout the period of study (Table 9-2). We consider that the testing eliminated was unnecessary.

We can now examine ways to control testing that were implemented and the effect on specific laboratory tests.

PRINCIPLES OF MANAGEMENT

Much of our behavior is automatic and is not based on scientific data. Therefore, as a management principle, we believed that change was permissible whenever the existing policy was based only on tradition or parochialism. For instance, a program for the calculation of various parameters of renal function had been incorporated into our ICU programmable calculator. Unnecessary widespread usage in normal patients was identified and mentioned daily. There was a significant decrease in the number of ordered urinary creatinines, osmolarities, and electrolytes as a result of the "spotlight" approach—identifying the patient and discussing indications and need.

We suspected in contrast to others[2] that a lot of "little ticket" items would make a significant impact; therefore, we resolved to examine each detail of care to uncover areas for potential small savings. Our Pathology Department had acquired an automated cell counter (ACC) that they used to perform what had traditionally been called a complete blood count (CBC). We had not been aware that the terminology had changed so that CBC included a differential (DIFF) white blood count (WBC) with an extra $10 charge. Accordingly, we emphasized the substitution of ACC for CBC in

TABLE 9-2. Description of Population

	BEFORE	AFTER
CLASS IV		
No. of Patients	10	12
TISS (24°)	39	40
Deaths	2	4
CLASS III		
No. of Patients	32	30
TISS (24°)	27	25
Deaths	3	4
CLASS II		
No. of Patients	8	8
TISS (24°)	12	15
Deaths	0	0
TOTAL		
No. of Patients	50	50
TISS (24°)	28	27
Deaths	5	8

Number in each class and TISS were compared by T-tests for two means. Mortality between groups was compared by chi-square test. There were no differences. Before = 1983, and after = 1984 samples. TISS scores were calculated 24 hr after admission.

routine circumstances. The augmented numbers of ACCs and diminished CBCs translate into diminished charges of approximately $25,000 per year.

Finally, we promulgated the phrase that "thinking, not screening, detects rare abnormalities." Calculation of the amylase:creatinine clearance ratio had been proposed to help detect subtle cases of pancreatitis. However, the indications for this screening technique were gradually broadened in our unit to include many stable, postoperative patients, which increased the number of tests without finding unsuspected cases of pancreatitis. Once recognized, this practice was spotlighted and the screening eliminated. The effects of these principles are shown in Table 9-3.

DELETION OF STANDING ORDERS FOR TESTING

Routine use of "standing orders" was designed to eliminate a number of problems. An inexperienced person, responsible for writing orders, might overlook an important test. A busy practitioner, performing the same procedure frequently, might save a great deal of time by having preprinted orders to cover the usual postoperative situations. Preprinted orders would also increase the likelihood that they could be deciphered. On the other hand, imprecise thinking in the past might become codified as "tradition," and laboratory testing might proliferate. Arterial blood gases (ABGs) are the most frequently ordered test in intensive care.[12] Our unit was no exception, resulting in the frequency of 9.3 blood gases per patient per day, or 45 during

TABLE 9-3. Tests Related to Management Principles

	BEFORE	AFTER	CHARGE ($)	SAVINGS ($)
CHANGE WHEN NO SCIENTIFIC SUPPORTING DATA				
Creat (U)	4.7	0.7	22	88.00
Osm (U)	2.2	0.9	18	23.40
Elec (U)	3.0	1.2	44	79.20
EACH DETAIL OF CARE EXAMINED				
ACC	5.2	7.5	23	−52.90
CBC with diff	5.5	2.3	33	105.60
THINKING, NOT SCREENING, DETECTS ABNORMALITIES				
Amylase (S)	3.7	1.2	27	67.50
Amylase (U)	2.5	0.1	27	65.80
K	7.0	2.6	21	92.40

Mean number of tests/ICU admission/patient in 1983 (before) and 1984 (after). Groups compared using t-test for two means. All values were significant.
Savings in dollar charges to patient.
Creat = creatinine; osm = osmolarity; elec = electrolytes; U = urinary; S = serum; ACC = automated cell count; CBC = complete blood count with differential.

the average ICU stay.[6] This frequency reflected our standing order to obtain a blood gas for every change in the patient's condition and after each change in ventilatory support. In practice, blood gases were also obtained at the end of each nursing shift and before morning and evening medical report. All could be justified under our standing orders. Blood gases were then ordered individually with an initial decrease of 19 blood gases per patient. Encouraged by these early results, we continued to stress test-by-test evaluation; the present frequency is approximately three blood gases per patient per day. We hope that continuous arterial and mixed venous oximetry will permit further containment of "routine" sampling.

STRUCTURED DECISION TREES TO SELECT TESTS

One intention of standing laboratory orders was to decrease the likelihood that a fatigued or inexperienced staff member might overlook a clinically relevant test. Since our gross overutilization seemed to be an unanticipated result, standing orders for testing were deleted. We substituted structured decision trees to help select appropriate tests in commonly encountered situations such as the "fever work-up" and nutritional support monitoring. These decision trees were also created to aid in the initial selection of laboratory testing depending on the source of admission: elective preoperative admissions for invasive hemodynamic monitoring, routine postoperative admissions, and emergency admissions. For instance, elective preoperative admissions usually have all the necessary testing completed before admission to the ICU. No useful purpose had been served by the routine repetition of these tests just because the patient's *location* in the hospital had changed (*i.e.,* routine nursing care area to ICU) rather than his or her physiologic status.

Routine postoperative patients were slightly more complex. These patients often remained intubated, had new catheters inserted into the central circulation, may have had hypotension or dysrhythmias during the operation, received many blood transfusions, or had had oliguria. "Blanket" testing had been applied in our unit to nearly all postoperative patients since at least one or more of these conditions usually applied. In Table 9-4, however, these conditions are separated with our "suggestions" for appropriate ordering. This separation into specific clinical indications results in a decreased overall frequency of individual tests because they were no longer grouped (Table 9-5).

With respect to emergency admission, the decision tree included an admonition to check for prior laboratory orders since most, if not all, available tests are often ordered during the initial assessment of the multiple injury or severely ill patient in the emergency room. Repetition of the same tests is not necessary after ICU admission (usually only an hour later) but was a common practice.

NO ORDERS FOR REPEATED TESTING

When efforts are designed to avoid omissions, initial orders are often repeated at specified time intervals. Even if necessary initially, it is unlikely that all such repetitions are necessary; in this case, we "encouraged" a new order to be entered after reassessment and review of available information. Combinations provided by the laboratory, such as our Profile 8, fell into this class, as did repetitive testing of coagulation parameters in many patients who had no evidence of a coagulation disorder (Table 9-6).

We believe that control of laboratory testing serves as a convenient model to examine bedside practice. We discovered many habits and traditions that even a moment's thought eliminated. Perhaps the very intensity of our prior activity precluded any chance or need for close scrutiny. Our experience led to the hope that the diminished activity could have salutary effects. Physicians and nurses can return to decision-making and thinking instead of frenetically ordering, reacting, and intervening—Robin's informational overload.[14] Examination of laboratory testing may have application in other ICUs, although potential overutilization may take expression in different forms. Necessary, even if costly, elements can be preserved so that quality is maintained. Our task is to recognize overutilization resulting in overload so that efficiency can be improved while charges are diminished.

With the relationships between overall concepts of outcome, goals of ICUs and cost-control measures as a basis, we can examine the quantitative methods to assess severity and predict survival.

TABLE 9-4. *Schematic for Selecting Laboratory Tests*

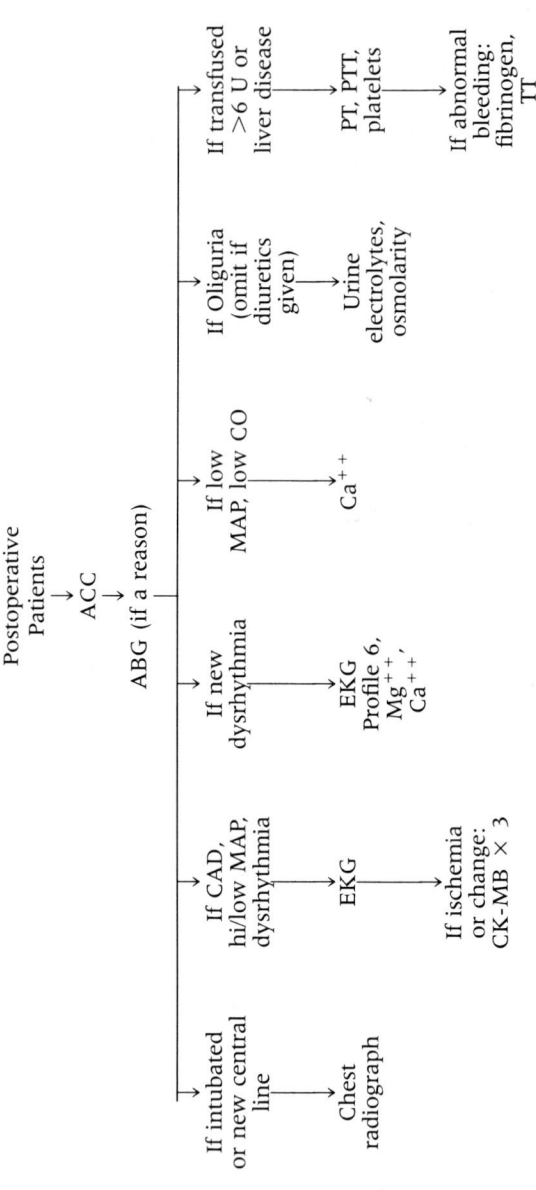

ACC = automated cell count (Hct, Hb, WBC); CAD = coronary artery disease; MAP = mean arterial pressure; ABG = arterial blood gas; TT = thrombin time; CO = cardiac output; PTT = partial thromboplastin time; PT = prothrombin time.

TABLE 9-5. Structured Decision Trees to Select Test

	BEFORE	AFTER	CHARGE ($)	SAVINGS ($)
CARDIAC ENZYMES	2.3	1.2	30	33.00
CK-MB	2.2	1.4	30	24.00
LIVER ENZYMES	2.2	1.5	48	33.60
CA^{++}	3.5	2.8	24	16.80
MG^{++}	3.3	1.3	23	46.00

Average number of tests/patient during ICU admission in 1983 (before) and 1984 (after). Groups compared using t-test for two means. All values were significant.

TABLE 9-6. No Orders for Repeated Testing

	BEFORE	AFTER	CHARGE ($)	SAVINGS ($)
PROFILE 8	2.8	1.1	45	76.50
PT/PTT	5.4	2.4	54	162.00
PLATELETS	5.5	1.7	23	87.40
FIBRINOGEN	1.0	0.4	28	16.80
OSMOLARITY	2.9	0.4	20	50.00

Average number of tests/patient during ICU admission in 1983 (before) and 1984 (after). Group comparisons performed using t-test for two means. All values were significant. PT = prothrombin time; PTT = partial thromboplastin time.

CLASSIFICATION OF QUANTITATIVE INDICES

Predictive indices can be classified as based on patient–disease interactions, perceptions of physicians, and requirements for nursing care. Each may be examined from the standpoint of basis, development, advantages, and disadvantages.

PATIENT–DISEASE INTERACTIONS

The first type concerns the interrelationship of patient and disease. Shoemaker and coworkers have concentrated on cardiorespiratory patterns and oxygen transport variables.[16] Rather than focusing therapy on normalizing values, their perspective reflected Claude Bernard's observation that the bodily responses to injury and illness are compensatory and have survival value. They believed that the values of patients who survived life-threatening cardiorespiratory problems were more appropriate to be applied to the critically ill patient and devoted their efforts to an analysis of the cardiorespiratory patterns of patients who survived and died. For classification purposes a region of survivability, a region of lethality, and a region of overlap (including

TABLE 9-7. *Cardiorespiratory Variables: Units, Calculations, Normal Values, Preferred Values*

VARIABLES	UNITS	MEASUREMENTS OR CALCULATIONS	NORMAL VALUES	PREFERRED VALUES
Volume-related				
Mean arterial pressure (MAP)	mm Hg	Direct measurement	82–102	>84
Central venous pressure (CVP)	cm H$_2$O	Direct measurement	1–9	<5
Central blood volume (CBV)	ml/m^2	CBV = MTT × CI × 16.7	660–1000	>925
Stroke index (SI)	ml/m^2	SI = CI/HR	30–50	>48
Hemoglobin	g/dl	Direct measurement	12–16	>12
Mean pulmonary artery pressure (MPAP)	mm Hg	Direct measurement	11–15	<19
Occlusion pressure (OP)	mm Hg	Direct measurement	0–12	>9.5
Blood volume (BV)	ml/m^2	BV = PV(1 − Hct) × surface area	Men 2.74 Women 2.37	>3.0 >2.7
Red cell mass (RCM)	ml/m^2	RCM = BV − PV	Men 1.1 Women 0.95	>1.1 >0.95
Flow-related				
Cardiac index (CI)	liters/min/m^2	Direct measurement	2.8–3.6	>4.5
Left vent stroke work (LVSW)	g m/m^2	LVSW = SI × MAP × 0.0144	44–68	>55
Left cardiac work (LCW)	kg m/m^2	LCW = CI × MAP × 0.0144	3–4.6	>5
Right vent stroke work (RVSW)	g m/m^2	RVSW = SI × MPAP × 0.0144	4–8	>13
Right cardiac work (RCW)	kg m/m^2	RCW = CI × MPAP × 0.0144	0.4–0.6	>1.1
Stress-related				
Systemic vasc resist (SVR)	dyne sec/cm^{5}m^2	SVR = 79.92(MAP − CVP)/CI	1760–2600	<1450
Pulmonary vasc resist (PVR)	dyne sec/cm^{5}m^2	PVR = 79.92(MPAP − OP)/CI	45–225	<226
Heart rate (HR)	beats/min	Direct measurement	72–88	<100
Rectal temperature	°F	Direct measurement	97.8–98.6	<100.4

Oxygen-related				
Hemoglobin saturation	%	Direct measurement	95–99	>95
Arterial co_2 tension	mm Hg	Direct measurement	36–44	>30
Arterial pH	pH	Direct measurement	7.36–7.44	>7.47
Mixed venous o_2 tension	mm Hg	Direct measurement	33–53	>36
Arterial–mixed venous o_2 content difference	ml/dl	$Ca_{O_2} - C\bar{v}_{O_2}$	4–5.5	<3.5
O_2 delivery	ml/min m²	$\dot{D}_{O_2} = Ca_{O_2} \times CI \times 10$	520–720	>550
O_2 consumption	ml/min m²	$\dot{V}_{O_2} = C(a-\bar{v})O_2 \times CI \times 10$	100–180	>167
O_2 extraction rate		$O_2\text{ext} = (Ca_{O_2} - C\bar{v}_{O_2}/Ca_{O_2})$	22–30	<31
Perfusion-related				
Red cell flow rate		RCFR = CI × Hct	0.6–1.8	>1.3
Blood flow/volume ratio		BFVR = CI/BV	0.6–1.8	>1.7
O_2 transport/red cell mass		OTRM = $\dot{V}_{O_2}$/RCM	0.06–0.18	>0.25
Tissue O_2 extraction		TOE = C(a−$\bar{v}$)O_2/RCFR	0.8–6.6	>5.7
Efficiency of tissue O_2 extraction		ETOE = C(a − $\bar{v}$)O_2/RCM	0.06–0.18	>1.3
O_2 tranport/red cell flow		OTRF = $\dot{V}_{O_2}$/RCFR	1–7	<3

(Adapted from Shoemaker WC, et al: *Am J Surg* 1983; 146:43) values of both survivors and nonsurvivors) were defined for each variable. Results of several variables were combined to develop predictors thought to have possible relevance to therapy. Approximately 13.5% of the variables gave a correct prediction, whereas 86.5% fell into the large region of overlap and were thus indeterminant. By analyzing the number of right and wrong predictions and combining the results for all variables, Shoemaker and colleagues achieved an average correct prediction of 85%. The clinical evaluation produced a correct percentage of 67%. Later, they reported a prospective test of the accuracy of this predictive index as well as an evaluation of the efficacy of using median values of survivors as therapeutic goals.[17] The system was based on 12 directly measured cardiopulmonary variables as well as on 20 derived calculations (Table 9-7). Within the overlap or indeterminant region, they defined a classification point that would represent the best separation of data into survivors and nonsurvivors. The predictive score for each variable was determined by comparing the observed value for each variable with the 10th and 90th percentile shoulders of the curve of distribution and the classification point. The predictive score of each variable was combined into a single overall predictive index. The predictive indices were 93% correct when calculated from the last available data set. Of the patients who died, 85% were correctly predicted. Patients were then managed by a protocol based on the goal of attaining survivors' values. The mortality rate in this group was less than that in the group considered as a control. Commonly monitored variables, including heart rate (HR), central venous pressure (CVP), systemic vascular resistance (SVR), hematocrit (Hct) value, and mean arterial pressure (MAP), were among the least relevant to predict outcome. They did not delineate the therapeutic approach in either control or protocol patients, however. They then developed an automated method for the evaluation of the cardiorespiratory data that distilled a large number of complex variables (Table 9-8) into a simple index reflecting overall severity.[18] Patients were monitored during the intraoperative and immediate postoperative periods. Again, a high percentage of patients (96%) were correctly predicted from the last available cardiorespiratory record. It is not clear whether values obtained on ICU admission had similar accuracy.

One advantage of this method is that the data are readily available, given a decision to use invasive monitoring and laboratory testing. Automation and on-line statistical analysis for providing clinicians with target values seem reasonable and desirable. The disadvantages, however, recognized by the authors, reflect the fact that cardiorespiratory causes are not the only determinants of outcome. Also the system would be expensive to initiate. The ability to predict survivors after elective surgery should be quite high since mortality rates for most elective surgery are quite low. An error rate of 15% in patients who ultimately were predicted to die is excessive in terms of serving as a basis for decisions for continuing or discontinuing therapy.

Phillips and coworkers tried to establish whether outcome could be predicted at an early stage so as to determine why patients died in order to concentrate diagnostic and management resources in those areas, and to establish criteria for withdrawal of therapy in patients who did not meet established criteria for brain death.[19] In contrast to the optimistic outlook expressed by Shoemaker's group, they did not find any absolute predictors of outcome. Low-prevalence, high-impact factors were identified such as renal failure and coma, but they did not identify variables that would support the exclusion of certain patients before ICU admission. With respect to discontinuing life support in the absence of brain death, they ultimately outlined a process based on comprehension of the nature of the illness, an adequate time interval for care, and a hopeless prognosis accepted by all nurses, physicians, and the patient's relatives, rather than a predictive model.

Another approach to the patient–disease interaction has been based on diagnosis or identification of "complications" or "conditions" in patients admitted to ICUs. One such approach was called the Complications Impact Index[20] and another termed the Condition Index Score.[21] The Complications Impact Index was based on a list accumulated from analysis of observable diagnoses and complications classified by organ system. The name reflected the hope that the initial impact of all diagnoses and complications would be the unique determinant of outcome. There was no weighting or discrimination between the various complications in an individual organ system in the statistical analysis. Rather, each of eight systems was considered in addition to the patient's age in a multivariant analysis. A severity weight for each organ system was derived from a multiple linear regression technique. These observed weights were used in a simple equation containing a constant, the severity weights for each system, and the number of complications actually observed. Correct predictions were noted to be 85%. Again, a high percentage of patients who survived could be predicted to survive.

Snyder and coworkers assigned a weight to each of 225 complications so that a Condition Index Score or Prognosis Index could be objectively calculated.[21] Cardiovascular and respiratory conditions are listed in Table 9-9. They used a linear probability equation to define the conditional probability of death after some amount of time in an ICU. The technique had a reliability ($r^2 = 0.72$) that was higher than other efforts, but the authors considered that there was still much room for improvement.

The advantage of these approaches was that they were based on observed conditions in the ICU at admission. Disadvantages included the difficulty in delineating definitions because of overlap and misclassification. Finally, trained nurse researchers were required to abstract the charts in both the Complications Impact Index and Condition Index Score methods.

More recently, Lemeshow and his colleagues described another method for predicting survival and mortality of ICU patients using a multiple logistic regression (MLR) model.[22] They collected a few and easily obtained variables (Table 9-10) and analyzed them by a statistical technique known as maximum likelihood. The result was expressed as a probability rather than a score. Using 0.5 as a cutoff for predicting mortality, 87% and 85% of the patients were correctly classified at admission and at 24 hours, respectively.

TABLE 9-8. Empirically Derived Ranges of Highest Survival

VARIABLE	NORMAL	POSTOPERATIVE 0–2 hr	POSTOPERATIVE 96 hr
Vital signs			
MAP (mm Hg)	82–102	80–100	85–100
Temperature (°C)	36.5–37.2	36–37	37–38
Heart rate (beat/min)	70–88	62–99	64–80
Respiratory rate (breath/min)	10–15	10–18	10–15
Hematocrit (%)	35–45	30–38	33–40
Systemic hemodynamics*			
Cardiac index (liters/min m^2)	2.8–3.5	2.6–7	3.5
CVP (mm Hg)	1–9	2–12	1–8
LVSWI (g m/m^2)	44–68	32	44
LCWI (kg m/m^2)	3–4.6	4.8	4.2
SVRI (dyne sec/cm^5 m^2)	1760–2600	2000–3000	1500–2500
Pulmonary hemodynamics*			
MPAP (mm Hg)	11–15	11–23	10–20
Occlusion pressure (mm Hg)	0–12	9–15	4–6
PVRI (dyne sec/cm^5 m^2)	45–225	60–215	40–150
Blood gas and oxygen metabolism*			
pH	7.36–7.44	7.35	7.4–7.5
Pa$_{CO_2}$ (mm Hg)	36–44	32–40	36–42
Arterial O$_2$ saturation (%)	96–99	84–99	95–99
Mixed venous O$_2$ tension (mm Hg)	35–50	34–45	34–40
C(a−v̄)O$_2$(ml/dl)^2	4–5.5	2.1–4.2	3.5–5
O$_2$ delivery (ml/min m^2)	520–720	500–1160	500
O$_2$ consumption (ml/min m^2)	110–160	120	140
O$_2$ extraction (%)	22–30	12–30	20–30
Pulmonary shunt (%)	1–6	6	

(Adapted from Bland R, et al: *Crit Care Med* 1985; 13:91)
*LVSWI = left ventricular stroke work index; SVRI = systemic vascular resistance index; MPAP = mean pulmonary artery pressure; PVRI = pulmonary vascular resistance index; C(a−v̄)O$_2$ = arteriovenous O$_2$ difference; LCWI = left cardiac work index.

In a later study using a prospective series, similar results were reported.[23] The authors believe that this technique is superior because it is based on statistically derived weights for its variables rather than subjectively determined values common to APACHE and TISS (see below). The data are easy to gather, and the variables are few in number, which would make it easier to use as a general predictive index, but the variables include high-impact but low-prevalence conditions such as cardiopulmonary resuscitation (CPR) before admission and coma. Again, similar to all other systems, the very well

TABLE 9-9. Selected Cardiovascular and Respiratory Conditions from Condition Index Score

	INCIDENCE (455 PATIENTS)
CARDIOVASCULAR	
(1) Dysrhythmias—major (VT, VF, PAT > 180 with ↓ BP or ↓ CO)	29
(2) CAD, fully compensated (by hx, or previous MI, CHF, digitalis)	136
(3) CHF (clinical signs of admission; PAOP 12–20; rales, radiograph)	53
(4) Cardiac surgery, patients with MI or critical emergency	5
(5) Cardiac arrest (primary respiratory, resuscitation < 5 min)	2
(6) Cardiac arrest (primary respiratory, resuscitation > 5 min)	5
(7) Cardiac arrest (primary cardiac)	34
(8) Low output status, judged severe—BP < 80 or < 2/3 of usual	94
(9) Pressor or antihypertensive infusion started on ICU day 0–4	113
(10) Intra-aortic balloon pump (required, not prophylactic)	4
(11) Hypertension—diastolic 110, by hx or requiring therapy	106
RESPIRATORY	
(1) Mechanical problems—flail chest, hypercapnia, (P_{CO_2} > 50 or > 10 above normal level), obstructed airway, dysphagia, aspiration risk	55
(2) Pulmonary resection, fibrosis or other restrictive disease, or mild obstructive disease	45
(3) Atelectasis—radiograph, segmental or lobar	20
(4) Pneumonia (fever, radiograph, positive culture, ↑ WBC; 3 of 4 signs needed)	40
(5) Prophylactic PEEP: PEEP applied when not required by blood gas criteria	44
(6) Prophylactic vent: mechanical ventilation not for pulmonary parenchymal failure	118
(7) Respiratory failure requiring mechanical ventilation; PEEP not used	100
(8) Respiratory failure requiring mechanical ventilation; PEEP used	113

(Adapted from Snyder JV, et al: *Crit Care Med* 1981; 9:598)
VT = ventricular tachycardia; VF = ventricular fibrillation; PAT = paroxysmal atrial tachycardia; BP = blood pressure; CO = cardiac output; hx = history; MI = myocardial infarction; CHF = congestive heart failure; WBC = white blood cells; PEEP = positive end-expiratory pressure; PAOP = pulmonary artery occlusion pressure; CAD = coronary artery disease.

TABLE 9-10. Demographic and Discrete Variables at Time of ICU Admission

VARIABLE	VITAL STATUS AT HOSPITAL DISCHARGE	NUMBER	%	MEAN	(SD)	p VALUE*
Age	Alive	592	(79.8)	56.9	(19.10)	<0.001
	Dead	150	(20.2)	68.6	(16.28)	
SYSTOLIC BLOOD PRESSURE	Alive	593	(79.9)	139.2	(29.83)	<0.001†
	Dead	149	(20.1)	118.1	(38.13)	
HEART RATE	Alive	574	(80.6)	95.7	(24.15)	<0.001†
	Dead	138	(19.4)	106.2	(30.50)	
NUMBER OF ORGAN FAILURES	Alive	593	(79.8)	1.4	(0.71)	<0.001†
	Dead	150	(20.2)	2.3	(1.19)	

VARIABLE CODING	ALIVE		DEAD		p VALUE‡
	Number	(%)	Number	(%)	
Service at admission (medical/surgical)	207	(69.7)	90	(30.3)	<0.001
	386	(86.5)	60	(13.5)	
Infection at admission (no/probable)	400	(88.1)	54	(11.9)	<0.001
	193	(66.8)	96	(33.2)	
CPR before admission	580	(83.0)	119	(17.0)	<0.001
	13	(29.5)	31	(70.5)	
Type of admission (elective/emergency)	215	(95.1)	11	(4.9)	<0.001
	378	(73.1)	139	(26.9)	
P_{O_2} (mm Hg) (>60/≤60)	555	(81.3)	128	(18.7)	0.002
	38	(63.3)	22	(36.7)	
Bicarbonate (meq/liter) (≥18/<18)	569	(80.7)	136	(19.3)	0.13
	24	(63.2)	14	(36.8)	
Creatinine (mg/dl) (≤2.0/>2.0)	573	(80.8)	136	(19.2)	0.004
	20	(58.8)	14	(41.2)	
Level of consciousness (coma or deep stupor/not)	584	(84.6)	106	(15.4)	<0.001
	9	(18.4)	40	(81.6)	

(Lemeshow S, Teres D, Pastides H, et al: A method for predicting survival and mortality of ICU patients using objectively derived weights. Crit Care Med 1985; 13:519)
* Based on Student's t-test.
† Because homogeneity of variances was significant at the α < 0.01 level, a separate variance estimate was used.
‡ Derived using chi-square tests for dichotomous variables.

TABLE 9-11. Therapeutic Intervention Scoring System

4 POINTS
(a) Cardiac arrest or countershock within 48 hr
(b) Controlled ventilation with or without PEEP
(c) Controlled ventilation with intermittent or continuous muscle relaxants
(d) Balloon tamponade of varices
(e) Continuous arterial infusion
(f) Pulmonary artery line
(g) Atrial or ventricular pacing
(h) Hemodialysis in unstable patient
(i) Peritoneal dialysis
(j) Induced hypothermia
(k) Pressure-activated blood infusion
(l) G-suit
(m) Measurement of cardiac output
(n) Platelet transfusions
(o) IABA (intra-aortic balloon assist)
(p) Membrane oxygenation

3 POINTS
(a) Hyperalimentation or renal failure fluid
(b) Pacemaker on standby
(c) Chest tubes
(d) Assisted respiration
(e) Spontaneous PEEP
(f) Concentrated K drip (> 60 meq/liter)
(g) Nasotracheal or orotracheal intubation
(h) Endotracheal suctioning (nonintubated patient)
(i) Complex metabolic balance (frequent intake and output, Brookline scale)
(j) Multiple ABG, bleeding, and stat studies
(k) Frequent infusions of blood products
(l) Bolus IV medications
(m) Multiple (>3) parenteral lines
(n) Vasoactive drug infusion
(o) Continued antidysrhythmia infusions
(p) Cardioversion
(q) Hypothermia blanket
(r) Peripheral arterial line
(s) Acute digitalization
(t) Active diuresis for fluid overload or cerebral edema
(u) Active Rx for metabolic alkalosis or acidosis

2 POINTS
(a) CVP
(b) ≥2 IV lines
(c) Hemodialysis for chronic renal failure
(d) Fresh tracheostomy (less than 48 hr)
(e) Spontaneous respiration by endotracheal tube or tracheostomy
(f) Tracheostomy care

1 POINT
(a) EKG monitoring
(b) Hourly or neuro vital signs
(c) "Keep open" IV route
(d) Chronic anticoagulation

(Continued)

TABLE 9-11. Therapeutic Intervention Scoring System (Continued)

- (e) Standard intake and output
- (f) Frequent stat chemistries
- (g) Intermittent IV medications
- (h) Multiple dressing changes
- (i) Complicated orthopedic traction
- (j) IV antimetabolite therapy
- (k) Decubitus treatment
- (l) Urinary catheter
- (m) Supplemental oxygen (nasal or mask)
- (n) IV antibiotics

(Cullen DJ, Civetta JM, Briggs BA, et al: Therapeutic intervention scoring system: A method for quantitative comparison of patient care. *Crit Care Med* 1974; 2:57)

and the very sick are easily distinguished; also, approximately 15% of the patients are misclassified.

Acute Physiology and Chronic Health Evaluation (APACHE) will be discussed under systems based on perceptions.

INDICES BASED ON PHYSICIAN PERCEPTIONS

In 1973, Civetta described the three groups of intensive care patients used at the beginning of this chapter by subjectively estimating the amount of care.[24] Later, Cullen and associates presented TISS as a method for quantitating categories of ICU patients.[25] This was an outgrowth of the anecdotal "tube sign" in use among the surgical resident staff at the Massachusetts General Hospital in the 1960s: the higher the number of "tubes" used, the less likely was survival. The basic premise of TISS was that the more seriously ill patient required more therapeutic interventions independent of a specific diagnosis, and the severity of illness could be quantitated by the interventions used. The interventions were weighted from 1 to 4 points (Table 9-11). However, this presumed that physicians seeing a similarly ill patient would prescribe the same therapy which, empirically, is not the case. However, TISS separated the four classes of patients, with class I representing a patient receiving routine postanesthesia care. Classes II, III, and IV represented observation only, extensive nursing care, and intensive physician care groups, respectively. In subsequent years, TISS has been used most frequently to describe the class IV patients for purposes of analysis of expenditures, outcome, and results of intensive care (Table 9-12).[26] In fact, there have been few reports using the entire perspective of the four distinct classes of patients, presumably because the quantitation added nothing to the subjective classification. That the patients in whom extensive interventions were used should be studied is entirely appropriate, and, indeed, the use of the term "class IV patients" conjures up a similar picture in the minds of most intensivists today.[27] Nearly 10 years later, the TISS system was updated due to changing perspectives regarding therapeutic interventions (Table 9-13).[28] The updated

(Text continues on p. 162.)

TABLE 9-12. *TISS Class IV Patients Divided into Eight Categories of Disease Processes*

	TISS POINTS	1-YEAR SURVIVAL (%)	COST OF HOSPITALIZATION ($)	COST TO ACHIEVE ONE SURVIVOR ($)
ELECTIVE OPERATION FOR MALIGNANCY	45	6	13,619	232,523
MASSIVE TRAUMA	50	53	12,420	23,287
NEUROSURGERY AND HEAD TRAUMA	35	24	9,820	46,507
EMERGENCY MAJOR VASCULAR SURGERY	47	17	15,191	88,107
ELECTIVE MAJOR VASCULAR SURGERY	45	64	15,564	24,210
UNEXPECTED COMPLICATION OF ELECTIVE SURGERY	43	46	12,811	27,951
GASTROINTESTINAL BLEEDING, CIRRHOSIS, AND PORTAL HYPERTENSION	44	10	16,523	170,738
EMERGENCY ABDOMINAL CATASTROPHIES, NONBLEEDING	45	27	16,074	59,568
SURVIVORS	43	—	15,077	
NONSURVIVORS	44	—	14,012	
TOTAL	44	27	14,304	52,140

(Adapted from Cullen DJ: *Anesthesiology* 1977; 47:203)

TABLE 9-13.   Therapeutic Intervention Scoring System—1983

4 POINTS
(a)   Cardiac arrest or countershock within past 48 hr*
(b)   Controlled ventilation with or without PEEP*
(c)   Controlled ventilation with intermittent or continuous muscle relaxants*
(d)   Balloon tamponade of varices*
(e)   Continuous arterial infusion*
(f)   Pulmonary artery catheter
(g)   Atrial or ventricular pacing*
(h)   Hemodialysis in unstable patient*
(i)   Peritoneal dialysis
(j)   Induced hypothermia*
(k)   Pressure-activated blood infusion*
(l)   G-suit
(m)   Intracranial pressure monitoring
(n)   Platelet transfusion
(o)   IABA (intra-aortic balloon assist)
(p)   Emergency operative procedures (within past 24 hr)*
(q)   Lavage of acute gastrointestinal bleeding
(r)   Emergency endoscopy or bronchoscopy
(s)   Vasoactive drug infusion ($>$ 1 drug)

3 POINTS
(a)   Central IV hyperalimentation (includes renal, cardiac, hepatic failure fluid)
(b)   Pacemaker on standby
(c)   Chest tubes
(d)   Intermittent mandatory ventilation (IMV)* or
(e)   Continuous positive airway pressure (CPAP)
(f)   Concentrated K^+ infusion by central catheter
(g)   Nasotracheal or orotracheal intubation*
(h)   Blind intratracheal suctioning
(i)   Complex metabolic balance (frequent intake and output)*
(j)   Multiple ABG, bleeding or stat studies ($>$ 4/shift)
(k)   Frequent infusions of blood products ($>$ 5 U/24 hr)
(l)   Bolus IV medication (nonscheduled)
(m)   Vasoactive drug infusion (1 drug)
(n)   Continuous antidysrhythmia infusions
(o)   Cardioversion for dysrhythmia (not defibrillation)
(p)   Hypothermia blanket
(q)   Arterial line
(r)   Acute digitalization—within 48 hr
(s)   Measurement of cardiac output by any method
(t)   Active diuresis for fluid overload or cerebral edema
(u)   Active Rx for metabolic alkalosis
(v)   Active Rx for metabolic acidosis
(w)   Emergency thora-, para-, and pericardiocenteses
(x)   Active anticoagulation (initial 48 hr)*
(y)   Phlebotomy for volume overload
(z)   Coverage with more than 2 IV antibiotics
(aa) Rx of seizures or metabolic encephalopathy (within 48 hr of onset)
(bb) Complicated orthopedic traction*

2 POINTS
(a)   CVP
(b)   2 peripheral IV catheters
(c)   Hemodialysis—stable patient
(d)   Fresh tracheostomy (less than 48 hr)

TABLE 9-13. Therapeutic Intervention Scoring System—1983 (Continued)

(e) Spontaneous respiration by endotracheal tube or tracheostomy (T piece or trach mask)
(f) Gastrointestinal feedings
(g) Replacement of excess fluid loss*
(h) Parenteral chemotherapy
(i) Hourly neuro.vital signs
(j) Multiple dressing changes
(k) Pitressin infusion IV

1 POINT
(a) EKG monitoring
(b) Hourly vital signs
(c) 1 peripheral IV catheter
(d) Chronic anticoagulation
(e) Standard intake and output (q 24 hr)
(f) Stat blood tests
(g) Intermittent scheduled IV medications
(h) Routine dressing changes
(i) Standard orthopedic traction
(j) Tracheostomy care
(k) Decubitus ulcer*
(l) Urinary catheter
(m) Supplemental oxygen (nasal or mask)
(n) Antibiotics IV (2 or less)
(o) Chest physiotherapy
(p) Extensive irrigations, packings, or debridement of wound, fistula, or colostomy
(q) Gastrointestinal decompression
(r) Peripheral hyperalimentation/intralipid therapy

(Keene AR, Cullen DJ: Therapeutic Intervention Scoring System: Update 1983. *Crit Care Med* 1983; 11:1)

* Therapeutic Intervention Scoring System explanation code:

4-Point Interventions: (a) Point score for 2 days after most recent cardiac arrest. (b) This does not mean intermittent mandatory ventilation which is a 3-point intervention. It does mean that regardless of the internal plumbing of the ventilator, the patient's full ventilatory needs are being supplied by the machine. Whether or not the patient is ineffectively breathing around the ventilator is irrelevant as long as the ventilator is providing all the patient's needed minute ventilation. (c) For example, D-tuborcurarine chloride, pancuronium (Pavulon), metocurine (Metubine). (d) Use Sengstaken–Blakemore or Linton tube for esophageal or gastric bleeding. (e) Pitressin infusion via IMA, SMA, gastric artery catheters for control of gastrointestinal bleeding, or other intra-arterial infusion. This does not include standard 3 ml/hr heparin flush to maintain catheter patency. (g) Active pacing even if a chronic pacemaker. (h) Include first 2 runs of an acute dialysis. Include chronic dialysis in patient whose medical situation now renders dialysis unstable. (j) Continuous or intermittent cooling to achieve body temperature less than 33°C. (k) Use of a blood pump or manual pumping of blood in the patient who requires rapid blood replacement. (p) May even be the initial emergency operative procedure—precludes diagnostic test (*i.e.*, angiography, CT scan).

3-Point Interventions: (d) The patient is supplying some of his own ventilatory needs. (g) Not a daily point score. Patient must have been intubated in the ICU (elective or emergency) within 24 hr. (i) Measurement of intake/output above and beyond the normal 24-hr routine. Frequent adjustment of intake according to total output. (x) Includes Rheomacrodex. (bb) For example, Stryker frame, CircOlectric.

2-Point Interventions: (g) Replacement of clear fluids over and above the ordered maintenance level.

1-Point Interventions: (k) Must have a decubitus ulcer. Does not include preventive therapy.

TABLE 9-14. Acute Physiology Score, Weighting of Physiologic Measurement, Weighted Score

POINTS	+4	+3	+2	+1	0	+1	+2	+3	+4
Cardiovascular									
Heart rate ventricular response	180 or >	141–179	111–140		70–110		56–69	41–55	40 or less
Mean blood pressure (mm Hg)	160 or >	131–159	111–130		70–110		51–69		50 or less
R atrial pressure/CVP (mm Hg)			26 or >	16–25	1–15	<1			
CK-MB or EKG evidence of acute MI	Yes				No				
EKG-dysrhythmias		Atrial dysrhyth-mias + hemody-namic instability	Atrial dys-rhythmias alone					>6 PVCs/min	Ventricular tachycardia or fibrillation
Lactate meq/liter (serum)	>8	3.5–8			0–3.4				
pH (blood)	7.7 or >	7.6–7.69		7.51–7.59	7.33–7.5		7.25–7.32	7.15–7.24	<7.15
Respiratory									
Respiratory rate total nonventi-lated	50 or >	35–49	26–34		12–25	10–11	7–9		6 or less
P(A−a)O$_2$(100%) or*	>500	351–499		200–350	<200				
Pa$_{CO_2}$	70 or >	61–69	50–60		30–49		25–29	20–24	<20
Renal									
Urine output/day			5 liters or >	3501–4999 ml	700–3500 ml		480–699 ml (20–29 ml/hr)	120–479 ml (5–20 ml/hr)	<120 ml/day (5 ml/hr)
Serum BUN	>150	101–150	81–100	21–80	10–20		<10		
Serum creatinine	>7	3.6–7	2.1–3.5	1.6–2	0.6–1.5	<0.6			
Gastrointestinal									
Serum amylase (international units)	2000 or >	500–1999			500 or >				
Serum albumin	>8	15 or >			3.5–8	2.5–3.4	<2.5		
Bilirubin (total)				5.1–14.9	0–5				
ALKP-alkaline phosphatase (serum) international units				>160	0–160				
SGOT			1500 or >	101–1499	0–100				
Anergy (skin tests)†	Total		Relative		None				

Physiologic Variable	+4	+3	+2	+1	0	+1	+2	+3	+4
Hematologic									
Hematocrit	>60	51–60		47–50	30–46		20–29		<20
WBC (total)	>40,000	20,001–40,000		15,001–20,000	3000–15,000		1000–2999		<1000
Platelets		>1,000,000	600,001–1,000,000		80,000–600,000		20,000–79,999		<20,000
Protime (in sec > control) no anticoagulants	>12	5.1–12		3.1–5	0–3				
Septic									
CSF-positive culture	Yes				No				
Blood-positive culture	Yes				No				
Fungal-positive culture	Blood or CSF	2 sites other than blood or CSF		1 site other than blood or CSF	None				
Temperature °C (rectal)	>41.0°	39.1–41.0°		38.6–39.0°	36.0–38.5°	34.0–35.9°	32.0–33.9°	30.0–31.9°	29.9° or less
Metabolic									
Serum calcium mg/100 ml	16 or >	14–15.9	11.1–13.9		8–11.0		5.0–7.9		<5
Serum glucose	>800	500–800	251–499		70–250		50–69	30–49	<30
Serum sodium	>180	161–180	156–160	151–155	130–150		120–129	110–119	<110
Serum potassium	>7	6.1–7		5.6–6	3.5–5.5	3–3.4	2.5–2.9		<2.5
Serum HCO₃	>40		31–40		20–30	10–19		5–9	<5
Serum osmolarity	>350	321–350	301–320		260–300		240–259	220–239	<220
Neurologic									
Glasgow coma score	3	4–6	7–9	10–12	13–15				

(Knaus WA, Zimmerman JE, Wagner DP, et al: APACHE—Acute physiology and chronic health evaluation: A physiologically based classification system. *Crit Care Med* 1981; 9:591)

* $P(A-a)O_2 = [FiO_2 (713) - PaCO_2 - PaO_2]$.

† Total anergy—no response to all provocative skin tests including mumps and fungal. Relative-reduced response to skin tests indicative of compromised cellular immunity.

CVP = central venous pressure; BUN = blood urea nitrogen; SGOT = serum glutamic oxaloacetic transaminase; CSF = cerebrospinal fluid; PVC = premature ventricular contraction.

system also contained some general guidelines so that other investigators could perform TISS calculations in a standardized fashion. There was no difference in overall point score using the updated system.

One advantage of TISS is its simplicity to perform because it lists interventions easily recognized at the patient's bedside. It also serves to quantitate the physician's perception of the illness, which translates into requirements for nursing care and other aspects of total patient care. Its basic, fundamental, and most important limitation is that the physician's perception of illness can change over time, and there is no current method of deciding that different physicians faced with the same patient and same illness would agree on the same intervention.

More recently, objective physiologic indicators were added to the TISS system.[29] Although the percentage of abnormal TISS indicators did not discriminate between patients who died and those who lived, the results were said by the authors to demonstrate the extremely abnormal physiology and need for massive support in class IV critically ill patients when compared to the other classes.

First introduced in 1981, APACHE has been described as a physiologically based classification system, consisting of two parts: the acute physiology score (APS) and the chronic health evaluation (CHE).[30] The APS is a weighted sum of each of 34 physiologic measurements obtained from the patient's clinical record within the first 24 hours of ICU admission (Table 9-14). If a physiologic variable is not measured, it is assumed to be normal or not necessary to estimate the severity of illness. The second portion is a four-category designation of preadmission health status (Table 9-15). A major difference between the systems described under disease–patient interaction and APACHE is that the physiologic variables collected under APACHE are then weighted from 0 to 4 according to a group consensus as to the perceived significance of abnormality, similar to the *a priori* judgments contained in TISS. Thereafter, the data were subjected to logistic multiple regression adding age, sex, operative status, and indication for admission. A risk of death was calculated and used to determine the number of expected deaths in an attempt to relate outcome to the initial severity of illness as assessed by APACHE. When this method was applied in different hospitals, the authors found substantial differences in the severity of acute illness among the hospitals, but projected death rates were similar to the observed deaths in each hospital.[31] Their studies then compared intensive care in the United States and France.[32] Patients admitted to French ICUs were significantly younger, remained in the ICU twice as long, and had hourly vital sign monitoring and invasive hemodynamic monitoring at half the rate of U.S. patients. The probability of hospital death at any given APS score was the same in both countries. APACHE has since been proposed for quality review in intensive care.[33] The authors emphasize that the APS of the APACHE classification system is measured on admission to the ICU so that the impact and appropriateness of subsequent ICU care can be evaluated. Survival or death was considered the most important outcome variable. APACHE was considered

TABLE 9-15. Calculation of APACHE: Determination of Preadmission Health Status

QUALIFYING QUESTIONS	CHRONIC HEALTH	BRIEF DESCRIPTION
Did the patient have weekly visits to a physician? Was the patient unable to work because of illness? Was the patient bedridden or institutionalized because of illness? Had the patient suffered a relapse after systemic treatment for carcinoma?	D	Severe restriction of activity due to disease; includes persons bedridden or institutionalized due to illness.
Was the patient's usual daily activity limited? Did symptoms occur with mild exertion? Had the patient received treatment for neoplasm with remission or uncomplicated hemodialysis?	C	Chronic disease producing serious but not incapacitating restriction of activity.
Did the patient see a physician monthly? Did he take medication chronically? Was he mildly limited in his activity level because of illness? Had the patient had diabetes mellitus, chronic renal failure, a bleeding disorder, or chronic anemia?	B	Mild-to-moderate limitation of activity because of a chronic medical problem.
(Negative response to all of the above questions.)	A	Prior good health; no functional limitations.

(Knaus WA, Zimmerman JE, Wagner DP, et al: APACHE—Acute physiology and chronic health evaluation: A physiologically based classification system. *Crit Care Med* 1981; 9:591) to be useful to identify low-risk monitored patients.[34] The authors proposed that collection of APACHE data could identify those patients having no further significant risk of complications after 24 hours of intensive care. In their studies, these patients were commonly treated 2.1 days, and they proposed that this might be cut in half, resulting in a savings of approximately 4% of all intensive care days. These data are similar to those cited earlier in which 110 elective patients were discharged after their first ICU day without calculation of APACHE scores.[5] Statistical validation of APACHE, when reported in terms of total correct classification, was 81% using the decision rule that 50% predicted risk of death resulted in death.[35] In the validation set, 79% of patients were correctly classified. Then, in 1985, APACHE II was described, which compressed the APS from 34 to 12 routine physiologic measurements plus age and previous health status.[36] The original APACHE set of 34 variables was modified in a number of different ways. For instance, infrequently measured physiologic variables such as serum osmolarity, lactic acid, and skin testing with antigens were deleted, as were potentially redundant variables. Other reductions were accomplished by deleting the measurements (based on clinical judgments) and then evaluating that decision using a multivariant comparison of the original APACHE system with each proposed revision. Ultimately, the smallest number of variables that maintained statistical precision was 12 (Table 9-16). Of subsequent ICU admissions, 87% had all physiologic measurements available. Creatinine and ABGs were most commonly missing: these patients were considered to have been admitted for monitoring only, and ABGs and creatinine were not essential for their care. Again, mortality was closely correlated to increasing APACHE II score. The number of patients correctly classified was 85.5%. In the validation study performed in 13 tertiary care hospitals, the author used the same methodology that was used previously to validate APACHE.[37] In the first studies, APACHE was considered validated because there were similar observed death rates to expected rates provided by the predictive APACHE model.[31,32] In the validation of APACHE II, actual and predicted death rates were compared using group results as a standard.[37] When one hospital had significantly better results and another significantly inferior results, failure of validation was not mentioned. In its place, the differences were interpreted: the authors concluded that these were related more to the interaction and coordination of each hospital's intensive care staff than to the unit's administrative structures, amount of specialized treatment used, or the hospital teaching status. Unfortunately, the interpretations have been widely quoted in both the medical and lay press. That APACHE II did not meet the authors' previous validation standard[31,32] has generally escaped notice.

The advantages of APACHE and APACHE II, especially, are that the measurements are usually easy to obtain from the patient's chart and that the statistical methods have been extensively tested. APACHE and APACHE II appear to measure the severity of illness present at admission; indeed, they can be expected to measure only that which is actually present. The disadvantages include the perceptual bias induced by the decision to rank severity

TABLE 9-16. *The APACHE II Severity of Disease Classification System*

PHYSIOLOGIC VARIABLE	HIGH ABNORMAL RANGE				0	LOW ABNORMAL RANGE			
	+4	+3	+2	+1		+1	+2	+3	+4
(1) Temperature—rectal (°C)	≥41°	39°–40.9°		38.5°–38.9°	36°–38.4°	34°–35.9°	32°–33.9°	30°–31.9°	≤29.9°
(2) MAP mm Hg	≥160	130–159	110–129		70–109		50–69		≤49
(3) Heart rate ventricular response	≥180	140–179	110–139		70–109		55–69	40–54	<39
(4) Respiratory rate (nonventilated or ventilated)	≥50	35–49		25–34	12–24	10–11	6–9		≤5
(5) Oxygenation: (A − a)D_{O_2}, or Pa_{O_2} (mm Hg)									
(a) FI_{O_2} 0.5 record (A − a)D_{O_2}	≥500	350–499	200–349		<200				
(b) FI_{O_2} 0.5 record only Pa_{O_2}					$P_{O_2} > 70$	P_{O_2} 61–70		P_{O_2} 55–60	$P_{O_2} < 55$
(6) Arterial pH	≥7.7	7.6–7.69		7.5–7.59	7.33–7.49		7.25–7.32	7.15–7.24	<7.15
(7) Serum sodium (mM/liter)	≥180	160–179	155–159	150–154	130–149		120–129	111–119	≤110
(8) Serum potassium (mM/liter)	≥7	6.6–9		5.5–5.9	3.5–5.4	3–3.4	2.5–2.9		<2.5
(9) Serum creatinine (mg/100 ml) (Double point score for acute renal failure)	≥3.5	2–3.4	1.5–1.9		0.6–1.4		<0.6		
(10) Hematocrit (%)	≥60		50–59.9	46–49.9	30–45.9		20–29.9		<20
(11) WBC (total/mm³) (in 1,000s)	≥40		20–39.9	15–19.9	3–14.9		1–2.9		<1
(12) Glasgow Coma Score (GCS) Score = 15 minus actual GCS									

(Adapted from Knaus WA, et al: *Crit Care Med* 1985; 13:818)

similarly to the ranking of therapeutic interventions in TISS. The 15% misclassification rate, common to every system, it seems, means that it cannot be applied to individual patients. Two additional limitations are not inherent in the system itself but rather seem to depend on the interpretations of the authors. First, APACHE II has been promulgated as a useful tool in clinical trials or in nonrandomized or multi-institutional studies of therapeutic efficacy. The authors believe that APACHE II scores will help investigators determine whether control and treatment groups are similar. They also plan to compare the expected death rate with the actual death rate as a test of therapeutic efficacy; however, an incorrect classification rate of 15% makes achievement of this goal unlikely. They also subsequently used differences in observed-to-expected death rates to point out differences in the functioning of an ICU staff, not differences in therapy.[37] The "strength" of calculating APACHE II in the first 24 hours—to eliminate the effects of treatment—also ignores that subsequently developed complications and illnesses determine outcome of the patients who are most "critical" (midway along the severity spectrum). Further, the latest data that were expected to validate APACHE II showed that observed and expected death rates differed significantly in certain hospitals.[37] APACHE II then did not meet the standard of validation demonstrated for APACHE.[31,32] However, the author believes that APACHE II should be used to answer questions concerning restriction of intensive care services from patients who are too healthy or too sick to benefit from aggressive care, despite the fact that APACHE previously demonstrated that neither group consumes significant resources.[38]

NURSING CARE INDEX

Nursing care forms the third perspective for viewing the patient–disease interactions. A quantitative approach to categorization of care, specific activities, and types of patients was presented by Hudson and colleagues.[39] Forty-seven activities in seven categories were timed and converted to a similar point scale. The vital sign and measurement category is listed in Table 9-17. This is discussed in detail in Chapter 15, titled "Allocating Nursing Care." Three classes were subsequently defined based on the number of nursing hours generated by the perceived acuity of illness and the physician's orders. The three groups represented 12 hours of nursing care or fewer and were deemed serious; 13 to 24 hours, critical, and more than 24 hours of nursing care per 24-hour day, crisis. Since nursing tasks are based on both the physician's and nurse's perception of the patient's illness, it is clear that changes in delivered care would be possible. Subsequent groups of patients studied in 1979[40] and 1984[41] demonstrated significant differences in the distribution of patients by nursing classification although both TISS and APACHE scores remained the same. In fact, nursing hours per patient have been reduced by approximately 50% without affecting outcome. This is not surprising if we recognize that intensive care is a young discipline and the "traditional" methods of ICU nursing date back only a few years. In the

TABLE 9-17. Intensive Care Nursing Requirements: Vital Sign and Measurement Category

TYPE	SPECIFIC ACTIVITIES	POINTS/HR OR AS SPECIFIED
Basic vital signs	Blood pressure, pulse, respirations, hypo/hyperthermia, CVP (H_2O manometer), EKG monitoring, AV shunt patency, and checking peripheral pulses	Every: 1 hr = 16 2 hr = 8 3 hr = 4
Neurologic vital signs	Examination/assessment of pupils, level of consciousness, movement of extremities, reaction to stimuli	Same as above
Peripheral arterial line	Routine maintenance: calibration, measurements, and catheter irrigation	4/shift
	Catheter insertion: setup transducer system, assisting MD with procedure, calibration, measurements	8 each
Central venous line	Routine maintenance: as above	4/shift
	Catheter insertion: as above	8 each
Pulmonary artery catheter	Routine maintenance: as above	8/shift
	Catheter insertion: as above	12 each

(Adapted from Hudson J, et al: *Crit Care Med* 1979; 7:69)

United States, hourly vital signs were considered "mandatory" in the ICU and a nurse:patient ratio of 1:1 was considered "ideal." One aspect of the French–United States comparison of APACHE revealed that only half the patients in French ICUs received hourly vital signs compared to nearly 100% of patients in the United States.[33] Since outcome was the same for a given APACHE score, it is apparent that *recording* hourly vital signs is not a critical element of ICU care. The value of the nursing care categorization became evident during personnel shortages and when the cost-containment focus arose. Because nursing care could be adequately quantitated, modification and change in bedside practice could be attempted to eliminate these "traditional" nursing tasks that actually had little, if any, effect on outcome. It was through this "change and measure" technique that the total number of nursing care hours could be diminished.

VALUES AND LIMITATION OF PREDICTIVE INDICES

It is interesting to note that the creators of most of the indices list essentially the same objectives and potential uses for the system described. Indeed, prediction of the potential usefulness of intensive care for an individual patient is a lofty objective. Most easily separate patients at the ends of the severity spectrum. It is unlikely that any index completed at the time of the patient's admission can do this for the problematic long-term patient (Table 9-18). When sequential APACHE II calculations were made in long-term ICU patients, separation of the scores of the patients who actually died from those who actually survived occurred after 1 week of ICU care (Table 9-19). Further, calculations of APACHE II made 24 hours before death actually occurred revealed a score associated with a predicted 65% survival. With respect to TISS scores (Table 9-20), there were no significant differences for the first 2 weeks, and the mortality predicted in the group that expired was only 12% on the day before death. TISS scores decreased over time even in patients who died. This would underscore the basic premise that TISS represents a physician's perspective of the patient's illness reflected in the choice of interventions. The patients die of MOSF and not of acute catastrophic cardiorespiratory failure; the latter alone is highly weighted in TISS and APACHE. All indices can and will fail to predict outcome in long-term patients because the data that will determine outcome are either not known or not abnormal on admission. It is interesting that all of the systems evaluated have approximately a 15% misclassification rate. It is of further interest that this is exactly the same rate found in studies of clinical judgment.[42,43] Indices based on physiologic assessment quantitate clinical judgment but do not improve upon it. The value of indices, therefore, cannot be derived from the ability to predict events that have not yet occurred but rather to provide a quantitative categorization of patients by physiologic systems at varying times after the initiation of illness and admission to the ICU. Subsets of patients who are truly severely ill on admission may be identified for sub-

TABLE 9-18. Severity of Illness Judged by Duration of ICU Stay

	RAW AII		PREDICTED MORTALITY BY AII		RAW TISS		PREDICTED MORTALITY BY TISS	
	1 Day	Long-Term	1 Day	Long-Term	1 Day	Long-Term	1 Day	Long-Term
ACTUAL SURVIVORS	8.6	12	6%	12%	19.1	30.6	5%	15%
ACTUAL DEATHS	31.6	16.5	72%	20%	37.8	31.6	26%	18%

Living and dying patients who spend 1 day in unit represent opposite ends of severity spectrum.
Long-term patients (> 13 days) are midway along spectrum (56% hospital mortality).
APACHE II (AII) and TISS calculated on first ICU day.

TABLE 9-19. *Repetitive APACHE II Calculations in Patients with Prolonged ICU Stay*

SURVIVORS—AFTER PROLONGED ICU STAY (> 13 DAYS)							EXPIRED—AFTER PROLONGED ICU STAY (> 13 DAYS)						
DAY	1	2	3	5	7	14	F	DAY	1	2	3	5	7	14	F
APACHE II*	12	10.8	9.9	12.9	11.4	9.4	7.6	APACHE II*	16.5	14.7	16	14.6	16.4	20.9	21.6
% MORTALITY PREDICTED	12	12	12	12	12	6	6	% MORTALITY PREDICTED	20	20	20	20	20	35	35

F = Day before ICU discharge.
* = APACHE II, Knaus WA: *Crit Care Med* 1985; 13:818.

TABLE 9-20. *Repetitive TISS Calculations in Patients with Prolonged ICU Stay*

SURVIVORS—AFTER PROLONGED ICU STAY (> 13 DAYS)							EXPIRED—AFTER PROLONGED ICU STAY (> 13 DAYS)						
DAY	1	2	3	5	7	14	F	DAY	1	2	3	5	7	14	F
TISS*	30.6	26.2	24.4	22.8	23.9	20.1	14.7	TISS*	31.6	29.7	28.4	26.8	27.4	28.2	27
% MORTALITY PREDICTED	15	11	10	7	7	5	0	% MORTALITY PREDICTED	18	15	14	12	12	14	12

F = Day before ICU discharge.
* TISS, Civetta JM: *Ann Surg* 1985; 202:254.

sequent treatment protocols. However, it is unlikely that the systems, as currently described, will contribute to the decision-making process with respect to limitation of therapy for patients who have no reasonable chance of survival. None of the indices currently available accurately describes the outcome of these patients. An important direction for further investigation is to identify early markers of the later determinants. Clearly, the isolated catastrophic event or iatrogenic occurrence will never be predictable, but these events change patients deemed survivable into patients who die, rather than the opposite.

Most investigators have proposed that indices be used for interunit comparisons. The present indicators should be useful to assess the care of patients whose outcome is determined by elements present at admission. Qualitatively, this can be viewed as a mortality function curve relating the index to an observed mortality (Fig. 9-3). The curves for each hospital could be calculated and compared. This would improve discrimination caused by differing degrees of illness and relate performance/outcome to the classes of patients (observation, nursing care, and physician care). One can postulate that a "good" hospital should achieve a lower mortality at any given degree of severity as opposed to an average hospital. Perhaps only a tertiary care hospital could achieve survivals in extremely critically ill patients. Although this might be impossible to attain in a community hospital where personnel and equipment are not available, a "good" community hospital could achieve the same expected mortality for lower degrees of severity. On the other hand, a "bad" hospital would have a higher than expected mortality for all degrees of severity. This type of investigation should be possible given present physiologic predictors. Indices then will be most useful to quantify initial illness

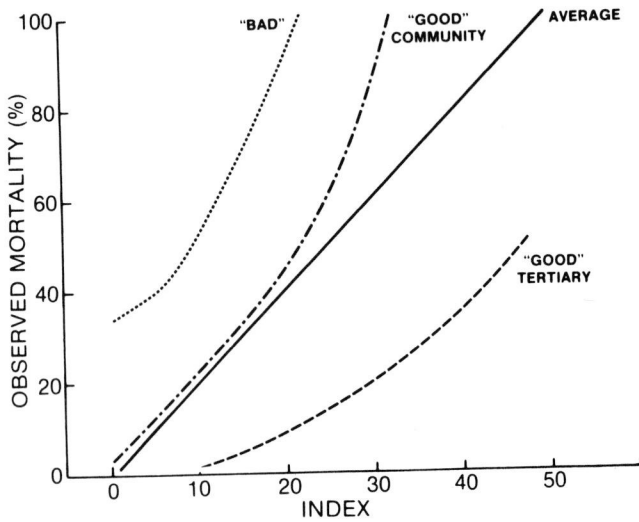

FIGURE 9-3. Mortality function curves relating the predictive index to an observed mortality.

and identify short-term objectives with respect to evaluating current therapy and resource allocation rather than the prediction of outcome for an individual patient.

REFERENCES

1. Stern RS, Epstein AM: Institutional responses to prospective payment based on diagnosis-related groups: Implications of cost, quality, and access. *N Engl J Med* 1985; 312:621
2. Showstack JA, Stone MH, Schroeder SA: The role of changing clinical practices in the rising costs of hospital care. *N Engl J Med* 1985; 313:1201
3. Klarman HE: Application of cost-benefit analysis to health systems technology. *J Occup Med* 1974; 16(3):172
4. Critical Care Medicine, Consensus Development Conference Summary, National Institutes of Health, 1983; 4(6)
5. Civetta JM, Hudson–Civetta J, Nelson LD: Costly care: Data problems and proposing remedies (abstr.) *Crit Care Med* 1986; 14:357
6. Civetta JM, Hudson–Civetta JA: Maintaining quality of care while reducing charges in the ICU: 10 ways. *Ann Surg* 1985; 202:524
7. Thurow LC: Medicine versus economics: Special article. *N Engl J Med* 1985; 313:611
8. Butler PW, Bone RC, Field T: Technology under medicare diagnosis-related groups prospective payment: Implications for medical intensive care. *Chest* 1985; 87:229
9. Welch HG, Larson EB: Dealing with limited resources: The Oregon decision to curtail funding for organ transplantation. *N Engl J Med* 1988; 319:171
10. Engelhardt HT Jr: Shattuck Lecture—Allocating scarce medical resources and the availability of organ transplantation: Some moral presuppositions. *N Engl J Med* 1984; 311:66
11. Schelling T: The life you save may be your own. In Chase SB (ed): *Problems in Public Expenditure Analysis*, p 127. Washington, DC, the Brookings Institute, 1966
12. Drucker WR, Gavett JW, et al: Toward strategies for cost containment in surgical patients. *Ann Surg* 1983; 198:284
13. Campion EW, Mulley AG, Goldstein MA, et al: Medical intensive care for the elderly: A study of current use, costs, and outcomes. *JAMA* 1981; 246:2052
14. Robin ED: A critical look at critical care. *Crit Care Med* 1983; 11:144
15. Robin ED: The cult of the Swan–Ganz catheter: Overuse and abuse of pulmonary flow catheters. *Ann Intern Med* 1985; 103:445
16. Shoemaker WC, Pierchala BS, Potter Chang, et al: Prediction of outcome and severity of illness by analysis of the frequency distribution of cardiorespiratory variables. *Crit Care Med* 1977; 5:82
17. Shoemaker WC, Appel P, Bland R: Use of physiologic monitoring to predict outcome and to assist in clinical decisions in critically ill postoperative patients. *Am J Surg* 1983; 146:43
18. Bland R, Shoemaker W: Probability of survival as a prognostic and severity of illness score in critically ill surgical patients. *Crit Care Med* 1985; 13:91
19. Phillips GD, Austin KL, Runciman WB: Deaths in intensive care. *Med J Aust* 1980; 424
20. Civetta J: The ICU milieu: An evaluation of the allocation of a limited resource. *Resp Care* 1974; 21:498

21. Snyder JV, McGuirk M, Grenvik A, et al: Outcome of intensive care: An application of a predictive model. *Crit Care Med* 1981; 9:598
22. Lemeshow S, Teres D, Pastides H, et al: A method for predicting survival and mortality of ICU patients using objectively derived weights. *Crit Care Med* 1985; 13:519
23. Teres D, Lemeshow S, Spitz Avrunin J: A validation of an objectively weighted mortality prediction model for intensive care unit patients. *Crit Care Med* 1986; 14:399
24. Civetta JM: The inverse relationship between cost and survival. *J Surg Res* 1973; 14:265
25. Cullen DJ, Civetta JM, Briggs BA, et al: Therapeutic intervention scoring system: A method for quantitative comparison of patient care. *Crit Care Med* 1974; 2:57
26. Cullen DJ: Results and costs of intensive care. *Anesthesiology* 1977; 47:203
27. Silverman DG, Goldiner PA, Kay BA, et al: The therapeutic intervention scoring system: An application to acutely ill cancer patients. *Crit Care Med* 1975; 3:222
28. Keene AR, Cullen DJ: Therapeutic Intervention Scoring System: Update 1983. *Crit Care Med* 1983; 11:1
29. Cullen DJ, Keene R, Waternaux C, et al: Objective, quantitative measurement of severity of illness in critically ill patients. *Crit Care Med* 1984; 12:155
30. Knaus WA, Zimmerman JE, Wagner DP, et al: APACHE—Acute physiology and chronic health evaluation: A physiologically based classification system. *Crit Care Med* 1981; 9:591
31. Knaus WA, Draper EA, Wagner DP, et al: Evaluating outcome from intensive care: A preliminary multihospital comparison. *Crit Care Med* 1982; 10:491
32. Knaus WA, Wagner DP, Loirat P, et al: A comparison of intensive care in the U.S.A. and France. *Lancet* 1982; 62:642
33. Knaus WA, Draper EA, Wagner DP: Toward quality review in intensive care. The APACHE system. *QRB* 1983; 9:196
34. Wagner DP, Knaus WA, Draper EA, et al: Identification of low-risk monitor patients within a medical–surgical intensive care unit. *Med Care* 1983; 21:425
35. Wagner DP, Knaus WA, Draper EA: Statistical validation of a severity of illness measure. *Am J Public Health* 1983; 73:878
36. Knaus WA, Draper EA, Wagner DP, et al: APACHE II: A severity of disease classification system. *Crit Care Med* 1985; 13:818
37. Knaus WA, Draper EA, Wagner DP, et al: An evaluation of outcome from intensive care in major medical center. *Ann Intern Med* 1986; 104:410
38. Knaus WA: When is intensive care inappropriate: New "prognostic" measures provide answers. *Hosp Med Q* 1986; 14
39. Hudson J, Caruthers TE, Lantiegne K: Intensive care nursing requirements: Resource allocation according to patient status. *Crit Care Med* 1979; 7:69
40. Hudson–Civetta J, Caruthers T, Civetta JM: Redistribution of intensive care as to patient status. *Crit Care Med* 1981; 9:226
41. Civetta JM, Hudson–Civetta JA: Cost effective use of the ICU. In Eisman B (ed): *Cost Effectiveness in Surgery,* pp. 3–13. Philadelphia, WB Saunders, 1987.
42. Rodman GH, Etling T, Civetta JM, et al: How accurate is clinical judgment? *Crit Care Med* 1978; 6:127
43. Civetta JM, Carruthers TE: Does clinical judgment correctly allocate surgical intensive care? *Crit Care Med* 1983; 11:236

Part II

People

Joining the Team 10
Mary F. Murtha
Lisa Regueiro

PERCEPTIONS

"After all my years of training, I do not think a nurse could tell me much about managing critically ill patients." "I would prefer that the nurses just take care of the patients, give medications, hang IVs, take vital signs, you know, the things they are good at, and let the doctors manage the patients."

These are some of the comments we received from physicians who at one point in their career rotated through the ICU. Yet, eventually, most physicians thought that their rotation was a positive, enjoyable experience. They believed that they learned a tremendous amount about the pathophysiology of the critically ill patient, about death and dying, *and* about getting along with their co-workers.

We also polled nurses working in ICUs, and some of their comments follow: "I've worked this ICU for 5 years, I've seen what works and what doesn't." "I'm with my patients every minute for 8 hours, and I can tell when something is different." "I think the residents could be more open to suggestions and not so afraid of having their egos bruised."

Do these different attitudes merely reflect real differences of opinion? It would seem that if we all were working toward a common goal, if we all were working as a team for the benefit of the patient, there would be no conflict. This, however, is very idealistic. It is true that we, the nurses and physicians, have the same goal; however, dealing with many different personalities requires a delicate blend of tact and diplomacy. Remembering that those who work in an ICU setting are working under a great deal of stress and tension will help us to manage better one another's idiosyncrasies. Only then can we accomplish our goal in caring for the critically ill.

Greenburg, Civetta, and Barnhill describe an ICU as a high-tension environment where uncertainty about survival is coupled with uncertainty about the random appearance of catastrophic events or unpredictable clinical crises. "Uncertainty produces anxiety and anxiety readily translates into stress."[1]

Perhaps these expressed comments reflect this stress—defenses set up to protect "new" physicians, at least as they enter the established ICU for the first time, and nurses, who perhaps feel a need to express the proprietary "rights" of the establishment—the "permanent" ICU staff. Physicians may, justifiably, be somewhat fearful because they are unfamiliar with procedures and with the environment—independent of the recognized gaps in their medical knowledge about the care of the critically ill.

Nurses, too, feel protective, ostensibly for the patients and to ensure that "protocols" are adhered to. But again, the order and structure can greatly help them to cope with the activity, acuity of illness, and interpersonal stressors. Thus the protection has great value for the nurse as well.

Although the stressors in an ICU cannot be eliminated, recognition and understanding will reduce anxiety and the perceived stress. It follows that awareness of the meaning of these attitudes should allow us to go beyond— to recognize the attributes and characteristics necessary to mold a team so that misperception can be replaced by trust and isolation by communal spirit, and thus the good to be gained can be effectively attained.

Knowing how we handle stress and how it handles us can only benefit the new ICU physician—and all members of the ICU team. We must understand that we all handle stress differently. Some laugh and joke, others are very solemn. Still others will shout, and some become very quiet and withdrawn. Initially the new ICU physician will be unaware of everyone's stress-releasing mechanisms, just as his/her co-workers will be unaware of his or hers. Recognition and respect of the human elements in this equation underlie all attempts to learn about total ICU care. The emphasis of teamwork should be on *what* is right, not necessarily *who* is right. Factors influencing the ability of the team to perform satisfactorily include a clear understanding of the team's objective, role delineation, perceptions of team members' roles, nurse–physician collaboration, and communication skills.

In the following pages, we hope to help the new ICU physician integrate easily into the ICU setting by identifying the team, roles of team members and how they function in the unit, and potential stressors. Perhaps with this information, the ICU rotation will be a positive, enjoyable experience.

FUNCTIONS OF THE TEAM

A team functions best when the members work toward one common goal. Objectives must be clear and each member's role clearly delineated. As with any team, there is one captain or leader, who would not be able to accomplish the team's objectives without the assistance and support of the other team members. If we compare the ICU team to a football team this will become clear. The quarterback does not win the game alone. Each team member must be aware of his/her task, as well as the roles of the other team members.

The same is true in the ICU. Caring for patients is a team effort. The ICU physician can be looked upon as the quarterback. The other team members look to him/her for the plan of therapy—decision-making—and support for their cause—taking care of the patient. The team includes nurses, respiratory therapists, junior residents, and other ancillary personnel. If all work together and support one another, their goal can be easily met. It is easy to fall back on learned patterns of behavior, even if they have failed—and this failure may even be recognized. As junior residents, the goal was to complete the daily "scut sheet"—this was expected, and no one asked how it was to be accomplished. One learned quickly to rely solely on oneself and to take care of each detail. In critical care, this is not only impossible but also undesirable. The quarterback does not block, throw, and catch the pass. In the uncertainty of transition to the ICU world of divided and graded responsibility, the attitude of "I'd rather do it myself" is a carry-over from earlier, perhaps, simpler days.

The goal of an ICU is the safe delivery of coordinated medical care. Using observational skills and advanced technical equipment, the clinician can assess the patient's status in new, more detailed ways. All the team members are important, contributing their skills and expertise to complete this objective.

A system of checks and balances is used. Fellows, junior residents, nurses, and respiratory therapists must be aware of the daily plan of care. Each member is responsible for individual tasks but will continually monitor the entire patient care process to ensure that daily goals are being achieved. Therefore, inquiries about therapy are generally not meant to question an individual's judgment, but to ensure that the rationale is understood and the plan of care is consistent—by the questioner as well as the questioned.

ORGANIZATIONAL FACTORS

Critical care areas often use primary nursing techniques as their patient care methods because they foster a continuum of practice and enhancement of the team relationship. Because there is a specific nurse responsible for a given patient's care, communication is simplified, and thus increased working contact should encourage trust. Team spirit develops in this type of practice, enhancing morale for nurses and physicians in caring for a specific group of patients. This is a firm foundation for further development. The team, which can rely on individual commitment to a common goal, thereby establishes understood behaviors and expectations such as honesty, sound judgment, satisfactory job performance, an attitude of caring, a strong desire to do what is right for the patient, an attention to detail, and an acknowledgment that the team is important. This team spirit may become difficult to maintain if any dissension develops. For instance, new team members (physicians) are almost always tested by members who perceive themselves as constants (nurses). Team membership has to be "earned." This requires recognition of the importance of the other team members, decision-making skills, judgment, and honesty, all demonstrated by adhering to group-approved behavior. This behavior, the unwritten rules of the game, is based on the desires of the organizational hierarchy. Initially, it is easiest to accept the unit's "correct" way in order to earn a spot on the team roster. Later, one's ideas can be evaluated on their merit. The opposite, starting off by correcting "errors" or by introducing new (and better?) ways, leads only to defensiveness, isolation, and hostility instead of trust and acceptance. Participation in unit activities demonstrates acknowledgment of the team and its importance in the overall functioning of the unit, even if some particular procedures seem wrong. Specific procedures or policies are truly inconsequential compared to the importance of morale; they should be considered manifestations of team consensus, and thus of the team itself. Deviance from established policy is considered an unwillingness to be part of the team, not evidence of a superior way of doing a task, and is disruptive to morale, can heighten organizational stress, and ultimately can obstruct the delivery of optimum health care.

ROLES OF TEAM MEMBERS

The medical director or attending of the ICU may coordinate, supervise, and evaluate the care given to all ICU patients or serve as an administrator/arbiter. If any controversy should arise in terms of the plan of patient care, the attending can become involved to clarify these objectives. Promptly involving the attending in particular situations can alleviate some of the stress created by uncertainty, and this will aid the new ICU physician.

The ICU fellow has the most grueling task of all. Responsibilities include not only the management of the patients, but also being educator for the junior residents, administrator, and, sometimes, counselor for patients' family members.

In most units, the fellow is responsible for the minute-to-minute decisions governing patient care. The fellow must pay close attention to each detail of patient status. Decisions on initiating therapy, changing therapy, or deleting it are commonplace. He/she may also have to contend with the input from outside sources (surgeons, anesthesiologists, and various medical services) and synthesize the opinions to form a decision. Since time is essential, the ICU fellow should rely on other team members for assistance. He/she must be able to delegate certain responsibilities to the other health care providers.

As the quarterback of the ICU team the fellow not only must make decisions and plans for therapy but also may be asked, at times, to explain the rationale. Do not look upon this as a criticism of judgment but as an opportunity for teaching new ideas and reinforcing old information. This will ensure that all team members have the same plan of therapy in mind.

As an educator to the junior residents, the fellow will be sharing knowledge and technical expertise by supervising line insertions, intubations, and other procedures specific to the ICU areas.

As an administrator, he/she may be asked to devise a call schedule, make a formal evaluation of junior residents, and inform proper unit personnel of potential problems that may hinder patient care (*i.e.*, necessary equipment that is unavailable or improperly functioning equipment).

Finally, the ICU fellow will be asked to speak with family members and inform them of their relative's progress, whether favorable or poor. This can be very difficult at times, but the gratitude received from the family will compensate for this difficult task.

In summary, the ICU fellow has numerous responsibilities. Without the assistance and support of the rest of the team, he/she would find it extremely difficult to keep an organized plan of care. Everyone on the team works together, sharing information, communicating goals of therapy, and supporting one another to achieve a high standard of patient care.

The nurse is another important member of the team. He/she too has numerous responsibilities and could not complete the goals satisfactorily without the help of other team members. He/she also acts as an educator, administrator, and counselor. His/her responsibilities include direct patient care and documentation of that care along with gathering of data, including vital signs, intake and output, and laboratory values. He/she may be the most informed member of the team in terms of the actual status of the patient. Flow sheets set up to organize the data that he/she has been gathering facilitate communication and sharing of the information. The information needed to make an assessment should be on the flow sheet. If it is not, the nurse is the best resource. He/she may also be helpful to the new ICU fellow in guiding him/her through the various systems of a particular institution. The nurse may be able to assist in expediting test results or in identifying whom to call to get a test scheduled. If anyone on the team is unsure about how to complete a task, he/she probably should check with the nurse; most likely, he/she will save time and energy by asking him/her.

Nurses are generally at the bedside throughout their entire shift. Because of this he/she may be the first to notice a change in the patient's condition. Communication of this information to the ICU fellow is one of the more important aspects of the nurse's role. This type of communication and interaction between the fellow and nursing personnel can foster a trust that will be the basis for a good working relationship. It is rare that this trust will occur immediately. Each member of the team will be analyzing other members until each has verified that the "new" member can be safely included in the team. This can and will be frustrating at first, but the benefit of having that trust and working *with* one another is invaluable. Communication among team members is and must be the most important tool in the team concept.

Nurses also deal with the patient's family. It is important that the family receive the same messages concerning the patient's progress. Again, communication plays a major role. Family members are also dealing with stress and generally hear only what they want to hear—or are capable of hearing. For this reason, simple and clear language should be used. The nurse and fellow can speak with the family together or separately, but the same content should be maintained. This can alleviate yet another stressor for the fellow and the nurse because family members who cannot accept a poor prognosis often confront team members separately in desperate attempts to alter outcome through manipulation.

The important factors in achieving nurse–physician collaboration and communication are the creation of a system which recognizes that nurses render the direct patient care and allows both formal and informal exchanges between nurses and physicians. The outcomes in such a system are an enhanced quality of patient care, increased patient satisfaction with the care they receive, and increased satisfaction of nurses and physicians with both the care they provided and their practice experiences.

FACTORS CONTRIBUTING TO COLLABORATION

A number of factors potentially affect the establishment and maintenance of reciprocal relationships between team members within a critical care unit. These factors can basically be broken down into personal and organizational groups.

Personnel Factors. The nurse's educational background today may be quite varied, ranging from a hospital diploma or associate's degree to a baccalaureate or master's degree. Physicians should learn about the different backgrounds to avoid stereotyping and to be able to enhance collaboration.

The nurse's length of experience is also a factor: Greater experience in critical care generally provides more skill and confidence and greater opportunities to build working relationships with physicians. On the other hand, rigidity and independence may result from unpleasant experiences with inexperienced yet autocratic physicians.

The physician's educational background and his/her social or family background will play a part in his/her acclimation to the critical care environment and ability to adjust easily and quickly to new people. The physician becomes acutely aware of the demands placed on him/her to be an active team member—in fact, one of the leaders within the team. The other members look to him/her for support of their cause, direction for specific patient care, and overall unit function and communication of ideas and plans. The communication issue appears initially to pose a threat to new members of the team. New physicians on the unit often speak of continually being questioned as to their particular plan of therapy or thought process in providing interventions. Members attempting to pursue this type of communication (*i.e.*, asking why, how this will work, what did the attending say) are often considered, by the new physician, to be questioning his/her judgment or ability to make the correct decision. In the best of circumstances, the questioner is simply attempting to understand the rationale for therapy and to learn from the physician's previous experiences. He/she is looking for evidence that the team is a reality, that all members understand where they are going and why. He/she is also looking for pleasure and stimulation in working as part of the team. This communication differs from, say, general care areas where team members are usually not involved in acute situations or the focus is not concentrated on one or two patients. This is not to say that, at times, judgments are not questioned. They are, and, although this is a delicate situation, the questioning may be necessary. Ultimately, trust, the backbone of the team management approach, will evolve—and we must trust the process of its evolution. An ability to be open with perceptions and to validate them is vitally important. Major problems in communications can often be avoided if one can say, tactfully, what one feels. (Example: "I feel as if you think I've not made the correct decision.") The real issue—which only you can decide for yourself—is, do you want to do your work as part of a team, or do you want to be an independent practitioner explaining your actions only if you wish? If the latter, it will be extremely difficult to mobilize the best possible efforts from the necessary members to provide optimal health care for your patients, for this attitude is often perceived as defensive, condescending, supercilious, or outright antagonistic—none of which encourages whole-hearted cooperation. Intensive care units are composed of a relatively small number of people. Each member will affect the group as a whole, whether intended or not. In choosing to be part of a critical care unit today, one must understand, or at least be willing to try, participatory management to learn what improvements in patient care and cost efficiency have occurred. The ideal working relationship between team members should be an equitable, joint practice. If an organization does not provide adequate support for its staff in terms of the necessary authority, responsibility, and resources, professionals will become disenchanted and not invest the energy needed to function as part of a team. Also, if organizational channels become unwieldy, staff physicians and nurses will adjust by diminishing their efforts to function as a team. Feedback mechanisms are established within critical care units that help to enhance the team functions. Participation in feedback sessions is vital in establishing good communication. Verbalizing one's thoughts within a group allows for growth of each team member. Verbalization also causes the individual, and therefore the team, to become more vulnerable. Group interaction such as this can occur only when some degree of trust has been established. This is when growth as a team can truly occur.

Respiratory therapists, nursing assistants, and unit secretaries are also members of the team. All have varying roles from institution to institution, but all are important members of the team, necessary for the care of the critically ill patient.

We hope that the approach and information provided can assist the new ICU physician in acclimating himself to the ICU. Further, we hope that the physician's rotation will be a positive learning experience.

REFERENCES

1. Greenburg AG, Civetta JM, Barnhill GW: Neglected components of intensive care. *J Surg Res* 1979; 26:494
2. Webster S, Kelly L, Johst B, et al: A method of stress management: The support group. *Nurs Manage* 1982; 13:26

ICU Fellowship: Blending Science and Art

11

Louise Dion

INTRODUCTION

Everyone knows the ICU is stressful; however, we should remember Selye's observation, "Stress is the spice of life . . . the complete freedom from stress is death."[1]

One of the most important goals of an ICU fellowship is an increase in self-knowledge and understanding. This may be of greater value than the increase in medical knowledge and skills commonly associated with successful completion of the fellowship.

Perspective is all-important; you are neither the first nor the last, and, probably, neither the best nor worst. It may be difficult to maintain perspective and even a sense of humor when you are fatigued and overworked, when new crises develop and your shift seems endless. Remember to enjoy yourself; no matter how bad things seem, "Tomorrow always comes (and someone else will take over!)."

Functioning as an ICU fellow certainly requires scientific knowledge but also includes the art of interacting with a multitude of persons. No matter what specialty training served as preparation, it will not be adequate during the first days in the new position. There are many unavoidable adjustments to the new environment and successfully "fitting in" requires willpower from you and help from those already in place. As the fellow becomes more confident in his or her new role, he or she can develop into a "central pivot," the focal point of information and action for the team of nurses, medical students, interns, and residents. He or she becomes an important link between the patient and the primary care team, assuming, at times, even a political role in resolving the many nonmedical "crises" common in the busy hospital. This role is, most of the time, full of gratification but occasionally is overwhelmingly frustrating. For instance, at times delegating responsibilities to the junior staff can become a challenge but is probably a good stepping stone to becoming an attending.

INITIAL ADJUSTMENT

It is safe to say that a new ICU fellow, no matter what his or her prior specialty training, will find the new environment to be very different in many ways. Anesthesiologists, used to a one-on-one relationship with their patients, have to learn to treat many patients simultaneously. Fully trained general surgeons have to deal with the fact that the closest they will actually come to performing surgery, for a whole year, may be putting in a chest tube. Preoperative and postoperative care now will totally occupy their time. Internists in a multidisciplinary unit may be exposed to surgical patients for the first time–and be responsible for their care.

Arriving in a new hospital, often a new city, with perhaps a different spectrum of patients, diseases, and even different cultures, can easily become overwhelming. Listening to others, who have successfully completed their training, and asking the nursing staff (who have certainly been there longer than the new fellow) help to smooth the way while you try to learn the "tricks of the trade" at least for *that* (soon to become *your*) ICU. As the fellow acquires experience and self-confidence, things do become easier.

"Tous les chemins menent à Rome" is a phrase often heard in the French language. Each unit does believe, strangely, that it too, is the central place, that its ways are the "best"; in a way you are reinforcing this perception, for you did go there for training. The new fellow is the "new kid in town" and, early on, has to learn how things are done in that particular unit. It is wise to spend the first few months filling one's head with knowledge, like a dry sponge absorbing water, and learning the unit's routine. Freedom for personal variations on the treatment of certain problems can come only after many months of training and mastering the basics. This freedom, like money in the TV ads, is usually obtained in the old-fashioned way, you "earn it."

ORIENTATION

A good orientation before truly becoming the fellow in charge in the ICU would be ideal. Adjusting to the physical environment, the topography, the equipment, the different teams, nurses, respiratory therapists, and even the phone numbers, can make the transition easier for everyone. Much is expected of the new fellow who, unfortunately, is taking over after a very competent individual has just finished a full year of ICU training. Comparisons inevitably are made. Of course, no one remembers how the predecessor functioned on his or her first day; the memories are of the last days, after much had been learned. Spending a full week learning about the types of ventilators, functioning of the special equipment, on-going protocols in the unit, and techniques for line insertion can avoid heartache. Spending the day with the "on-call" fellow with some experience is the best way of learning the routines. It is evident that the learning process should be on-going but an orientation period would give the new fellow an idea of what to expect before actually being confronted with the responsibility of patient care. Ideally, he or she should be introduced, in addition to the ICU staff, to the different chief residents, attendings, and to the emergency room staff. All of these individuals, with their different personalities, will be interacting with the fellow, and proper introductions make the interaction smoother. Rotations rarely do overlap, making this ideal difficult to accomplish. It is well worth the effort to make some arrangements to spend more time (vacation or electives) to provide this exposure for yourself.

EVOLUTION OF GOALS AND OBJECTIVES

The year of ICU training can be divided into four 3-month periods, in order for the fellow and attendings to be able to evaluate his or her performance and for responsibilities and self-confidence to increase progressively. The newcomer usually evolves from feeling almost totally helpless and calling for advice about almost everything to being almost totally autonomous and calling to let the attending know that he or she is handling a particularly complicated problem. This implies a process through which trust on the part of the attending and a self-awareness of one's own limitation on the part of the fellow have developed. There should be sessions with the fellow and the attendings during which his or her performance is discussed and constructive criticism given. This should preferably occur every 3 months, or sooner if problems arise, so that aspects of the fellow's work can be improved and meaningful learning achieved.

The emphasis in the first 6 months should be to review basic science concepts, which during medical school and residency, are often learned for the sole purpose of passing an exam and then are put away in some remote part of the brain. Because much of ICU care is based on a thorough knowledge of physiology, all physiologic concepts should be reviewed, updated, and made available in quick reach of conscious recall. Pharmacology and drug interactions are also part of everyday ICU life and should be subjected to the same processes. Once all of these concepts are fully integrated, they can be put to good use with full understanding of their implications. During these first 6 months, the fellow will also gain self-confidence and learn–and accommodate to–different practice styles among responsible physicians both within and outside the ICU staff.

The next 3 months should be spent developing skills in handling different problems and emergencies according to one's own style–with guidance. The last 3 months will be spent perfecting that style which usually is composed of a blending of the various styles and personalities encountered during the fellowship. The last day of fellowship and the first day as an attending should be a continuum, a smooth transition rather than a giant step in one's professional life.

It is important for the fellow to understand the actual distribution of authority and responsibility in the ICU. This varies almost infinitely but, today, a faculty member or attending physician is ultimately responsible for the patient's care. This responsibility for care must be combined with the responsibility to teach. Thus, the supervisor must facilitate a sensitive and evolving process of maintaining overall responsibility for the patient yet relinquishing direct control to the fellow. This is also true of the fellow who must learn throughout the year to delegate responsibility to the junior staff to the extent of their capabilities. It is important to communicate information well and to learn when information should be passed on to the attending. This more artistic goal of an ICU fellowship is often more difficult to attain. If uncertain, it is important always to remember to ask for advice *before* rather than *after* the fact. This recommendation will be useful throughout one's career, from the medical student to the full professor.

ORGANIZATION ACCORDING TO TASKS

A very simplistic yet realistic view of the fellow's main task in the unit is to stay in control of everything and ensure smooth operation of the unit as a whole. He or she must become a *reliable* resource for giving advice and information and for handling emergencies. Another task is to become the major "repository of information," gathering, collating, and processing all the data collected by many people from multiple sources, inside and outside the unit. The "junior" ICU physicians, ICU nursing staff, emergency room charts, and referring or primary physicians (including chief residents, senior residents, and attendings), and operating room and anesthesia records have valuable information that the fellow must learn. Processing this data so that it can be documented in the chart is the fellow's responsibility and often requires patience and skill.

Interacting with families of critically ill or dying patients is a part of everyday life for the fellow. No matter what method of communication or hierarchy of responsibility is conceived, the families of the long-term patients always get to know the ICU fellow and rightfully perceive the fellow as a valuable source of information. Unfortunately, prior medical training may not have dealt with the issues of dying nor how to discuss it. Developing these arts during ICU fellowship is done "on the job" but, as difficult as this task may be emotionally, it is a necessary and real part of being a physician and will only make one a better and more caring human being. Death and dying are everyday occurrences in an ICU, even with the best of care; thus, both the issue and the communication must become part of the everyday routine.

When a critically ill patient becomes acutely unstable, delegating responsibility for the emergency measures to the junior staff becomes impossible. Emergency right heart catheterization, central line insertion, and intubation should be handled by the most experienced person, often the ICU fellow. Routine line insertion and patient care can and should be handled by the junior staff: thus, supervision is part of the fellow's training and responsibility. Bedside teaching of physiology and pathophysiology as well should be part of the fellow's responsibilities.

The junior staff may often include different level physicians, ranging from the medical student to the senior resident. Responsibilities should be different for the most junior and the most senior personnel, and they should be tailored not only to the level of training but also to the interest of the individual. Some individuals learn faster than others, others need "spoon feeding" for a longer period of time during this training, still others are on "required" rotations and may have little interest (and even less enthusiasm). The fellow must recognize that too much freedom of action may be dangerous if the resident is not ready or interested. Equally damaging for overall unit function is being too restrictive with more senior residents who may then lose interest and ruin a precious learning experience.

One of the fellow's most important roles is orientation of the junior members. Newcomers in an ICU should sit down with the fellow who should explain the daily schedule, describe what is expected, and answer their questions before they are confronted with working in the unit. Knowing what to expect alleviates anxiety and makes for better and easier working relationships.

PRIORITIZATION

Being organized is one of the keys to success. Planning the workday in an ICU is important, especially since the frequent unpredictable events will add confusion to the best organized schedule. Having an idea of what needs to be accomplished and setting priorities will help bring some sense to the chaos that can be created during the day. I believe that my general approach, though derived in a specific ICU, can be used to relieve some of the uneasiness, if not the real chaos, created by unavoidable simultaneous emergencies.

Assignment of the patients for junior residents should be done *before* rounds as the team "coming on" will pay more attention to the specifics of their own patients when the team "going off" gives report. All of the details of disease and management must be presented and discussed among the responsible physicians, depending on the organization and hierarchy of each unit. Whatever the hierarchy, it is crucial that a single care plan results and is understood by all involved. This may or may not occur at the bedside, but should include the nurse in charge who is responsible for providing the nursing care *and* also may offer important information and insights into the care, the patient, and the family. If these rounds are not made at the bedside, I like to make work rounds which are important in organizing the day at the bedside with the team "coming on." Interacting with the nurse, making sure that the junior staff understands the treatment plan, writing pertinent orders, and reviewing laboratory results, IV fluid orders, and cultures will assure that everyone has the relevant information to facilitate the daily care. This should be done at each patient's bedside and usually takes from 1 to 2 hours in our 12- to 15-bed unit. After these rounds are completed, the junior staff should proceed to study new patients, perform the steps outlined, and gather any additional relevant information.

The time after work rounds is usually best to perform planned line insertions, such as nutritional support, arterial lines, or pulmonary artery catheters before elective (surgical) or emergency admissions arrive. Nurses should preferably have been notified of line changes during bedside work rounds so that they have the necessary materials ready. It is also a good time, depending on visiting hours, to talk to families, answering any of their questions and collecting pertinent information from them. The goal is to accomplish as many routine or daily tasks before new admissions arrive, either scheduled from surgery or unscheduled from the floors, emergency room, or surgery. When they arrive, the pace of activity will increase (see Chap. 17, "Accepting a New Admission"). This can become a busy period, trying to coordinate on-going care of the current ICU patients with many new admissions arriving in a short time. The ICU team will usually be busy until the late afternoon or early evening.

Because many ICU patients are septic, obtaining the results of numerous culture specimens from different sites in the patients on different days and even in different places in the hospital can become a nightmare. Developing an easy yet thorough system for getting this information back to the unit is an achievement. The routine work has to be tailored to each hospital and each unit and, from experience, may take many years to function adequately. Inadequate, sketchy, or "hearsay" information concerning organisms cultured and antibiotic sensitivities definitely adds to confusion in the process of making a diagnosis and selecting appropriate treatment for the septic patients. Time invested in developing a reliable system in the long run is time well spent.

The "on call" schedule may be determined by many factors, including the number of fellows, their responsibilities, or historical precedent. The 24-hour rotation, despite its time-honored history is not as desirable, in my opinion, as 12-hour shifts, alternating days and nights. In a very busy unit, patients obviously do not stop being sick during the night. The last 12 hours of the 24 are more difficult because of fatigue and increasing inefficiency. The 12-hour shift permits a new and rested individual to tackle the night chores and assures around-the-clock patient care (Table 11-1). For example, on a 24-hour call schedule, extubating a patient may be delayed until morning when everyone is more alert and will react more rapidly if a problem arises. On a 12-hour call schedule, extubation can be performed when the patient is deemed "ready" and can safely be done at any hour.

This 12-hour work schedule requires that a complete report be given from the "going off" to the "coming on" fellow. This can easily be accomplished in 30 to 60 minutes, discussing the day's major events, laboratory results, and plans for the following 12 hours. We often make use of a three-way phone call including the responsible ICU attending to transfer the "call" responsibility and update management plans at the same time. The new fellow should, once again, make work rounds at the bedside with the junior staff, reviewing the data and establishing a treatment plan for the night. If things are quiet, everyone may be able to get a little sleep but, most of the time, our ICU patients continue to require acute care 24 hours a day. Most fellows learn to live without sleep during the night, much facilitated by the 12-hour shift concept.

*TABLE 11-1. Four-Week Schedule**

| | WEEK 1 | | WEEK 2 | | WEEK 3 | | WEEK 4 | |
	Day	Night	Day	Night	Day	Night	Day	Night
Monday	1	2	3	4	2	1	4	3
Tuesday	1	2	3	4	2	1	4	3
Wednesday	3	4	1	2	4	3	2	1
Thursday	3	4	1	2	4	3	2	1
Friday	1	2	3	4	2	1	4	3
Saturday	1	2	3	4	2	1	4	3
Sunday	1	2	3	4	2	1	4	3

*A rotation for four fellows working 12-hour shifts which provides continuity of care, changes diurnal patterns every 2 weeks, and has reasonable weekend scheduling.

DOCUMENTATION

Adequate recordkeeping is crucial for medical-legal purposes and also for transmitting information from one care giver to another (see also Chap. 8, "Avoiding Legal Problems"). It is important that all techniques done to a patient are thoroughly documented with their complications if they arise. It is also useful to write an admission note on each new patient, to summarize the patient's course and medications before admission to the unit from either the floor, the operating room, or the emergency room. In order to write a good note, containing information, assessment, and plan, the material must be gathered and processed in the mind of the writer. Good documentation, then, is a stimulus to good thinking and evidence of it. It also provides an up-to-the-minute presentation of the patient, which serves as a good reference for yourself, for others, and for comparisons later on in the course. On a busy day, it is too easy to forget who has had what done, and a good admission note is a marvelous help for a fatigued and failing memory. Progress notes should be written at least every 24 hours, preferably in the early morning hours when all laboratory data is available, radiographs have been seen, and fluid balances have been calculated on the nursing flow sheet. A good well-processed note may take 15 to 20 minutes to complete, even more if the patient's course has been complex or unstable.

The best planned or organized schedule may be difficult to accomplish because of multiple on-going emergencies. Establishing priorities becomes imperative. This sometimes proves difficult because each nurse, team, or attending considers his or her own problem to be the most acute and important. Resolution of conflicts is yet another of the arts of the ICU fellow.

The ICU is a stressful environment, often with more than one person requiring attention and with more than one person wanting to ask a question at the same time. It becomes an interesting and necessary exercise in self-control to stay on top of the situation and in control of one's own emotions and temper, especially when tired. Yet, understanding and controlling one's reactions to this level of stress may be one of the most important objectives and accomplishments of the fellowship and should be discussed openly. Ultimately, we realize that many have gone through the same reaction and that they are, for the most part, healthy.

CONCLUSION

I believe that an ICU fellowship is a worthwhile, sometimes thrilling, sometimes overwhelming experience. Understanding and applying basic physiology to patient care is the scientific aspect of the fellowship.

Humanizing patient care, interacting with families, nurses, and different medical teams, and developing a sense of organization and priority can be called the more artistic side of the fellowship. It may be difficult to remember that behind the ventilator, at the end of the pulmonary artery catheter and all the IV lines, is a human being with a family. This perspective is the most important to recognize to maintain an active and long-term role in bedside ICU patient care.

Interest in ICU training and care has boomed in the past 15 years. A stimulating ICU fellowship for someone willing to go through an additional year of training makes it easy to understand why the interest is so great.

Finally, in the words of Elliott Hubbard, "Don't take life too seriously. You'll never get out of it alive."[2]

REFERENCES

1. Selye H: *Stress Without Distress*, p 20. New York, The New American Library, 1974
2. Peter LS, Dana B: *The Laughter Prescription*, p 133. New York, Ballantine Books, 1982

Getting Along in the ICU: Physician Interrelationships

12

Peter Angood

THE SURGEON AND THE ICU

As surgical and anesthetic techniques and postoperative care continue to improve, surgeons will continue to expand indications for operation and include more severely compromised patients. Before the development of intensive care units (ICUs) and "intensivists," surgeons directed the entire postoperative course of their patients. Since surgeons pioneered the development of physiologic perioperative care in the past, they were also intimately involved in the care of their patients during the ICU portion of a patient's hospital admission. This practice has, of necessity, changed in the last number of years. The patients in the ICU are now generally more ill and have major physiologic changes occurring with increased frequency. At the same time, the surgeons are spending longer hours in the operating rooms doing more extensive operations, doing patient consultations, or performing often lengthy outpatient procedures. They are also spending more time on documentation and paper work for these procedures. Overall, this makes them less available for the minute-to-minute requirements of patient care in the ICU. The evolution of this aspect of health care has resulted in the presence of full-time ICU personnel, with specialized training in critical care, to care for the patients in the surgeon's absence. This has also naturally led to the capacity, and need, for the ICU environment to become a center of on-going education at many different levels. Obviously, there are now many people caring for the patients, whereas, in the past only a handful were involved.

This blossoming of personnel in the ICU has many benefits for the patient in terms of continual care, but at the same time carries many potential problems in patient management. The surgeons themselves are at risk for losing control and contact with their patients in the ICU, while just the opposite should be occurring during this most dynamic phase of the hospital stay.

I shall discuss many aspects of how the operating surgeon and the ICU must interact to maintain optimal patient management; in addition, relationships with other physicians create different needs that will be described as well. The interaction with surgeons will be highlighted because the surgeon's role is usually perceived as more active, direct, and personal because of the relationship created in the operating room. There must be well-understood responsibilities for each member of the teams involved, as well as an efficient communication network so that both the surgical and the ICU teams are aware of the degree of illness or wellness of the patients. The system should facilitate effective patient management and allow for achievement of the expectations the teams have for each other and for the patients' outcomes.

MEMBERS OF THE TEAMS

The identification of various members on both the surgical and ICU teams is important before further discussion of their roles can be undertaken (Fig. 12-1).

The ICU fellow should be considered the central figure with whom most other team members come into contact for patient information, and he or she carries the most responsibility for communicating the patient's status to the others. Although the attendings on both the surgical and ICU teams have ultimate legal responsibility for the patients, the interaction between the ICU fellow and the surgical team seniors is the level on which many decisions reflecting changes in management occur. The fellows and team seniors (both surgical and non surgical) are responsible for recognizing which decisions need confirmation by their respective attendings and then to gain

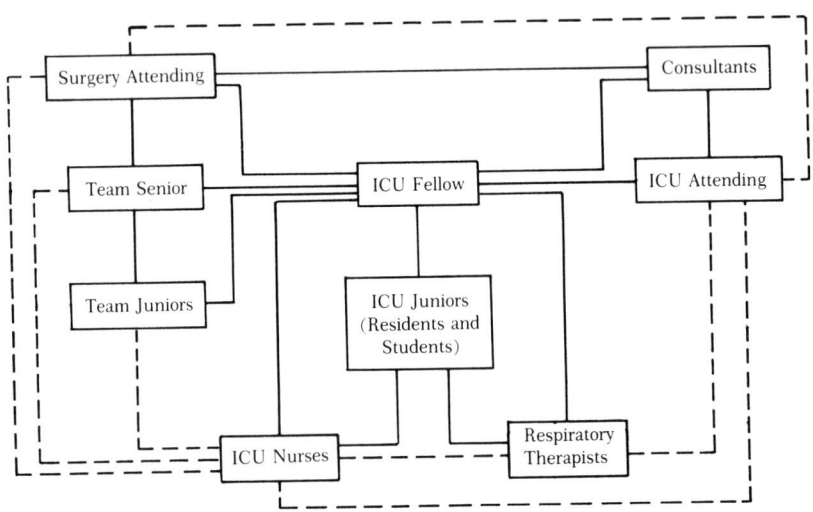

FIGURE 12-1. *Diagram illustrating the interrelationships among ICU personnel. Communication is centralized in the Fellow. Solid lines indicate commonly used routes; dotted lines signify available avenues that are used less frequently.*

feedback in those instances. The consulting services are just that, consultants, but they may be brought into the patient's management at the request of either the ICU or surgical team. The nurses in the ICU are vital not only for nursing care of the patient but also for keeping the ICU fellow abreast of the patient's condition. The same holds true for the respiratory therapists and the ICU fellow in terms of the goals for respiratory management. Although given the least responsibility as far as patient management decisions, the junior members of both the surgical and ICU teams are important. They are in the early stages of their careers and training, and it is often their seemingly naive or innocent questioning that many times leads the "elders" to change perspectives on a patient's care.

ROLES, RESPONSIBILITIES, FREEDOMS, AND LIMITATIONS

For patient management to remain complete and efficient in a busy ICU setting, each member of a team must understand the responsibilities, freedoms, and limitations of his or her own role and those of the others as well. Functioning in these roles is often learned "on the job" through gradual familiarization with the local "unwritten rules and customs." Given the larger number of personnel involved in ICU care nowadays, however, better delineation of roles is important to avoid confusion, overlap, and even confrontation in patient management. The understanding of these roles enables all involved physicians to form realistic expectations of each other's capacities, not only in tasks performed, but also in achieving a successful patient outcome. A *brief* description of these roles, responsibilities, freedoms, and limitations follows, recognizing, of course, that variations occur in most institutions. The fundamental principles by which we operate are that responsibility is shared, that unilateral or arbitrary decisions compromise the overall quality of care, and that communication not only avoids confrontation but also, more importantly, allows varied input which often serves to clarify difficult management decisions.

THE SURGICAL ATTENDING

In terms of overall patient responsibility, the surgery attending is the *most* important. His or her role should be to provide the patient with the most continual care and valid information so the patient can understand what to expect during the course of the illness. The attending should orchestrate the patient care, direct the technical aspects of the surgery itself, and educate all those helping manage the patient.

For private patients, the surgery attending usually has the first patient contact in the office preoperatively and is ultimately responsible for the patient's pre-, intra-, and posthospital care, as well as the long-term follow-up. For the nonprivate patients, he or she is also ultimately responsible to guarantee the best management of those patients cared for through the hospital clinics. These responsibilities should not be dismissed once the patient enters an ICU. Communication from the surgical attending to the ICU team on the goals for a patient's care is vital. This allows the ICU team members to be cognizant of those goals and allows their input as to the success or failure of the goals. The acceptance of these responsibilities by the surgery attending has even more ramifications in today's litiginous society.

Given the important role, the surgical attending should, therefore, have a healthy degree of freedom for directing care in those patients who require ICU management. Given the responsibility, the attending should exercise the control and provide goal orientation during rounds on these patients at least daily and through regular communication with the ICU team. This interaction aids in realistic expectations on both sides as to the best care for a patient from surgical and critical care perspectives.

Although control of patient care by the surgical attending is of prime importance, some limitations should be exercised. Critical care has progressed rapidly in recent years, and some aspects of a patient's management should be left to the ICU team, whose knowledge of critical care equipment, techniques, and pharmacology is usually more detailed and current. Therefore, they are more aptly qualified to make the many adjustments in daily patient intensive care.

THE SURGERY TEAM SENIORS

The role of the senior residents (usually considered to be in the fourth and fifth years) on a surgery team is varied. They are the instruments through which the surgical attendings can maintain minute-to-minute management of the patients without needing to be physically present. The senior residents should be continually aware of all their patients' status and able to manage the problems without an excess of supervision. Their interaction with the ICU team is, therefore, vital. They provide an essential link between the ICU team and the surgery attending. They are also able to provide assistance in managing the many minor surgical problems as they arise (*e.g.*, opening an infected wound and doing the initial dressing changes).

We believe that the responsibilities of team seniors should include twice daily rounds on the ICU patients, writing admission/discharge orders on ICU patients, reviewing surgical medications (antibiotics), arranging for nonroutine investigations or consultations, communicating needs for admissions and scheduling of surgical procedures (both in main operating rooms or at the ICU bedside) to the ICU physicians, and coordinating with the nurses on issues such as the timing of complex dressing changes. They should always be readily available for consultation on the ICU patients and should respond to the paging system promptly when called by the ICU.

Being so closely involved with the ICU patients should naturally allow the team seniors much freedom in the ICU. As they have progressed through their training program, the General Surgery residents usually have a good understanding of a team senior's range of duties with respect to the ICU.

Their intimate association with the patients and ICU team is usually good-natured, often based on the camaraderie developed during their own ICU rotations. The senior residents from the subspecialty services are less involved with the ICU on a regular basis and often need prompting to recognize these freedoms and the necessity to be involved with the patients in the ICU.

The limitations senior residents have in the ICU are similar to those of the surgery attendings. They should not expect to order intensive care-type interventions directly (*e.g.*, dopamine infusions) without first discussing it with the ICU team, nor should they expect to be able to wander into the ICU at a moment's notice to perform bedside procedures without forewarning. The arrangements necessary to send a patient for special procedures, including transportation and support from nurses, respiratory therapists, and junior staff, need to be discussed beforehand to ensure the patient is stable for, and during, transfer and that the manpower is available.

THE ICU ATTENDING

An ICU attending has a diversified role. He or she should have a strong understanding of physiology and pathophysiology, be well grounded in the knowledge of managing critical care patients, have background knowledge of the technical aspects of the monitors and equipment, be a stimulating researcher and an effective educator on multiple levels, be a diplomatic manager and politician, and have the empathy required to deal with dying patients and their families.

Coupled with this diverse role are many responsibilities. The ICU attending has the ultimate responsibility for the patients during their stay in the ICU and, therefore, must have knowledge of not only the medical care, but also the nursing and respiratory care of patients. He or she should be able to maintain an appropriate degree of supervision for his or her delegates of patient care (ICU fellows) and yet not be meddlesome in their educational experiences. The attending must always be ready to discuss management with his or her delegates, the surgery teams, the nurses, the respiratory therapists, and the patient or families. He or she is usually ultimately responsible for decisions relating to admissions or discharges to the ICU. He or she may be involved in specific management decisions of the extremely ill patients and be able to settle any disputes among the various teams or ICU members.

We believe that the ICU attending should have the final say in the management of the ICU and its patients. He or she must be able to effect this position, not arbitrarily, but diplomatically through accessing and processing information and forming judgments, otherwise he or she will soon be deemed an ineffective manager. This also, necessarily, puts the attending in the position of having to be involved, at least to some degree, in hospital policy planning and formation so the ICU's function and integrity are not lost to the hospital administration.

Despite having seemingly unlimited freedoms, the ICU attending should recognize some limitations in responsibility. Most importantly, he or she should be able to *not* become overly involved in the minute-to-minute management of patients or the ICU itself. There is a necessity for the ICU fellows, surgery teams, nurses, and ICU juniors to have some freedom to get educational value from their ICU experiences. An effective ICU attending is in essence, therefore, an effective manager.

THE ICU FELLOW AND THE SURGICAL TEAM

As noted above, the ICU fellow is the pivotal figure in the ICU in most respects. The other aspects of fellowship and the fellow's functions in the ICU are well discussed in Chapter 11, "ICU Fellowship: Blending Science and Art." A brief description of the fellow's interaction with the surgical team follows.

The primary role of the ICU fellow is to effect the plan of care for *the surgeon's patients* and to keep the surgical team informed of the anticipated or unanticipated changes the patients manifest. He or she accomplishes this overall objective with the assistance of the ICU attending as required.

The responsibilities, freedoms, and limitations of this role are continually changing for the ICU fellow as more knowledge and experience are gained throughout the fellowship period. Of utmost importance, however, is ongoing communication and assessment with the ICU attending responsible for the ICU. Any difficulties between the fellow and the ICU or surgical teams necessitates immediate resolution to guarantee patient safety and smooth functioning of the unit.

CONSULTANTS

A consultant's role should be to answer the specific questions that are asked by the ICU or surgical teams. This expectation can be realized only if specific questions are formulated *and* communicated directly. Relying on a hastily written consult form in the chart will usually result in unnecessary and even unwanted and/or unwarranted opinions about other aspects of management and no real answer to the problem. The ICU and surgical teams have a better understanding of the patient's overall condition and usually just require assistance on specific problems or need specific skills associated with a consulting specialty. Initiation of a consult from the ICU is also done to ensure proper long-term management or follow-up of a patient's condition (*e.g.*, chronic ischemic heart disease).

A responsible consulting service should evaluate the new consults expeditiously and then provide regular follow-up, as needed, without further prompting. The consultation results should be brought to the attention of the ICU fellow. The service should also have senior members of their team doing the ICU consults and not the most inexperienced members. This saves not only time, but often a great deal of confusion. As for procedures to be done by a consulting team, they are responsible for notifying and coordinating the best time of the procedure with the ICU. They should also coordinate the assembling of all needed equipment.

The consultants have the obvious freedom to suggest whatever they deem required for a patient. However, they should not expect this to occur without discussing the pertinent aspects of their suggestions with the ICU team. Today, it is preferable to have the discussion orally before committing remarks to the legal record (the patient's chart). They are consultants and should not expect to have all their suggestions followed.

As implied above, the consult teams have strict, but necessary, limitations on their actual input to patient management. This screening process not only avoids confusion in patient care but also helps guarantee that the results of a consultation are communicated to the responsible physicians.

THE ICU JUNIORS

The role of the juniors on rotation through an ICU is straightforward. They are in the ICU to learn the basics of caring for a critically ill patient and recognizing the physiologic abnormalities. They learn some of the management skills for these patients primarily through passive association, data collection, and supervised procedures.

Their responsibilities are few. The juniors should be expected to participate in the formal daily teaching rounds and to spend on-call periods in the ICU. During the on-call periods, they are assigned patients, and they are then responsible for collecting data, analyzing it, and formulating an assessment and management plan. Even though their management plan may not be implemented in its entirety, the juniors are able to develop some of the cognitive skills required in managing critically ill patients. They should give formal presentations of their patients during the teaching rounds the following day and receive immediate feedback on their understanding, assessment, and skills.

The junior ICU staff have limited freedoms and many limitations. This is a reflection of their inexperience and should be a built-in design factor to ensure patient safety—at the same time allowing them access to the patients for educational purposes. They should have a strictly defined and limited role in both care and communication because of the limited comprehension which is an anticipated accompaniment of their limited knowledge and experience.

THE SURGERY TEAM JUNIORS

In our institution, these people have essentially no role in the ICU. They learn of the patients often at the surgery team's service rounds and only occasionally come to review a patient on their own, perhaps reflecting other demands on their time or lack of initiative since an active role has been precluded. This system is not necessarily correct but the tradition is hard to change. The surgery team juniors should be encouraged, however, to visit the patient during the ICU course of a patient's hospital admission. This will provide them with a more complete picture on the course of a patient's illness, for they will be returned to a more active role in the patient's care once the patient is discharged from the ICU.

THE NURSES

The nurses in an ICU have important roles not only in each patient's nursing care, but also in the overall function of the ICU. A full discussion of the roles, responsibilities, freedoms, and limitations for nursing in the ICU is beyond the scope of this chapter. Suffice it to say, the surgeon should include communication with the ICU nurses in the daily assessment and management of his or her patients. The nurses can provide valuable information on a patient's general physiologic response to illness, as well as the responses of the family and patient according to their perception of the illness.

THE RESPIRATORY THERAPISTS

Again, a full discussion on the functions of the respiratory therapists in the ICU is beyond the scope of this chapter. These people interact with the ICU physicians more than physicians from outside the unit, but if approached, may offer information on the respiratory status of a patient or information on the ever-changing modes of ventilatory support and types of equipment.

COMMUNICATION

The smooth functioning of any system is dependent on effective communication. This is the keystone in critical care patient management, and its importance needs only to be underscored by the reality that mistakes resulting from miscommunication may be life-threatening and lethal.

The various teams and the ICU team should be in regular contact throughout any particular day. The amount of communication required among the various members will vary with the positions, personalities, and capabilities of the team members. Coming to understand which individual requires which degree of interaction can only be learned through experience.

The ICU fellow has the central role in coordinating all the communications because he or she has the most information on the patients. The strongest communication links are with the ICU attending, the team seniors, and the nurses. Lesser degrees of communication, but equally important links, exist between the ICU fellow and virtually all other members of all teams.

The ICU attending depends heavily on the ICU fellow for on-going updates on the patients and together they make management decisions. Prior to these decisions, the ICU attending often interacts with other attendings or the team senior to clarify problems or institute therapy not discussed previously. In general, ordinary and familiar care rarely requires special discussion. On the other hand, when problems are encountered, it is generally in everyone's best interest (starting with the patient) that discussion occurs before decisions are finalized.

The attending physician has not too dissimilar a function from the ICU attending. He or she is dependent on the team senior for updates on patient care and often must seek out the ICU fellow or attending for clarification of ICU management plans. Their delineation of goals and plans for total management is essential so that the ICU team can optimize patient care. In coordination with these goals, for instance, the multiple trauma patient improving from respiratory failure should not be extubated the night before a planned orthopedic procedure under general anesthesia.

Interaction between the team seniors and ICU fellow provides much of the minor decision-making. These decisions often need not even be relayed to the attending level. The number and magnitude of such decisions should become greater as experience is gained. Moving from minor to major decision-making is encouraged in the teaching environment, if learning is to occur. Limits or boundaries should be expressed through communication with the attendings.

The actual content of communications between the ICU fellow and the team seniors will again vary with *who* the individuals involved are. In general, much of *what* is discussed is covered in the discussion above on roles and responsibilities, while the *where* of communicating can be almost anyplace. *When* to communicate may lead to problems unless all major deteriorations in a patient's condition are made known to all four of the above individuals, regardless of the time of day or night. Major improvements in a patient may at times be cause for celebration, but that information should usually be enjoyed over morning coffee. *Why* communicate? It helps guarantee the most effective patient management by ensuring all relevant data pass among these key individuals before decision-making in the patient's care.

The above four people are the quantum necessary for proper ICU management. Their interrelationships should be open and direct, forming a foundation of honesty and trust that can be relied on for many patients.

UNCOMMUNICATED EXPECTATIONS

Despite the effectiveness of a well-managed system with open communication, there are always unexpressed emotions and expectations present. In a critical care setting, these often arise when patients suffer technical or iatrogenic complications or in difficult patient management problems, especially when death is likely.

THE SURGEON'S EXPECTATIONS OF THE ICU

Having invested a great deal of time and effort on a patient's surgery and care, the surgeon usually has the highest expectations, often presenting an *optimistic* attitude on the patient's outlook. A patient's survival may be interpreted by the surgeon as a measure of his sense of self-worth—a dead patient equating with low or negligible self-worth. This sounds extreme, but only serves to emphasize how the surgeon may come to regard the patient whose condition is worsening. He or she may then develop seemingly unrealistic expectations for the ICU management of a patient. He or she wants to believe that intensive care management will guarantee a successful outcome. A surgeon many times will focus only on the positive aspects of a patient's status and seem to ignore the negatives. He or she can even come to feel the ICU team is pestering him with unwanted details if there are more negative than positive parameters on a patient. Clearly, if these perceptions and attitudes affect the overall direction of care, resolution must be achieved at the level of the surgical and ICU attendings so that the other team members are not drawn into conflicts or subjected to ethical problems.

THE ICU's EXPECTATIONS OF THE SURGEON

Because many long-term ICU patients die after similar courses of progressive multiple system failure and sepsis, the ICU team often has a *pessimistic* outlook on a patient's course. They may at times seem almost anxious to withdraw support on some patients and "spare" themselves (and the patients) the extra supportive efforts necessary to maintain a patient only to have the patient die anyway in the next few days or weeks. The ICU team may often wonder why a surgeon cannot realize that further interventions are futile, and in extreme cases may even wish that the surgeon would not appear in the ICU to see his patients because it leads to so many conflicting emotions and ethical uncertainties.

FINDING THE BALANCE

Obviously, there are many differences and possible disputes on the direction of care for a difficult patient problem. The importance of open communication and honesty resurfaces because on-going interaction is needed to resolve the issues, not avoidance of the issues. Specially scheduled conferences among the surgical and ICU teams, with the four key personnel (the ICU attending and fellow plus the surgical attending and senior) involved as a minimum, may be required to not necessarily solve all the issues, but to at least develop a unified, mutually agreeable approach to the patient's management. This not only enhances the patient's care but also provides uniformity in the information given to the patients and families. The wishes of the patient should directly (if competent) or indirectly through the family (if the patient is incompetent) be sought and included in the discussion between the surgical and ICU teams. Without this unified approach, the patient's best interests will not be served and, unfortunately, the miscommunications can serve to stimulate legal action, even in the absence of any negligence.

Perhaps the desire to create the numerous illness severity scoring systems rested on the hope that they might help in the management of these conflicts. Objective information would enable the surgeons and the ICU personnel to find common ground more readily as they approach the issues from their, at times, divergent orientations. Unfortunately, no such help is presently available for the very data included in these various systems are the basis for the repeated clinical assessments which do not reliably differentiate between survivors and nonsurvivors.

SPECIAL SITUATIONS

This section is not meant for descriptions or solutions of the infinite variety of special situations that arise between the various physicians involved and the ICU. They can usually be resolved by special attention to communication.

Much of which has been discussed so far, however, centers on the ICU team and the General Surgery teams. The subspecialty services are now using the ICUs more frequently as the benefits of the ICU have become recognized. Interaction of these services and the ICU is a special situation which deserves mention.

The subspecialty teams usually have a more restricted focus and less experience with overall patient management necessary in the ICU and tend, therefore, to "give-over" the care of the patient to the ICU team, ready to resume a direct role only at the end of the patient's ICU stay. This is healthy up to a point. The ICU team is comfortable with most critical care and general management problems as they arise, but often is uncomfortable with the specific problems related to the subspecialties (*e.g.,* balanced orthopedic traction or plugged, special-drainage catheters). The subspecialty teams should not "park" their patients in the ICU but should continue close follow-up throughout the ICU admission. They need to be aware of the progress of their patients and available to assist the ICU team with specific problems. On the other hand, the ICU team should recognize that fully autonomous management of these patients is beyond their capabilities and should continue to keep the subspecialty surgical teams posted on the developments with their patients. The ICU team must remember its involvement with a patient is usually transient, and it cannot provide continuity of care for a patient's entire illness.

CONCLUSION

Surgical patients being cared for in the ICU often will be extremely labile and have many complex physiologic and pathophysiologic processes in action. Management of these processes now is usually better in the hands of experienced critical care personnel who can remain physically present at the bedside. The patients, however, shall also continue to have difficult surgical management problems and complications. This requires the operating surgeon to maintain close contact with and input on the patient's management. The ICU has positive impact on patient care, but the ICU team must remember it is responsible for the patients on only a temporary basis. The operating surgeon has ultimate responsibility for the patient's hospital care and long-term follow-up. Close communication among the team members in open and honest relationships is the ideal and should ensure smooth function in this complex environment.

Patients of other physicians create similar situations that must be resolved by developing appropriate limits and freedoms. Many other physicians, too, interact with the ICU team. The most effective care will result from careful integration and mutual respect.

Understanding Reactions of Patient and Family

13

George L. Wallace–Barnhill

I believe it would be beneficial if the medical profession learned to recognize and accept the psychological dynamics that permeate the intensive care unit (ICU) environment. Physicians need to recognize that all injury, regardless of severity, but most certainly critical injury, is more than a *physiologic* event.

When patients and families are faced with the crisis of an ICU experience, few are prepared for the physical trauma or the often devastating psychological repercussions they must endure.

Advancements in medical technology, particularly with invasive monitoring equipment, have changed the process of dying in America. It is now estimated that of the people who will die within the next year, 80% will die in hospitals or nursing homes. This makes it important for physicians to understand and to communicate with patients and families, particularly during times of extended crises and uncertainty.

There is a great need to *humanize* the ICU and provide honest communication with patients and families. Our task is to provide an environment in which families can learn to cope with their emotions during these crises. Understanding these psychological factors can lead to more productive medical interventions in the broad sense, by not restricting our point of view to procedures and medications.

PSYCHOLOGICAL CONCEPTS

Most people are familiar enough with psychological terminology to recognize the term "defense mechanisms." However, most nonprofessional personnel do not comprehend the concepts behind defense mechanisms, or more importantly, what purposes they serve and why they are implemented.

Few experiences in life force us to recognize our humanness and vulnerability more than those which place us out of control of our lives or the life of someone we love. There is no better example of this than that of a family facing the crisis of having a loved one in an ICU.

Physicians are not aware of or even very knowledgeable about the psychological dynamics that permeate the ICU environment. However, there are some common psychological problems whose consequences could be tempered, if recognized and properly assessed by the health care team.

The impact of these psychological dimensions on families can be devastating. Fully comprehending the physical injury that has befallen a loved one can be enough to render even a well-adjusted family unstable, at least temporarily. During the first 24 to 48 hours of their crisis, families usually deal with feelings of denial, fear, and loss of control.

DENIAL

Denial is a common term used to define a personal mechanism of defense against the reality of a given situation. This deception (denial) is an attempt to disavow the existence of unpleasant reality. Among adults it is probably more accurately described as a resistance.

In addition, denial aids a person's efforts to filter information. Because of its use in limiting absorption to only positive information, people using this defense frequently make poor judgments. At best, this mechanism is only a temporary reprieve from the realities of the circumstances that stimulated the denial response. Therefore, denial provides a very useful albeit temporary purpose by allowing time to accept the reality of a given situation at a pace that is more tolerable to one's senses.

It is crucial for physicians to establish open lines of two-way communication with families. The initial interactions during this crisis are vitally important and determine the pattern and degree of communication through the ordeal. The manner in which the news of a life-threatening situation is presented to families is extremely important to subsequent treatment. Family members' initial reactions, including shock and denial, may interfere with the effective communication and clarity of understanding.

Although patients and families have difficulty totally comprehending bad news, it is *no* news that is the most difficult to assess. Therefore, even disheartening news *should* be presented. The manner in which it is presented is important, as is the attitude of the presenter. The attending physician primarily responsible for the ICU treatment should relay the initial information to the family and therefore set the tone for all subsequent family contacts. Families are usually most receptive if medical information is presented in a straightforward manner with carefully chosen, simple words.

FEAR

Regardless of how family members present themselves, whether stoic, seemingly unemotional and in control, or out of control and behaving hysterically, the most overriding concern is fear of death for their loved one.

The fear is related to accepting the reality of a loved one's near-death condition and is awesome. However, as family members begin to verbalize their fears, this should be viewed as an improvement over their use of denial. Their confrontation of these fears and anxieties should be supported by the

ICU team. Families should be encouraged to discuss openly their feelings regarding the uncertainty of the circumstances.

It is impossible to determine exactly how each family will respond to this stressful circumstance. Most families are well aware of their psychological dynamics, and they are cognizant of the extent to which these forces are in play, even if they are not aware of terminology. An emotionally threatened family can usually be reassured if ICU personnel simply accept their sometimes dramatic emotional shifts rather than rushing in to provide a resolution. The willingness of families to express their thoughts and feelings is directly related to how they perceive their acceptance by the ICU staff. In other words, family members will usually withdraw if they sense that it is unsafe for them to express their emotions openly. Often families control their feelings and behavior in such a manner as to protect the staff from being uncomfortable. If this situation continues, it may have a negative effect on the physician–family relationship throughout the course of treatment. Therefore, it is recommended that there be a personal exchange of honest information and emotions to reduce the level of fear inherent in every family during crisis.

Although certain emotional or psychological responses are to be expected, the actual process of dealing with these powerful feelings is unique to each family. Therefore, ICU personnel and physicians in particular should become involved with families as soon as possible and establish a supportive relationship of communication and care. With the exception of the knowledge that their loved one is receiving medical treatment, the physician's attitude is the second most important factor for families.

Physicians must become aware of their own personal feelings of discomfort and uncertainty in dealing with families. When families are offered the physician's human side with his or her doubts, fears, and frequently the inability to predict the outcome for loved ones, families' tensions are reduced. Effective management of their own discomfort is a first step for ICU personnel in supporting their patients' and families' emotional responses.

LOSS OF CONTROL

In addition to the initial shock, the need for temporary denial, and the fear engendered in a crisis, families feel *immobilized* by their inability to control the outcome of the patient's life. These feelings of helplessness exaggerate the alteration in the family homeostasis. A time period of family disintegration will ensue until some meaningful role or sense of worth can be established for each family member. There are many factors that affect the time required for this family adjustment. They include the following:

1. Age and importance of the patient to the family
2. Number of family members directly involved
3. Individual relationships within the family

4. Amount of interpersonal stress at the time of the crisis
   5. General psychological stability of the family unit.

Other less tangible familial factors include feelings of guilt or responsibility for things said or done, petty jealousy, competitiveness, hostilities, and interpersonal differences.

The ICU staff should learn to recognize and accept the onset of these dynamics among family members. Physicians and nurses should be concerned if there is an absence of emotion demonstrated by family members. There are many variations of emotional response among individual families and cultures with different ethnic and religious backgrounds. These differences make it impossible to prescribe an acceptable set of responses appropriate for all situations. Anger or even rage are common emotional responses among patients' families during acute periods of crisis. If unresolved, these feelings may cause further disintegration within a family struggling to stabilize itself. In extreme circumstances, these feelings may lead to the destruction of some relationships within the family structure. Although most people seem to believe that emergency or family crisis situations have a tendency to pull family members together, and to bring out the best in everyone involved, in actuality this assumption is usually only valid for families who already have strong, healthy relationships. For less stable families the crisis situation tends to exacerbate their problems and drive them further apart.

STAFF INVOLVEMENT WITH FAMILIES

Staff response to family members is crucial to the establishment of emotional and behavioral stability for all concerned. As family members gain access to more and more information about what is going on, it reduces, rather than increases, their anxieties and fears. Knowing what is happening to the patient, even if negative, is less frightening than not knowing. This direct involvement with families helps them cope more effectively with feelings of helplessness and addresses their sense of immobilization regarding the patient. This acceptance and involvement of the family by the ICU staff permits the family to focus their fears and concerns more constructively. In addition, it provides a psychological sense of communal spirit of purpose, and it gives the family a feeling not only of worth but of much needed hope.

Physicians and patients or their families should talk with each other honestly on a daily basis. Decisions should be made through meaningful dialogue and compromise. This patient–physician interchange is based on the concept that patients are not only the recipients of medical decision-making but active participants as well. Further, this decision-making approach is a process among the primary people involved and based on the premise that the best decisions and treatment for a particular patient are most likely to emerge from this process.

Even though patients and families are encouraged to participate as well as take serious responsibilities for critical care decisions, it is the physician's obligation to not only initiate but to guide the decision-making process.

The task of effectively representing the ICU's or hospital's position regarding what are often life-threatening circumstances should not be left to the least experienced personnel. The perceptions and impressions, real and imagined, that families glean from these meetings will have a powerful and lasting impact on all concerned.

Physicians need to accept families as a part of their treatment responsibility. Working with families for the benefit of the patient decreases the probabilities that disgruntled family members may react out of fear, threat, or ignorance and seek recourse by personal or legal means.

HOW TO INVOLVE FAMILIES

Dealing with families will become easier if the following suggestions are considered. The physician must honestly assess his or her personal reaction and feelings about a given family. If the personal feelings are positive it will be easier to talk with them. The family members will recognize that the physician likes them and conclude that this means he or she *cares* about the patient. This process of interaction is actually quite simple and may take only a short time. This initial receptiveness will reduce family members' initial fears and uncertainties substantially. Often, however, a physician's personal response to a given family may be neutral or at times even negative. On these occasions it is best to recognize and admit one's inward feelings are real, particularly if the feelings are negative. No one is a Pollyanna and, therefore, each of us will have some negative reactions. Acceptance of these feelings is very important. The more the physician permits himself or herself to experience these negative feelings without guilt or judgment, the more accepting he or she will become of himself or herself. This process further reduces any tension or hesitation on the part of the physician and allows him or her to interact with the family in a more relaxed attitude. In other words, his or her manner will not project those inner feelings of negativism to the family. Often physicians inadvertently deal directly with families without regard to or identification of these inner feelings. When this occurs, families respond to the negativism that is being displayed unwittingly by the physician. This type of interchange creates tension and mistrust between family members and the ICU physician. These initial impressions are very real and tend to be long-lasting. Therefore, close attention and some mental preparation can go far in promoting a healthier and more effective treatment approach for all concerned. Occasionally, it may be necessary and simpler to arrange for a substitute to communicate with a particular family. The establishment of a positive interchange with family members will directly improve their cooperation throughout the patient's course of treatment.

For example, with a family in which the above-mentioned *positive* rapport has been established, flexible visiting hours may be permitted. For

ICU patients, loss of physical and psychological contact with familiar surroundings and loved ones is stressful. Therefore, additional visiting time with family members may decrease emotional as well as physical stress and positively contribute to the recovery process. These family members will create fewer problems regarding interactions with other ICU personnel. In addition, this positive arrangement between physician and family permits the establishment of meeting times between a designated family representative and a staff person. This process saves staff time and effort trying to cope with many members of the same family.

Meeting with a family representative should be scheduled on a regular basis. A private office or room should be designated for this purpose. This not only helps to reinforce trust and confidentiality but also provides a meeting place where additional family members can be told the content of the meeting. Last, it provides a haven for family members to share emotions and console each other in times of grief.

Families who are provided this attention and personal as well as professional response are almost always better prepared to handle decisions regarding medical, legal, or ethical considerations such as termination of life support, discontinuing aggressive treatment, or do not resuscitate (DNR) orders. With these families it is often possible to discuss openly their contingency plans if death for the patient becomes imminent. In dealing with families it is crucial to remember that hope for survival of their loved one is the most important factor in their ability to cope, regardless of the medical odds. The ICU personnel should be as supportive and as reassuring as possible to the patients' families. Most people can eventually accept and deal with even the gravest of situations if they are given some hope. However, at times it is extremely difficult for staff members to accurately assess the psychological needs of each family member. There are families that are not prepared for or capable of accepting, hearing, or interpreting the truth. In this situation emotional tension between the family and the staff may develop. However, it is important for the ICU staff to recognize that a family's negative behavioral reactions are usually a reflection of feelings of uncertainty and dread, and should not, therefore, be taken personally. For these reasons it may be more helpful to limit the depth of information given to families unless details and more complete information are requested. Even though this may seem paradoxical, it is wise to keep in mind that although families outwardly say that they want to know everything, they secretly wish to hear only good news about their loved one. Remember, for families each hour of each day may be filled with hopes and expectations that are often totally unrealistic. The dreaded feeling that the disease or injury may ultimately prove fatal is constantly present, although rarely· expressed. Also, there are times when this combination of feelings that have them on a roller coaster ride are mixed with brief thoughts that perhaps the patient should die so that suffering would end. It is difficult to tolerate the constant pressure of seeing a loved one near death without having some degree of optimism. Family members must focus so much energy on maintaining a positive hopeful attitude that often discouraging news is either not heard or is denied so that a false sense of optimism may prevail.

There are families who are not receptive to even the most appropriate of staff responses. The interactions with these families are more complicated. It needs to be determined what factors are precipitating the negative responses. As described earlier, for the most part they are normal defense mechanisms which are incorporated into the families' behavior to provide a way to cope with the crisis. For example, family members realize that their loved one is not "getting well," and they cannot or will not accept the reality that the patient is dying. The next step may be to defend against the reality of this information by reasoning that if the patient were receiving the best medical treatment he would be getting well. Since he is not getting better then he *must not* be receiving the best treatment, and as a result of this "psychological rationalization" and factual distortion the family becomes verbally and behaviorally dissatisfied with the ICU staff. Recognizing and understanding this common phenomenon among patients' families may help prevent negative or inappropriate responses by ICU personnel. In other words staff must deal directly with the underlying problem (fear of their loved one's death) rather than focusing on the behavioral symptoms presented by the family. If staff can accept this temporary state of affairs, usually the uncooperative behavior will dissipate. When necessary, however, it may be prudent to have a mental health professional evaluate the family. We do not live in the best of all possible worlds, and "difficult" families do exist, despite our best, most learned, and most compassionate efforts. A consultant could evaluate the psychological dynamics of the family as a unit and assess their psychological strengths and weaknesses. They could also provide appropriate alternative approaches to dealing more effectively with the family. Last, if the family unit or any individual member of the family is seriously disturbed, appropriate recommendations and referral for treatment can be offered at this time.

THE PATIENT IN THE ICU

With the exception of a concentration camp there is probably no more terrifying situation than to be in an ICU. There is the constant fear of death, even though for some there is a temporary feeling of omnipotence for having survived the disease or injury that caused them to be admitted.

The modern ICU surrounds patients with a massive array of equipment that spouts forth a mountain of data in various shapes, sights, and sounds. The ICU environment requires *major* adjustments both mentally and emotionally. Having been thrust into an unknown environment for which they have no "frame of reference" requires a Herculean adjustment. Patients must struggle to gain any sense of stability and self-control. The reality is that they become almost totally dependent, that is, loss of control over their environment and personal well-being. They are no longer in charge of even the simplest body functions including respiration, urination, and defecation. The need for a constant stream of medical data requires constant subjugation to physical examinations and probing into even the most private parts. Routine functions like bathing, washing one's hair, and brushing one's teeth become someone else's assignment on the morning shift. This sudden and absolute state of total dependence on others for survival is usually devastating to ICU patients.

COMMON SYMPTOMS

Almost every ICU patient suffers from severe sleep deprivation. Often the members of the health care team are responsible for disrupting patients' sleep patterns. Although the importance of sleep is generally recognized by health professionals, priorities are dictated by life-threatening physiologic needs that outweigh the need for sleep. The conditions in an ICU are inadvertently conducive to mental alterations as well as critical illness itself. The environment is constant, with little outside stimulation; body movement is minimal; the temperature is usually constant; the noise level although initially quite abrasive becomes essentially "white noise" providing little alternative stimulation; personnel come and go; they of course must pay attention to individual body parts or specific machinery, and this many be perceived as not being aware of the whole patient. It is therefore most important to make special efforts to react to, talk to, and reassure patients in an attempt to ameliorate rather than contribute to the subtle but real slippage toward psychosis.

Intensive care psychosis is a diagnosis often applied to patients exhibiting acute agitation varying from mild confusion to advanced delirium. Patients' feelings may follow a pattern varying from intense fear and anxiety to denial and depression. If this sequence of spiraling emotions is not halted, it is followed by increased dependency leading to a state of paranoia with the patient fearing for his life and being temporarily disconnected from reality.

The assessment of this state of psychosis is varied. It has been referred to as "an acute organic brain syndrome" involving impaired intellectual functioning, and as nothing more than a convenient diagnostic catchall term that is meaningless and inaccurate.[1,2] There is agreement, however, that some form of mental aberration begins to appear in patients who spend more than 5 to 7 days in an ICU and the longer the stay the greater the risk.[3] The reported percentage of occurrence of this syndrome ranges from 2% to 70%.[4,5] Some of the inconsistency may be due to the terminology which ranges from mental aberration, perceptual distortion, illusions, and hallucinations to delirium.

Patients who have sustained severe trauma, prolonged surgical procedures, and lengthy anesthesia have a greater tendency to develop this diagnosis. The common features of this ICU syndrome consist of clouding of the consciousness, decreased ability to maintain attention, orientation difficulties, memory problems, and labile affect. Patients may display symptoms of altered time perception, lack of emotion, feelings of surrealism, a sense of detachment, loss of control, revival of memories, and a sense of ineffability.

The ICU patients face not only constant concern about death but also fears for loved ones and concerns for those dependent on them financially or emotionally. This stress, in addition to the reality of their physical state, can cause extreme despondency or depression. The accumulation of environmental and situational factors affects all ICU patients to varying degrees, depending on their personality characteristics, physical state, extent of physical trauma, degree and severity of any surgery performed and subsequent responses, and length of stay in the ICU.

The problem of communication for ICU patients is extraordinary. The inability to express one's thoughts verbally to ICU staff or to convey feelings to loved ones creates severe emotional distress. In addition, the experience of being attached to monitoring machines and particularly to the respirator for ventilatory support produces a real sense of personal paranoia. The ICU staff members and families must be aware that these reactions may occur. They should be prepared to deal with them appropriately. For example, these extraneous factors may occasionally cause patients to feign drowsiness or other symptoms to avoid frustration or embarrassment due to the inability to communicate in a conventional fashion. Family members may respond defensively to this dilemma by shortening their visits, *observing* the patient rather than talking to the patient, and behaviorally withdrawing from the patient. If these or other manifestations by families or patient are recognized by the ICU staff, it may prove helpful to openly present your assessment to the family. If given in a concerned helpful manner, the family may use this time to respond with their feelings of frustration and fear related to the situation, thereby providing an opportunity to directly reduce some degree of familial tension. Hopefully, together with the staff, a more effective personal approach can be suggested to help the patient.

The ICU physician may wish to respond to a patient's symptoms of depression or psychosis with medications. Though the symptoms are relieved, the patient is usually rendered inaccessible to his family members. This act of emotionally immobilizing a patient negates what time may be left the patient and his family. It bars them from precious time to discuss and relate those most intimate of feelings and decisions. If the patient is not in pain, then there should be no real reason to medicate him. If pain is present, it should be relieved with small doses, titrated to achieve success without oversedation, if possible. An alternative is to offer increased human contact and physical touching with a family member. Many ICU survivors do not recall their experiences, no matter how bad, after they have recovered. However, most pertinent to this discussion, is the importance of the lucid time spent with loved ones, especially for the patient who does not survive.

From my own personal experience living through months of an SICU stay with my brother, I can attest to its powerful importance. Robert survived for 2½ months following a car accident. He received multiple injuries, including aortic transection, ruptured spleen, lacerated liver, multiple rib fractures, and paraplegia secondary to ischemia of the spinal cord. In addition he suffered acute renal failure, left pleural effusion, atelectasis of the left lung, gastrointestinal bleeding secondary to stress ulceration, peritonitis secondary to breakdown of a pyloroplasty, and acute respiratory insufficiency requiring a tracheostomy. The normal visiting policy of 5 min/hr was suspended, and I was permitted to stay with him throughout the day. Until the last week before he died, Robert was mentally alert and awake for much of the time. There were days when he suffered from depression, and there were days that he suffered visual hallucinations. Robert often had to ask me to confirm if there were monsters floating above his bed. We would talk about his visions, and then he would laugh as if realizing the absurdity of his thoughts. When Robert suffered from severe depression, his hands would grasp my arm as I leaned next to him, and we would cry. Invariably, however, before I left for the night he would turn his face to look at me and then, with his hand, give me the "thumbs up" signal. Robert survived two additional surgical procedures before his last operation which revealed widespread peritonitis. He suffered from septic shock, complete renal failure, worsening respiratory failure, and coma. Shortly before his death, Robert's wife Kathe and I agreed to discontinue therapy.

If Robert had been chemically treated for his depression and periodic psychotic states, we would never have experienced the last 2½ months of his life with him.

WHEN DEATH IS IMMINENT

Families may respond with despair and disbelief on hearing from their loved one's physician that there is nothing more that can be done. Some families wish to continue treatment at any cost despite overwhelming odds against survival or continued life with dignity. Therefore, families and physicians not infrequently disagree over the appropriateness of specific therapy. Fortunately, such disagreements are usually resolved within the patient–physician–family triad. Physicians should not feel threatened when patients or families assume a greater role in decision-making regarding medical treatment. It should be recognized that in a moral, ethical, and legal sense, families should be and are empowered to participate in this decision-making. Although there will certainly continue to be situations that can be resolved only through the legal processes, it is quite possible that many such problems can be prevented by more effective communication by ICU physicians involved. When the inevitability of impending death is apparent, the medical staff must recognize and provide for family needs to allow the acceptance of death. Civetta believes that "providing an environment in which families can learn to cope with this unpleasant reality should, indeed, be one of physician's most important goals."[6] However, when confronted with the reality their loved one will not survive, families may not respond as expected. They are forced to give up the hopes and beliefs that have kept them together and helped them to tolerate this ordeal. Thus, regardless of prior discussion and counseling, physicians should expect reactions of denial and disbelief. Usually time is the main requirement for family members to adjust to and accept the reality of the death of their loved one. Most adjustments occur within 24 to 48 hours. If not, it is wise to secure the service of an experienced mental health professional before life-sustaining treatment is withdrawn. Unless all ICU beds are occupied and a critically ill or injured but potentially viable patient is waiting for a bed, any urgency to act quickly is ill advised. It is precisely during this time period that physicians should shift their efforts and attend to the needs of the family. This realignment of treatment objectives may allay feelings of antagonism and resistance that arise in the family in response to the imminent death of their loved one.

In circumstances where the death of the patient follows prolonged ICU treatment, the family may initially feel relieved. They may respond this way, not because their loved one has died but because the *ordeal* is finally over. Expressions of grief may be unspoken, inhibited by restrictions imposed by feelings of guilt. Nonetheless, it seems that the need for some sense of closure is greater than our ability to endure uncertainty.

During the time immediately following the death of a patient, ICU staff interactions with the family are needed and appropriate. Therefore the responsibility of the physicians and other ICU personnel should not terminate with the patient's death. In addition to responses to family members on an individual basis, more formal meetings should be arranged for all interested staff plus family members.

The meeting or meetings need not be strictly formal although some responsibility for comments and responses, both personally and professionally, should be presented by significant staff involved. These meetings provide a dual purpose for staff and family alike. Family members may want to know the exact manner in which the patient died. Was their loved one alone when he died? Was the death peaceful?

In addition these meetings provide an opportunity for families to communicate and share deep feelings of gratitude to the medical staff. Physicians and other ICU personnel are often left in doubt about the thoughts of family members. For example the staff may wonder what the family thought about how the patient was treated and cared for? Is the family angry? Does the family blame the staff? Do they think their loved one was tortured or do they think treatment was discontinued too soon or prolonged unnecessarily? Does the family understand that the ICU staff really cared and did their best? Answers to such questions may help foster acceptance of death for families and staff alike.

REFERENCES

1. Eisendrath SJ: ICU syndromes: Their detection, prevention and treatment. *Critical Care Update* 1980; 7(4):5

2. Cassem NH: Critical care psychiatry. In Shoemaker W, Thompson L, Holbrook P (eds): *Textbook of Critical Care,* p 981. Philadelphia, WB Saunders,1984
3. Kleck JL: Means to forestall ICU syndrome explored. *Anesth News* 1984:10:10
4. Noble J: Communications in the ICU: Therapeutic or disturbing? *Nursing Outlook* 1971; :195
5. Hackett TP, Cassem NH: *Handbook of General Psychiatry.* Boston, Mass. General Hosp, 1978
6. Civetta JM: Beyond technology: Intensive care in the 1980s. *Crit Care Med* 1981; 9:763

Behavioral Disturbances in the ICU

14

Michael G. Wise
Ned H. Cassem

This chapter outlines a practical clinical approach to evaluating and treating the behaviorally disturbed critically ill patient (Fig. 14-1). If these guidelines are followed, the reasons for many, if not most, behavioral disturbances in hospitalized patients will be apparent, and the problems can be rectified. Remember that in critically ill patients, disorders such as agitation and confusion are not specific diagnoses but rather behavioral manifestations of underlying problems. We hope to provide you with a road map to their elucidation.

Behavioral disturbances are common in the ICU. George Engle noted that 10% to 15% of the patients on acute medical and surgical wards suffer from delirium or confusional states during hospitalization.[1] The incidence of confusional states increases greatly in hospitalized patients over 60 years of age, and delirium occurs in almost all patients who have been burned over greater than 40% of the body surface area.[2] Other behavioral disorders resulting from a critically ill patient's fear, anxiety, denial, anger, depression, dependency, and personality are encountered daily by physicians and critical care nurses (Table 14-1). Regardless of your expertise, there are times when a psychiatric consultation is needed.

Physicians requesting psychiatric consultation must find a good psychiatrist. To qualify, the psychiatrist should have sound medical skills (i.e., use a mental status examination and a physical, especially basic neurologic examination). Most good medical training programs give their graduates these basic skills. Among the graduates who chose psychiatry, those who love medicine and relish the challenge of diagnosis and treatment make the best consultants.[3] They are able to integrate the current physiologic state of the patient with the psychosocial aspects of the situation, and to communicate this information in a clear, concise fashion to the requesting physician. There is no place for psychiatric jargon in this process. The psychiatrist must follow the patient until the problem is under control or resolved, and arrange psychiatric care for the patient following discharge, when it is necessary.

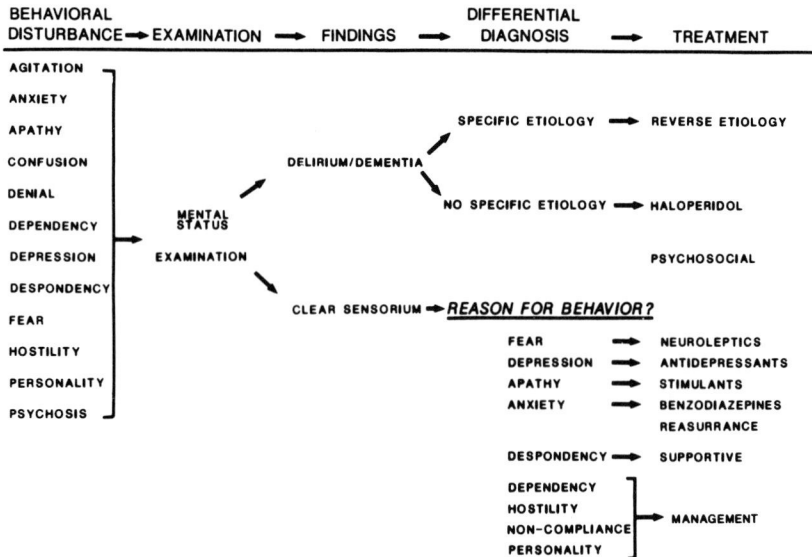

FIGURE 14-1. Overview of behavioral disturbances in the ICU.

WHAT TO DO FIRST

When faced with a patient who has a behavioral disturbance, the first question must be: "Is the patient delirious?" This is a crucial decision point in the evaluation (see Fig. 14-1). If a delirium or confusional state is present, the focus of the differential diagnosis must become the etiologic agent(s) causing the problem. The importance of discovering and correcting the underlying cause of a delirium cannot be overemphasized. Unfortunately, terms like "ICU psychosis," which infer a cause-and-effect relationship between the ICU setting and delirium, result in diagnostic apathy. Intensive care unit psychosis implies that the problem is somehow natural or expected when a patient is critically ill; therefore, delirium can be ignored. The evidence for such an etiology is flimsy. How many patients have been diagnosed as having "ICU fever" or "ICU dysrhythmia?" The brain's highly complex, multifactorial reaction to metabolic, anoxic, toxic, and infectious insults is delirium. Delirium is the tangible sign of cerebral insufficiency, just as angina is the ordinary warning sign of heart ischemia. The appearance of a delirium, which is often referred to as acute brain failure, should promote martialing of the same medical forces as failure of any other vital organ. Mortality associated with delirium is not trivial. From 20% to 76% of acutely ill patients diagnosed as delirious die within a few months.[4,5] Far from being a natural phenomenon or "disease of medical progress," brain failure is ominous, signaling a need for renewed concern and prompt attention.[6]

TABLE 14-1. Psychiatric Disturbances in the ICU

Agitation	Depression
Anxiety	Despondency
Apathy	Fear
Confusion	Hostility
Denial	Personality
Dependency	Psychosis

If cognitive impairment (delirium) is not present, the clinician can take an alternate approach to the patient's behavioral difficulties (see Fig. 14-1). Two lines of investigation are likely to illuminate the cause of the behavioral problem. These include examination of the patient's underlying areas of concern (these concerns are most often unrealistic expectations about their illness) and a thorough review of the patient's medications to ensure the behavioral disturbances are not drug-induced side-effects of medications.

CLINICAL FEATURES OF A DELIRIUM

Three good sources can be used to determine whether a patient is delirious. They are the medical record, particularly the nurses' notes, past and present observations of the family, and examination of the patient. A delirium has certain characteristics (Table 14-2). The patient often manifests prodromal symptoms such as restlessness, anxiety, irritability, or sleep disruption prior to the onset. One of the hallmark findings is rapid fluctuation in the degree of confusion. Patients may be grossly confused and hallucinating during the night and have brief lucid intervals interspersed with confusional periods during the day. They also have difficulty sustaining attention. During the interview, they typically are distracted by environmental events, such as a loud noise or a nurse checking the intravenous (IV) infusion, and forget the question asked. Their inability to sustain attention and preoccupation with

TABLE 14-2. Clinical Features of Delirium

Prodrome
Rapidly fluctuating course, reversible, lucid intervals
Altered arousal and psychomotor abnormality
Attention decreased
Sleep–wake disturbance
Impaired memory
Thinking and speech disorganized
Perceptions altered
Disorientation
Emotional lability
Dysgraphia/constructional apraxia/dysomic aphasia
Motor abnormalities

internal events undoubtedly play a key role in the severe memory impairment and orientation difficulties found in delirium.

Delirious patients, except for lucid intervals, are usually disoriented to time, often disoriented to place, but very rarely, if ever, disoriented to person. Following recovery from a delirium, some patients will be amnesic for the entire episode, others will have islands of memory, and a few will recall the entire period. Those patients who experience paranoid delusions with a relatively clear sensorium usually recall the ICU experience.

Another clinical feature of delirium deserves particular emphasis. Though usually aroused, the reticular activating system (RAS) of the brain stem in delirium may be hypoactive, in which case a patient appears apathetic, somnolent, and quietly confused. In most patients, RAS hyperactivity induces agitation, hypervigilance, and psychomotor hyperactivity. Some patients have a mixed picture that swings back and forth between hypoactive and hyperactive states. The medical staff often "diagnoses" the patient with a retarded (hypoactive) delirium as depressed. This diagnosis in an apathetic, quietly confused patient sometimes leads to inappropriate treatment with antidepressant medications.

The sleep–wake cycle of delirious patients is often reversed. They may be somnolent during the day and active during the night. Restoration of the normal diurnal sleep cycle is an important part of treatment. In addition, delirious patients' thought patterns are disorganized and their reasoning defective. They often experience misperceptions involving illusions, delusions, and hallucinations. These misperceptions often are woven into a loosely knit delusional, and frequently, paranoid system. Visual hallucinations are common and can involve simple visual distortions or complex scenes. During a delirium, they occur more frequently than auditory hallucinations. Tactile hallucinations are the least frequent. As the severity of the delirium increases, spontaneous speech becomes incoherent and rambling.

A number of neuropsychiatric signs accompany delirium, including dysgraphia, construction apraxia, and motor system abnormalities. Dysgraphia is one of the most sensitive indicators of a delirium. In Chedru's study, 33 of 34 acutely confused patients had writing problems ranging from motor (tremor to illegible scribble) and spatial (letter malalignment and line disorientation) impairments to misspelling and linguistic errors.[7] Construction apraxia also is a sensitive indicator of a confusional state and can be evaluated at the bedside, by asking the patient to draw a clock, showing a particular time, or a three-dimensional cube.

Motor system abnormalities such as tremor, myoclonus, asterixis ("liver flap"), or reflex and muscle tone changes can also be present. The tremor associated with delirium, particularly when toxic–metabolic in origin, is absent at rest but apparent during movement. Myoclonus and asterixis occur in many toxic and metabolic conditions. Symmetric reflex and muscle tone changes also are seen.

IS DELIRIUM PRESENT?

The bedside mental status examination for cognitive dysfunction is not difficult. Folstein's Mini-Mental State (MMS) examination (Fig. 14-2 A and B) provides a good screening tool for organicity and is also used to follow the patient's clinical course serially. The MMS examination tests for orientation, memory, attention, dysgraphia, and constructional apraxia. As noted earlier, these cognitive tasks are impaired in the delirious patient. A score of 15 or less out of a total of 30 on the MMS signals the presence of delirium or dementia.

The MMS also identifies demented patients as abnormal. A clinical history of chronicity found in the demented patient should be distinguished from the acute presentation found in the delirious patient. Demented patients have a lowered threshold for developing delirium, so both disorders can appear in the same patient. When they occur simultaneously, treatment of delirium improves the patient's behavior.

The electroencephalogram (EEG) is diagnostically helpful in difficult cases. Delirium is a clinical manifestation of global cerebral dysfunction. As mentioned earlier, one of the interchangeable terms for delirium is acute brain failure. The EEG characteristically, but not always, shows global cerebral slowing. Pro and Wells reported that EEG changes virtually always accompany delirium.[8] A low-voltage, fast-activity pattern as in delirium tremens also can be present.[9] Remember that the EEG appears worse than the mental status examination in the delirious patient; conversely, the mental status examination of the demented patient is usually much worse than predicted from simple review of the EEG (*i.e.*, the EEG is usually normal in dementia until the later stages).

IF DELIRIUM IS PRESENT, WHAT IS NEXT?

The differential diagnosis of delirium is extensive. Confusional states, particularly in the elderly, may have multiple contributory causes. An elderly, delirious patient can have a low hematocrit, multiorgan system disease (*e.g.*, pulmonary insufficiency, cardiac failure, or preexisting brain damage) and be taking multiple medications. Each potential contribution to the delirium

TABLE 14-3. Delirium—Differential Diagnosis of Urgent Items

Wernicke's encephalopathy/withdrawal
Hypertensive encephalopathy
Hypoglycemia
Hypoperfusion of CNS
Hypoxemia
Intracranial bleed
Meningitis/encephalitis
Poisons/medications

A

```
                                    Patient_____
                                    Examiner_____
                                    Date_____

                          "MINI-MENTAL STATE"*
```

Maxi-mum score	Score	
		Orientation
5	( )	What is the (year) (season) (date) (day) (month)?
5	( )	Where are we: (state) (county) (town) (hospital) (floor).
		Registration
3	( )	Name 3 objects: 1 second to say each. Then ask the patient all 3 after you have said them. Give 1 point for each correct answer. Then repeat them until he learns all 3. Count trials and record. Trials_____
		Attention and Calculation
5	( )	Serial 7's. 1 point for each correct. Stop after 5 answers. Alternatively spell "world" backwards.
		Recall
3	( )	Ask for the 3 objects repeated above. Give 1 point for each correct.
		Language
9	( )	Name a pencil, and watch (2 points) Repeat the following "No ifs ands or buts." (1 point) Follow a 3-stage command: "Take a paper in your right hand, fold it in half, and put it on the floor" (3 points) Read and obey the following:

Close your eyes (1 point)

Write a sentence (1 point)
Copy design (1 point)
Total score
ASSESS level of consciousness
  along a continuum _____
                    Alert   Drowsy   Stupor   Coma

FIGURE 14-2. A. The MMS examination.

needs to be pursued and, to whatever degree possible, reversed. A method for organizing the differential diagnosis of a delirious patient is helpful. This diagnostic system is found in Table 14-3 and is represented by the mnemonic WHHHHIMP. The diagnosis contained in the WHHHHIMP mnemonic can also help the clinician recall these critical items.

In hospitalized patients, prescribed medications are common causes of delirium (Table 14-4). A thorough medication history and review of the patient's medication records are essential. The doctor's order sheets can be misleading since drugs may have been ordered but not given. Correlation of changes in behavior with medication administration or discontinuation can be helpful in sorting through a difficult case.

A more comprehensive list of diagnoses that can cause delirium is

B   **Orientation**

(1) Ask for the date. Then ask specifically for parts omitted, e.g., "Can you also tell me what season it is?" One point for each correct.
(2) Ask in turn "Can you tell me the name of this hospital?" (town, county, etc.). One point for each correct.

Registration

Ask the patient if you may test his memory. Then say the names of 3 unrelated objects, clearly and slowly, about one second for each. After you have said all 3, ask him to repeat them. This first repetition determines his score (0-3) but keep saying them until he can repeat all 3, up to 6 trials. If he does not eventually learn all 3, recall cannot be meaningfully tested.

Attention and Calculation

Ask the patient to begin with 100 and count backwards by 7. Stop after 5 subtractions (93, 86, 79, 72, 65). Score the total number of correct answers.

If the patient cannot or will not perform this task, ask him to spell the word "world" backwards. The score is the number of letters in correct order. E.g., dlrow = 5, dlorw = 3.

Recall

Ask the patient if he can recall the 3 words you previously asked him to remember. Score 0-3.

Language

Naming: Show the patient a wrist watch and ask him what it is. Repeat for pencil. Score 0-2.
Repetition: Ask the patient to repeat the sentence after you. Allow only one trial. Score 0 or 1.
3-Stage command: Give the patient a piece of plain blank paper and repeat the command. Score 1 point for each part correctly executed.
Reading: On a blank piece of paper print the sentence "Close your eyes", in letters large enough for the patient to see clearly. Ask him to read it and do what it says. Score 1 point only if he actually closes his eyes.
Writing: Give the patient a blank piece of paper and ask him to write a sentence for you. Do not dictate a sentence, it is to be written spontaneously. It must contain a subject and verb and be sensible. Correct grammar and punctuation are not necessary.
Copying: On a clean piece of paper, draw intersecting pentagons, each side about 1 in., and ask him to copy it exactly as it is. All 10 angles must be present and 2 must intersect to score 1 point. Tremor and rotation are ignored.

Estimate the patient's level of sensorium along a continuum, from alert on the left to coma on the right.

FIGURE 14-2 (Continued) B. *Instructions for administration of the MMS.*

summarized in Table 14-5. The mnemonic used, I WATCH DEATH, may seem melodramatic, but the mortality rate within the first 3 months following the diagnosis of delirium is approximately 30%. We refer you to Tesar and Stern[10] or Wise[11] for recent complete discussions of the differential diagnosis of delirium.

In virtually every delirious patient, the evaluative process includes review of historical information, as well as basic and "advanced" laboratory tests (Table 14-6). When information concerning the patient's mental and physical status is combined with the basic laboratory battery, the specific etiology (etiologies) is usually apparent. If not, review the case and consider ordering further diagnostic studies.

TABLE 14-4. *Drugs Causing Delirium (Reversible Dementia)*

Analgesics
  meperidine (Normeperidine)
  opiates
  pentazocine
  salicylates
Antibiotics
  acyclovir (antiviral)
  aminoglycosides
  amodiaquine
  amphotericin B (antifungal)
  cephalosporins
  chloramphenicol
  chloroquine (antimalarial)
  ethambutol
  gentamicin
  interferon (antiviral)
  isoniazid
  rifampin
  sulfonamides
  tetracyclines
  ticarcillin
  vancomycin
Anticholinergics
  antihistamines
    chlorpheniramine (Ornade, Teldrine)
  antiparkinson drugs
    benzotropine (Cogentin)
    biperidin (Akineton)
  antispasmodics
  belladonna alkaloids
  diphenhydramine (Benadryl)
  phenothiazines (especially Thioridizide)
  promethazine (Phenergan)
  tricyclic antidepressants (especially amitriptyline)
  trihexyphenidyl (Artane, Pipanol, Tremin)

Anticonvulsants
  phenobarbital
  phenytoin (Dilantin)
  sodium valproate (Depakene)
Anti-inflammatory
  ACTH
  corticosteroids
  ibuprofen (Motrin, Advil)
  indomethacin (Indocin)
  naproxen (Naprosyn)
  phenylbutazone (Butazolidin, Azolid)
  steroids
Antineoplastics
  aminoglutethimide
  DTIC
  5-fluoruracil
  hexamethylenamine
  L-asparaginase
  methotrexate (high dose)
  tamoxifen
  vinblastine
  vincristine
Antiparkinsonian
  amantadine (Symmetrel)
  bromocriptine
  carbidopa (Sinemet)
  levodopa (Larodopa)
Cardiac
  beta-blockers
  captopril
  clonidine (Catapres)
  digitalis (Digoxin, Lanox)
  disopyramide (Norpace)
  lidocaine (Xylocaine)
  mexiletine
  methyldopa (Aldomet)
  quinidine (Quinidine Quinaglute, Duraquine)
  procainamide (Pronestyl)
  tocainide

Drug Withdrawal
  alcohol
  barbiturates
  benzodiazepines
Sedative–Hypnotics
  barbiturates (Miltown, Equanil)
  benzodiazepines
  glutethimide
Sympathomimetics
  aminophylline
  amphetamines
  cocaine
  ephedrine
  phenylephrine
  phenylpropanolamine
  theophylline
Miscellaneous Drugs
  baclofen
  bromides
  chlorpropamide (Diabinese)
  cimetidine (Tagamet)
  disulfiram (Antabuse)
  ergotamines
  lithium
  metrizamide (Amipaque)
  metronidazole (Flagyl)
  phenelzine
  podophyllin (by absorption)
  procarbazine
  propylthiouracil
  quinacrine
  ranitidine
  timolol ophthalmic

TABLE 14-5. Causes of Delirium

Infectious	Encephalitis, meningitis, syphilis
Withdrawal	Alcohol, barbiturates, sedatives–hypnotics, benzodiazepine
Acute Metabolic	Acidosis, alkalosis, electrolyte disturbance, hepatic failure, renal failure
Trauma	Heat stroke, postoperative severe burns, closed head
CNS Pathology	Abscesses, hemorrhage, normal pressure hydrocephalus, seizures, stroke, tumors, vasculitis
Hypoxia	Anemia, carbon monoxide poisoning, hypotension, pulmonary/cardiac failure
Deficiencies	B_{12}, hypovitaminosis, niacin, thiamine
Endocrinopathies	Hyper(hypo)adrenalcorticism, hyper(hypo)glycemia, parathyroid
Acute Vascular	Hypertensive encephalopathy, shock
Toxins/Drugs	Medications, pesticides, solvents
Heavy Metals	Lead, manganese, mercury

TABLE 14-6. Evaluation of the Behavioral-Disturbed Patient

MENTAL STATUS
Interview (assess level of consciousness, psychomotor activity, appearance, affect, mood, intellect, thought processes)
Performance tests (for memory, concentration, reasoning, motor and constructional apraxia, dysgraphia, dysnomia)

PHYSICAL STATUS
Brief neurologic examination (reflexes, limb strength, Babinski's, cranial nerves, meningeal signs, gait)
Review past and present vital signs (pulse, temperature, blood pressure, respiration rate)
Review chart (labs, abnormal behavior noted and if so when it began?)
Review medication records (correlate abnormal behavior with starting or stopping medications)

LABORATORY EXAMINATION—BASIC
Blood chemistries (electrolytes, glucose, Ca^{2+}-albumin, BUN, NH_4^+, liver functions, Mg^{2+}, PO_4^{2-}, thyroid function tests)
Blood count (hematocrit, white count, differential, mean corpuscular volume, sedimentation rate)
Drug levels (need toxic screen?; medication blood levels?)
Arterial blood gases
Urinalysis
EKG
Chest radiograph

FURTHER LABORATORY
EEG (seizures?, focal lesion?, confirm delirium)
CT (normal pressure hydrocephalus, stroke, space-occupying lesion)
Additional blood chemistries (heavy metals, thiamine and folate levels, lupus erythematosus, ANA, urinary porphobilinogen)
Lumbar puncture (if indication of infection or intracranial bleed)

Treatment

The goal of evaluation is to discover specific reversible causes for delirium. A delirious patient with a blood pressure of 260/150 and papilledema must immediately receive antihypertensive medications. The alcoholic patient having withdrawal symptoms must receive appropriate pharmacologic intervention with drugs such as thiamine and a benzodiazepine. If a specific cause for the confusional state cannot be found, a number of interventions are helpful in controlling unacceptable behavior.

Haloperidol is the drug of choice when you must treat a delirium of unknown etiology.[12,13] It is a potent antipsychotic, with virtually no anticholinergic or hypotensive properties, is not a respiratory depressant, and can be given parenterally. Intravenous haloperidol has been used in high doses for many years in seriously ill patients without harmful side-effects.[13,14] However, it is not approved by the Food and Drug Administration for intravenous use. If you wish to use intravenous haloperidol, we recommend that the hospital's human studies committee authorize use of the drug with careful monitoring of the results. Since haloperidol is the safest drug for control of agitation in the critically ill patient, it is certainly justifiable as an innovative therapy. After monitoring of the results is complete, the committee can authorize use of the intravenous haloperidol when necessary to care for the medically ill patient.

Although extrapyramidal side-effects are more likely with the higher potency antipsychotic drugs, the actual occurrence rate in medically ill patients, particularly with intravenous administration, is low. This observation may be related to the fact that medically ill patients frequently receive concomitant benzodiazepines or beta-blockers, which ameliorate extrapyramidal syndromes (EPS), or that psychiatric patients have a lower threshold for EPS.[15] Recommended dosages of haloperidol for the agitated patient are summarized in Table 14-7. The initial dosage for the elderly patient is at the lower end of the dosage schedule. It is repeated every 30 minutes until the patient is sedated or calm (remember, the oral dose is twice the parenteral dose). Also note that the calming effects of an antipsychotic drug are not immediate. The therapeutic delay may cause the physician and nursing staff to feel the medication is not effective. When calm is achieved, agitation then becomes the sign for a repeat dose. After confusion has cleared, *continue the medications for 3 to 5 days.* Abrupt discontinuation immediately following improvement is usually followed by recurrence of the delirium within 24 hours. A more rational approach is to taper the medication over a 3- to 5-day period, administering the largest dose before bedtime to help normalize the sleep–wake cycle. Small doses of intravenous lorazepam, particularly in patients who have not responded to high doses of haloperidol alone, are a useful adjunct.[16]

Other useful antipsychotic medications include thiothixene (Navane) and droperidol (Inapsine). Droperidol is used as a preanesthetic agent and for control of nausea and vomiting. It is a butyrophenone like haloperidol

TABLE 14-7. Guidelines for Intravenous Haloperidol

LEVEL OF AGITATION	STARTING DOSE
Mild	0.5–2.0 mg
Moderate	2.0–5.0 mg
Severe	5.0–10.0 mg

Note:
(1) Clear IV tubing with normal saline.
(2) For elderly, use starting doses in the low range.
(3) Allow 30 min between doses.
(4) For continued agitation, double previous dose.
(5) After 3 doses, give 0.5–1.0 mg of lorazepam IV concurrently or alternate lorazepam with haloperidol every 30 min.
(6) Once patient is calm, add the total mg of haloperidol and administer same number of mg over the next 24 hr.
(7) Assuming the patient remains calm, reduce dose 50% every 24 hr.
(8) Oral dosage is twice the IV dose.

and has comparable antipsychotic potency. Droperidol is approved for intravenous use but has the disadvantage of having a higher potential than haloperidol for causing hypotension. Less potent antipsychotic medications are thioridazine (Mellaril) and chlorpromazine (Thorazine). Because higher milligram doses are required, they are more likely to cause hypotension, have more anticholinergic side-effects, and should be used with caution in the unstable patient with cardiovascular disease. We recommend that you obtain psychiatric consultation before using thioridazine or chlorpromazine in critically ill patients.

Other interventions are also necessary. All nonessential medications should be discontinued. Increased observation by the nursing staff will permit closer evaluation of medical deterioration and frequent monitoring for dangerous behavior (crawling over bedrails or pulling out central venous or arterial catheters). Fluid input and output are monitored and good oxygenation is ensured.

Having a calm family member remain with a paranoid, agitated patient is reassuring and can prevent mishaps. In lieu of a family member, close supervision by reassuring staff is important. Both nurses and family members can frequently reorient the disoriented patient to date and surroundings. Placing a clock, calendar, and familiar objects in the room may be helpful. Adequate light in the room decreases frightening illusions at night. Despite recommendations to the contrary, a private room for the delirious patient is appropriate only if adequate supervision can be assured. A room with a window is helpful to orient the patient to normal diurnal cues.[17] If the patient normally wears eyeglasses or a hearing aid, improving the quality of sensory input by returning these devices is useful.

WHEN DELIRIUM IS NOT PRESENT

What should you do if the patient has a behavioral disorder, but the MMS examination and recent clinical history indicate that no cognitive dysfunction is present? The next step is to continue the examination with the goal of uncovering the concerns, realistic or not, that the patient has about his medical condition. Some patients can easily identify fears, anxiety, and depressive ideas concerning their medical condition, but this task is not always easy. Certain characteristic emotional responses are encountered in different intensive care settings (Table 14-8).

Although little research concerning the sequence of emotional and behavioral reactions in critically ill patients has been published, Cassem and Hackett have developed a useful hypothetical sequence of patient reactions to a coronary care unit (CCU) based on the timing of psychiatric consultations (Fig. 14-3).[18] The majority of behavioral problems during the first 2 days in the CCU are caused by fear and anxiety, most likely resulting from the threat to life posed by a heart attack (patients were healthy one hour and bedridden in an ICU the next). By the second or third day, they frequently convince themselves that nothing serious occurred and the physicians' and nurses' concerns are misplaced. During this period of denial, noncompliance with medical advice occurs and sign-out "AMA" is threatened. As evidence mounts that something did, in fact, injure the myocardium, patients become more depressed or appear demoralized and express pessimism about the future. Behavioral problems later in the course of illness often result from chronic personality traits. These patients are difficult to get along with and are often disliked by the staff.

When the critical care physician is called regarding a patient with a behavioral problem, the first concern is whether a change in medical status prompted the behavior (*e.g.*, shortness of breath prompts agitation). Concern of the physician for the patient's medical condition not only rules out problems but also helps to establish rapport. Once medical problems are discounted and rapport is established, the interviewer can ask open-ended questions about the current situation. The basic approach used is to uncover and correct the critically ill patient's unrealistic or distorted expectations. For example, "What is worrying you most right now?" If you cannot establish

TABLE 14-8. Frequency of Consultation Requests According to Type of ICU

CCU	SURGICAL ICU	RESPIRATORY ICU	MEDICAL ICU
Anxiety	Delirium	Depression	Delirium
Depression	Depression	Anxiety weaning	Management (suicide attempt)
Management	Anxiety weaning	from respirator	Depression
(AMA sign-out, dependency)	from respirator	Management (drug dependency, dependency)	Anxiety
Hostility			
Delirium			

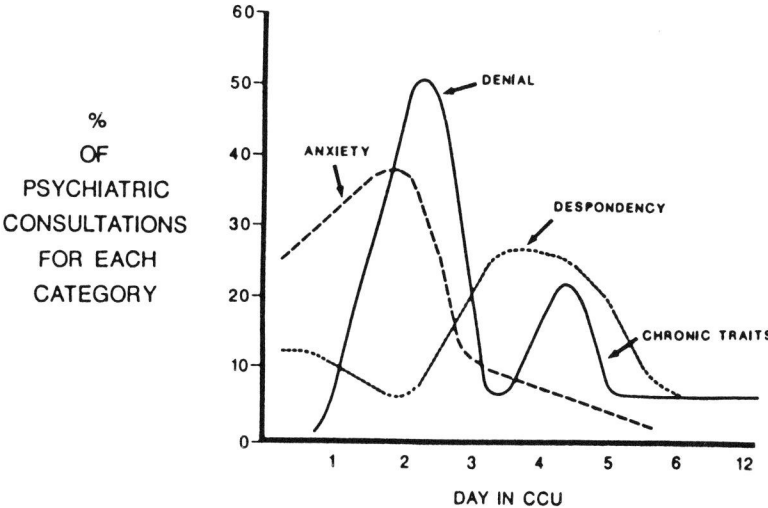

FIGURE 14-3. Hypothetical sequence of emotional and behavioral reactions in a CCU.

sufficient rapport, or if the patient is unable or unwilling to talk, request a psychiatric consultation.

Several behavioral disturbances deserve individual discussion, including agitation, depression and apathy, refusal to cooperate with treatment, hostility, and dependency.

AGITATION

Agitation is excessive motor activity resulting from a patient's internal discomfort. This discomfort may result from physical pain, anxiety, fear, or akathisia (an internal sense of discomfort often with motor restlessness that occurs as a side-effect of neuroleptic medications). As Tesar and Stern point out, "Agitation is usually a manifestation of a delirium."[10] If a delirium is not present, other sources for the agitation must be explored.

Physical pain in the critically ill patient can result in agitation. When pain is the cause of restlessness, the patient usually makes it known. The critical care nurse commonly asks about pain and administers a previously ordered narcotic. Agitated patients may not communicate pain severity when they are intubated. Prior to an analgesic trial, a brief mental status evaluation is recommended, since an underlying delirium, and therefore underlying medical problems, can be masked by narcotic analgesics. Sometimes, however, a trial of morphine is required.

For many critically ill patients, the cause of their anxiety and fear is the threat of death. In your conversations with the patient, if fears of dying are not mentioned, ask, "You look scared. How are you doing," or ask directly, "Are you worried that you may die?" If the patient answers that he/she believes he/she is dying, your response depends on the reality of those fears. If dying is an unrealistic possibility, reassurance and realistic explanations about the current situation markedly decrease the level of anxiety and fear. If dying is a likely or definite outcome of the illness, ask the patient, "What frightens you most about dying?" The patient may reply, "I'm afraid of the pain I will have" or "I have never been religious and don't know what to expect." In the former case, you can reassure the patient that he/she will be kept comfortable and free of moderate or severe pain. In the latter case, you can offer to arrange a consultation visit from a chaplain who can offer reassurance and advice.

Some critically ill patients inquire spontaneously whether or not they are dying. This direct question, especially if asked without much anxiety, means the patient wants to be told the truth. This patient usually suspects he/she is dying when the question is posed. The quick reply, "You'll be just fine," is usually frustrating and decreases hope of future communications about his/her predicament. Patients sometimes ask about dying with near panic. They really are asking for reassurance. Such patients often ask the nurse and usually avoid asking the physician. If you are in doubt about the patient's outcome, say "My focus is more on getting people well than on predicting death. You sound scared. What is it?" You can also mention that, "No one gets in this unit without being seriously ill. Why do you ask a question about dying now?" The patient can then clarify why the inquiry concerning death was made. Whenever anxiety seems to threaten overall stability, use medication judiciously or consult the psychiatrist.

Medications are helpful in treating anxiety and fear. Benzodiazepines reduce anxiety in most patients (Table 14-9). When you prescribe benzodiazepines for critically ill patients, considerations of the half-life of the drug, onset of action, drug interactions, and the route of metabolism are important. Diazepam produces a rapid, high level in the central nervous system (CNS) and is clinically useful when rapid tranquilization is desired. Drug interactions can result in behavioral changes. Cimetidine increases the half-life of longer-acting benzodiazepines, resulting sometimes in confusion or lethargy.[19] Short-acting benzodiazepines, such as oxazepam or lorazepam, are recommended in patients with liver damage to prevent build-up of drugs and their metabolites.

When anxiety is severe and is manifest as fear or panic, major tranquilizers (neuroleptics) are more efficacious. For example, a young man is admitted to the CCU to rule out myocardial infarction. He is noted to be extremely anxious with agitation, and oxazepam, 15 mg orally four times a day, is ordered. Despite the medication, he continues to be agitated, hypervigilant, and resists sleep. Inquiry into the patient's concerns reveals a strong family history of deaths associated with heart attacks. The patient is afraid to sleep "because I might not wake up," and he is "watching the monitors in case the alarms don't work." The patient, on a 0 (no anxiety) to 10 (terror) scale of anxiety, reports a 9.5 (*with* benzodiazepine treatment). He is then given perphenazine (Trilifon), 2 mg orally three times each day. His anxiety

TABLE 14-9. Antianxiety Agents: Benzodiazepines

DRUG	HALF-LIFE (HR)	ACTIVE METABOLITES IN HUMANS
SHORT-ACTING		
oxazepam (Serax)	5–15	none
lorazepam (Ativan)	10–20	none
temazepam (Restoril)	9–12	oxazepam
alprazolam (Xanax)	12–15	alpha-hydroxyalprazolam
triazolam (Halcion)	2–3	none
midazolam (Versed)	6	alpha-hydroxymidazolam
MODERATELY LONG		
diazepam (Valium)	20–80	N-desmethyldiazepam N-methyloxazepam (temazepam) oxazepam
chlordiazepoxide (Librium)	8–28	desmethylchlordiazepoxide demoxepam
halazepam (Paxipam)	14	N-desmethyldiazepam
clonazepam (Clonopin)	24	none
LONG		
clorazepate (Tranxene)	30–200	N-desmethyldiazepam
prazepam (Centrax)	30–200	N-desmethyldiazepam 3-hydroxyprazepam* oxazepam*
VERY LONG		
flurazepam (Dalmane)	96	N-desalkylflurazepam N-hydroxyethylflurazepam

* Found in low concentrations.

promptly drops to a self-rating of 3 out of 10, and all objective signs of emotional discomfort disappear. When panic emerges, as it did in this patient, low-dose major tranquilizers such as haloperidol, 1 or 2 mg twice each day; perphenazine, 2 mg orally three times each day; thiothixene, 1 or 2 mg three times per day; or trifluoperazine (Stelazine), 2 mg three times per day, can markedly reduce the level of anxiety.

Neuroleptic drugs, including droperidol, prochlorperazine (Compazine) and metoclopramide (Reglan), are associated with extrapyramidal side-effects such as akathisia. Patients usually report a sense of inner restlessness and sometimes manifest agitation. Akathisia is difficult to treat, and may or may not be improved by giving the patient diphenhydramine (Benadryl), benzodiazepines (usually diazepam), or anticholinergic drugs such as trihexyphenidyl (Artane) or benztropine mesylate (Cogentin). Propranolol may also reduce akathisia.[15] If symptoms do not remit, neuroleptics may have to be discontinued.

DEPRESSION OR APATHY

A medically ill patient is observed to lack energy and appears to have no interest in his medical condition. Is the patient apathetic or depressed? The question of depression versus apathy is important because the differential diagnosis and treatment are different.

Clinical depression consists of a depressed mood with a symptom constellation that includes sleep disturbance, decreased interests, increased sense of guilt, decreased energy, decreased ability to concentrate, decreased (or more rarely increased) appetite, altered psychomotor state (either decreased or increased), and suicidal ideation or preoccupation with death. The mnemonic in Table 14-10, SIG: E CAPS (prescribe energy capsules), may help you to recall these eight features of a clinical depression. If four of eight of these symptoms are present, the patient meets the American Psychiatric Association criteria for depression.[20] Many of these symptoms are difficult to interpret, since almost all seriously ill patients have problems with sleep, energy, and appetite, and some have difficulty with concentration. How, then, does one decide if a patient is depressed? The following characteristics help to identify critically ill patients who are also clinically depressed. These are sustained depressed mood, either increased (agitation) or decreased psychomotor movements, suicidal ideation, and, very importantly, a sense of helplessness and hopelessness about the current situation. The depressed patient also feels worthless. If the latter two symptoms are present, the patient requires treatment for depression. Failure to treat depression increases the mortality and morbidity of all medical illness.[21]

Apathy and depression do coexist in certain patients (*i.e.*, depressed patients often are apathetic about the future). Apathy, however, also exists as a separate entity. These patients are indifferent about the current medical condition and do not feel sad, hopeless, or worthless. They are not clinically depressed, although they may be misdiagnosed as depressed. One might say they are pseudodepressed.[22] Apathy in this group of patients is a product of brain dysfunction, probably in the frontal lobe. It occurs in hypoaroused, delirious patients, demented patients, and in some poststroke and brain-damaged patients. Nondepressed apathetic patients are not likely to respond to antidepressant medications. In fact, their mental status may worsen secondary to the anticholinergic side-effects of these drugs. A nondelirious subgroup may respond to stimulants. Methylphenidate (Ritalin) in doses of 10 mg twice per day, or dextroamphetamine 10 mg once per day, may energize the patient and improve rehabilitation.[23,24] The afternoon dose of

TABLE 14-10. Clinical Features of Depression

Sleep disturbance
Interests decrease
Guilt increases

Energy decreases

Concentration difficulties
Appetite decreases
Psychomotor alteration
Suicidal ideation

stimulants should be given before 3 PM so that the patient's ability to fall asleep is not impaired.

Certain medications are depressogenic.[25] Thus, review of the depressed patient's medication regimen is necessary. Frequent offenders are reserpine, methyldopa, propranolol, guanethidine, hydralazine, and clonidine.

REFUSAL TO COOPERATE

This problem can manifest itself as denial of serious illness, such as a threatened AMA sign-out, or refusal to follow a treatment plan, such as sneaking cigarettes or failure to remain in bed while on strict bed rest. As Hackett and Cassem suggest, "Although the threat to sign out can mean that the individual does not take the illness seriously (*e.g.*, is not frightened enough), the threat to sign out issued by an acutely ill patient should be assumed to be a reaction to panic unless proven otherwise."[18] Basically, when faced with flight or fight response to the severe stress of acute illness, the patient opts for flight.

We suggest several possibilities when you face this situation. If the patient seems incompetent (*i.e.*, is incapable of understanding the situation because of mental dysfunction), get a psychiatric consultation to document mental status. If the patient is competent and is demanding to leave against medical advice, try the following approach. Remain calm. Anger is a tempting response to this situation, but taking an adversarial stance rarely changes the patient's decision. In a calm, direct way, inform the patient about the medical difficulties, stressing the fact that the illness is manageable. Mobilize the patient's family. If certain members of the family can help to calm the patient, they are invaluable assets in this situation. If the family is as panicky as the patient, which is very rarely the case, keep the family and patient separated. As soon as possible, *medicate the patient* with a low-dose antipsychotic medication such as haloperidol, 1 or 2 mg, or perphenazine, 2 to 5 mg orally. Medication is important because, "If calm is achieved, it should not be expected to last."[18]

Patients who fail to comply with a medical regimen may also be frightened. The previously described young male patient in the CCU may not remain in bed. The usual translation of this behavior is something like, "My heart is not so damaged that I can't walk to the bathroom!" If you demand the patient return to bed, and do not understand the unspoken message, the behavior may be repeated to the increasing frustration of all parties involved. Instead of an adversarial statement, you can say, "Your heart is damaged and needs time to heal. The damaged part is like cement that is setting; right now it is soft and can be damaged more. If you allow the cement (scar) to harden, your heart will be as strong or stronger than before."

Many patients who refuse to comply with medical treatment are rebelling against dependency. The natural response of the staff to this rebellious behavior is to demand complete compliance. To do so is to fight a losing battle, with the staff attempting to function as the police and the patient feeling like a misunderstood criminal. The patient believes that his/her body has forsaken him/her by becoming ill, and now the medical staff is demanding total surrender. Certainly a fertile setting for rebellion! When faced with this situation, the staff should review the treatment plan and decide where flexibility can be allowed and where it is contraindicated. Use statements such as, "Would you like your sponge bath this morning or in the evening?" or "Your digitalis should be taken on schedule to keep your heart rhythm regular, but you can refuse your Valium. If you want the Valium later, just let us know." This gives the patient some sense of control in a situation where he/she is feeling totally powerless.

HOSTILITY

Anger in the critically ill springs from many roots. Patients may be frightened or feel threatened. They commonly ask, "What did I do to deserve this?" The nursing and physician staff may be the recipients of the resultant anger. If patients have complaints, hear them out, and correct the problem if appropriate. Empathize with the situation, "I know you are having a difficult time." For most patients, anger is a temporary state of affairs and will pass as they and the staff become adjusted to each other and to the situation. However, a few patients who exhibit chronic hostility have life-long difficulties with interpersonal relationships. A psychiatric consultation is indicated. These are difficult even for the psychiatrist to treat, and marginal control of the anger may be as much as can be achieved.

DEPENDENCY

Critically ill patients who regress to an infantile state during hospitalization (helpless behavior and unrealistic demands) irritate the medical staff. The latter may become so intent on controlling their own anger that they overcompensate and give in to the patients' demands. Unfortunately, acquiescence to unreasonable demands results in further regression and more demands. When dealing with a regressed patient, the staff must enforce reasonable limits and guide the patient towards rehabilitation. Firm demands for self-care and increased independence are recommended.

Transfer of the patient out of the ICU with a consequent reduced level of medical vigilance has both good and bad aspects. The patient is improving (good news), and the level of medical observation and monitoring are about to be reduced (bad news). The patient should be told in advance when transfer will occur and should be assured that less monitoring is appropriate because medical improvement has occurred. In some cases, a transitional status, such as a step-down unit, offers reassurance before transfer to a general medical ward.

CONCLUSION

The first task in the evaluation of a behaviorally disturbed, critically ill patient is to determine whether a delirium is present. A brief mental status examination, such as the MMS examination, should be used. If acute brain failure (delirium) is present, an immediate search for the etiology of the brain dysfunction is indicated. When a delirium is present but no clear etiology is found, haloperidol is the drug of choice to control confused behavior. If the behaviorally disturbed patient is not confused, the underlying emotional reason for the disturbance must be sought. Fear and anxiety are the most common causes. When dealing with behavioral problems in critically ill patients, there is no substitute for your ability to give calm reassurance and prescribe medications wisely. A good psychiatric consultant for difficult cases is essential.

REFERENCES

1. Engel GL: Delirium. In Freedman AM, Kaplan HI (eds): *Comprehensive Textbook of Psychiatry.* Baltimore, Williams & Wilkins, 1967
2. Lipowski ZJ: *Delirium (Acute Brain Failure in Man),* p 515. Springfield, IL, Charles C. Thomas Publishers, 1980
3. Glickman L: *Psychiatric Consultation in the General Hospital,* preface p x. New York, M Dekker, 1980
4. Epstein LJ, Simon A: Organic brain syndromes in the elderly. *Geriatrics* 1967; 22:145
5. Flint FJ, Richards SM: Organic basis of confusional states in the elderly. *Br Med J* 1956; 2:1537
6. McKegney FB: Intensive care syndrome: Definition, treatment and prevention of new "disease of medical progress." *Conn Med* 1966; 30:633
7. Chedru F, Geschwind N: Writing disturbances in acute confusional states. *Neuropsychologia* 1972; 10:343
8. Pro JD, Wells CE: The use of the electroencephalogram in the diagnosis of delirium. *Dis Nerv Syst* 1977; 38:804
9. Kennard MA, Bueding E, Wortis WB: Some biochemical and electroencephalographic changes in delirium tremens. *Q J Stud Alcohol* 1945; 6:4
10. Tesar GE, Stern TA: Evaluation and treatment of agitation in the intensive care unit. *J Int Care Med* 1986; 1:137
11. Wise MG: Delirium. In Hales RE, Yudofsky SC (eds): *The American Psychiatric Press Textbook of Neuropsychiatry,* p 89. Washington DC, American Psychiatric Press, 1987
12. Lipowski ZJ: Delirium updated. *Compr Psychiatry* 1980; 21:190
13. Cassem NH: Psychiatric and ethical issues in the critical care unit. In Parrillo JE (ed): *Current Therapy in Critical Care Medicine,* p 331. Philadelphia, BC Decker, 1987
14. Tesar GE, Murray GB, Cassem NH: Use of high-dose intravenous haloperidol in the treatment of agitated cardiac patients. *J Clin Psychopharmacol* 1985; 5:344
15. Lipinski JF, Zubenko GS, Cohen BM, et al: Propranolol in the treatment of neuroleptic-induced akathisia. *Am J Psychiatry* 1984; 141:412
16. Adams F: Neuropsychiatric evaluation and treatment of delirium in the critically ill cancer patient. *Cancer Bull* 1984; 36:156
17. Wilson LM: Intensive care delirium. *Arch Intern Med* 1972; 130:225
18. Cassem NH, Hackett TP: The setting of intensive care. In Hackett TP, Cassem NH (eds): *Massachusetts General Hospital Handbook of General Hospital Psychiatry,* p 319. St Louis, CV Mosby, 1978

19. Desmond PV, Patwardhan RV, Schenker S, et al: Cimetidine impairs elimination of chlordiazepoxide (librium) in man. *Ann Intern Med* 1980; 93:266
20. American Psychiatric Association: *Diagnostic and Statistical Manual of Mental Disorders*, 3rd ed, rev 2nd draft. Washington DC, 1986
21. Avery D, Winokur G: Mortality in depressed patients with electroconvulsive therapy and antidepressants. *Arch Gen Psychiatry* 1976; 33:1029
22. Murray: Personal communication, Massachusetts General Hospital
23. Katons W, Raskind M: Treatment of depression in the medically ill with methylphenidate. *Am J Psychiatry* 1980; 137:963
24. Kaufmann MW, Murray GB, Cassem NH: Use of psychostimulants in medically ill depressed patients. *Psychosomatics* 1982; 23:817
25. Klerman GL: Depression in the medically ill. *Psychiatr Clin North Am* 1981; 4:301

Allocating Nursing Care 15
Judith A. Hudson–Civetta

INTRODUCTION

In this cost-sensitive era, nurse and physician members of the ICU team are confronted daily with the mandate to deliver an increasing number of patient days (PD) of intensive care to older and sicker patients with the same or even decreased total health care resources. Unfortunately, no one in the bureaucracy tells those of us at the bedside how to do this. Since the costs of nursing personnel are known to be one of the highest in an institution,[1-3] and since there is limited availability of experienced ICU nurses,[4] we must evaluate, and where possible, change our practice so that we may begin to comply with this mandate and provide efficient, productive nursing care for the ICU patient while maintaining the quality of care. This chapter will review the allocation of nursing care in the ICU through discussion of the following areas: a brief description of the different role and care functions of the ICU nurse; the evolution of the study of nursing resource allocation in the ICU, developing categories of nursing care, quantitation of delivered nursing care, and improved nursing efficiency and productivity in equivalent illness; correlations between the severity of patient illness, the amount/type of nursing care required, and the role of the physician's preferences expressed through written orders; and descriptions of our nursing care classified according to the severity of illness and level of physician interventions.[5,6]

NURSING CARE FUNCTIONS

In most ICUs in this country, the nursing *care* is not limited to nursing *tasks* (measure and record). Appropriate ICU nursing addresses the whole patient and all disease processes: systematic determination of a patient's problems/needs, establishing the priority of those problems, making a plan to solve them, implementing that plan, and evaluating the extent to which the plan was effective in resolving the problems identified.[7] Given the limited number of residency positions and fellowships to train ICU physicians, it seems reasonable for physicians to learn about ICU nursing care during their ICU training since it is safe to predict that in the absence of physicians physically present in most ICUs, this description of nursing care will portray actual bedside ICU care in the physician's future practice for his or her patients. Within a patient day (PD) of 24 *possible* hours, the hours of nursing care that actually can be *delivered* to each patient are dependent on the nurse:patient ratio. For example, if this ratio is 1:2 in each nursing shift, then there are only 12 hours of nursing care available to each patient per 24 hours. Most commonly the nurse staffing allocations to an ICU, although idealized to be 1:1, are based on a projected 1:2 ratio.[4,8]

Nursing in the ICU is composed of dependent role functions, independent role functions, and a mixture of the two. The dependent role is most often actualized as the tasks necessary to complete and document the orders written by the physician, for example, the administration of an ordered medication and appropriate documentation. In the independent role, the nurse would initiate functions unrelated to the physician's orders, such as preventive skin care for a long-term immobile patient (turning, massage of reddened areas, initiation of range-of-motion exercises, careful skin hygiene). A mixture of independent and dependent roles is, perhaps, most common: a physician writes an order for wet-to-dry abdominal wound dressing every 8 hours. First, the order is transcribed and included in the patient's care plan (dependent). Each nurse assesses the status of wound healing, looks for evidence of infection, and evaluates the condition of the skin surrounding the wound (independent). The dressing is changed as prescribed (dependent). Finally, if excoriation is noted, the nurse will start the use of a skin protective substance such as karaya powder or zinc oxide (independent). From one perspective, the major goal of ICU medical therapy is, of course, to promote patient wellness and thus achieve positive patient outcome. Orders written by the physician are the most common method of communication used to outline and transmit the specific medical therapies that are deemed necessary to reach the goal of wellness. Yet, to prevent compromise of the quality of patient care, physician's orders should also have the following "nonmedical" goals: increase efficiency and productivity of patient care; support the independence of nursing assessment regarding the patient's physiologic stability; and control the costs of intensive care and thus impact on total hospital costs. The most important way to accomplish these ends is to think carefully to avoid the unnecessary.

ALLOCATION OF NURSING RESOURCES

In the past, we have perhaps confused activity with productivity and have allocated nursing resources with little regard for determining the patient's need for the tasks performed. A good example of this activity is the nearly universal "requirement" for hourly measurement and recording of vital signs and intake/output for the first, if not all, ICU days in all patients. This activity does not fulfill the physiologic need of every patient and serves only to waste valuable nursing resources.

In order to provide some scientific basis for nursing allocations in the ICU, we conducted staffing studies first in 1976-1977[9] and again in 1984[10] to quantitate the nursing care delivered in our own general surgical/trauma, adult ICU. In 1976, we could not find a method specific to the ICU to determine the number of nursing hours required to meet the needs of the patient. Although the Therapeutic Intervention Scoring System (TISS)[6] was available, this score reflects the tasks generated as a result of the physician's perceived severity of illness and personal bias about therapy. The score does not address the nursing time required to provide these interventions or, more importantly, the nursing time necessary to provide independent nursing care actions.

The first study, conducted prospectively, evaluated 61 PDs in 14 different patients. "Nursing time" was defined as the total hours actually delivered by the nurses to accomplish the necessary and ordered patient care. According to this methodology, if the sum of nursing time exceeded 24 hours, even a 1:1 nurse:patient ratio would be insufficient. Nursing care was divided into major categories and further subdivided into specific tasks/activities. The categories, activities, descriptions, and the average amount of time required to properly perform each activity are listed in the Appendix to this chapter. Procedures by different individuals were observed to determine the time required to perform each activity properly; the time required by less experienced nurses was combined with more proficient nurses to derive "average values". Supervisory nursing personnel then independently observed and confirmed the validity of the time quantitation. To collect information concerning each PD, the assigned nurses recorded all patient care procedures and their frequency on a form. Activities which would require variable amounts of time, for example, talking to a patient's family or patient teaching, were not included in the quantitation of nursing time in this early study. The results demonstrated that the average nursing care required per patient was 19.6 hours. We divided the patients into three classifications (Table 15-1): class 1, those patients requiring 12 hours or less of nursing care; class 2, those requiring 13 to 24 hours; and class 3, those requiring more than 24 hours of nursing care in a 24-hour PD in order to simulate nurse:patient ratios of 1:2, 1:1 and more than 1:1. Table 15-1 also contains the results of the 1984 study as well as TISS and Acute Physiology Score and Chronic

TABLE 15-1. Classification of Patients by Nursing Care Hours

		CLASS 1 ≤ 12 HOURS	CLASS 2 13–24 HOURS	CLASS 3 > 24 HOURS	TOTAL
% OF TOTAL PDs	1976	11%	69%	20%	61 PDs
	1984	66%	34%		148 PDs
NURSING HR/ PATIENT	1976	11.71 ± 0.6	19.1 ± 3.3	26 ± 1.39	19.6 ± 4.8
	1984	10.17 ± 1.4	14.9 ± 2.4		11.87 ± 2.97
TISS	1976	16.1 ± 2.9	26.8 ± 6.5	36.6 ± 3.3	27.6 ± 7.9
	1984	18.98 ± 6.7	32.6 ± 9.6		23.9 ± 10.2
APACHE II	1976	12.4 ± 4.9	12.5 ± 4.9	16 ± 2.7	11.9 ± 5.2
	1984	11.5 ± 5.96	18.3 ± 8.7		13.7 ± 8.3

Health Evaluation II (APACHE II)[11] scores, which were obtained retrospectively.

In 1976, according to our calculations, a nurse:patient ratio of 1:2 was inadequate for 89% of the PDs sampled. Not only was a 1:1 ratio "necessary," but the charge nurse had to have been free of a direct patient assignment to assist with the class 3 patients (those who required more than 24 hours of care per PD, more than one nurse could provide). After the study, we attempted to increase our nursing staffing to achieve a level of sufficient coverage to deliver the "required and ordered" care; no attempt was made to evaluate whether the *patient* actually physiologically *required* all of the nursing care delivered. Parenthetically, we learned that we, among others, often use the phrase, "The patient required ..." when we really mean, "We choose to use ...." The importance of this distinction rests in the awareness that if we realize that the latter is actually true, changes may then be made.

By 1984, two related problems had arisen which forced us to evaluate our nursing practice. First, there was a real shortage of *nurses* applying to our hospital for positions in any of the 12 ICUs, and second, there also was a shortage of nursing *positions* (full-time equivalents [FTEs] in the SICU table of organization) resulting from the nationwide and hospital-wide cost/reimbursement focus. We began, at first haphazardly and then systematically, to evaluate our nursing care practice and protocols. We asked if hourly *recorded* vital signs were really necessary for 24 hours after admission, *i.e.*, did the writing down of observed stable numbers add anything to the patient's care or improve outcome? This systematic evaluation was spurred by our realization that laboratory testing could be markedly decreased without affecting outcome or quality of care.[5] Also, we had noted a tremendous difference in the frequency of vital signs performed in an international study of APACHE: patients with the same score had the same outcome regardless of vital sign frequency.[12] The SICU nursing management and medical directors collaboratively changed our practice style and effected these changes by: changing or eliminating set frequencies defined in standing orders; substituting *observation* of continuously monitored vital signs for *recording* in all stable patients; simplifying intake and output recording; eliminating previously "routine" tasks that were of unproven value, such as daily prophylactic chest physiotherapy on all ventilated patients; diminishing laboratory work; and deleting repetition of other tasks or discarding tasks we redefined as unnecessary. The patient care protocols that evolved are discussed according to the simple patient classification (see Chap. 1, "Setting Objectives: Perspectives for Care"), derived from earlier studies,[6,13] with attendant implications for types of orders the physician may need to write. Although our personal preferences are used as examples, we propose only that the general principles and approach are worthy of investigation in other institutions. Finally, from April to June 1984, we repeated the staffing study with an updated list of categories, activities, and average times. Newly added activities which could not be abstracted from the flow sheet, such as time spent with the family, were recorded directly.

We had been able to effect a major reduction in the average number of nursing hours per patient per class and a redistribution of patients from the classes consuming a large number of nursing hours to the lowest category (Table 15-1). The effect on overall ICU function was to increase the number of PDs provided by 30% at a 10% increase in costs and an 8% increase in FTEs (Table 15-2). The major shifts in the distribution of patients according to class are, perhaps, most dramatically illustrated by the increase from 11% to 66% of patients now in class 1, requiring less than 12 hours of nursing care per PD, and the complete elimination of the patients requiring more than 24 hours of nursing care. There was no difference in mean APACHE II or TISS scores between the 2 years nor was there a significant difference in mortality. We infer that our overall patient population remained the same, at least as judged by the physician's perception of the degree of illness and therapy, physiologic status on admission, and outcome. Thus, we have achieved an increased productivity and efficiency of nursing care by collaborative practice change, which directed the elimination of nonessential but previously "required" tasks. Most of the eliminations were outgrowths of our unit's parochialism or arbitrary (often published) "standards" also based on opinion rather than data which had concretized into our daily practice, enforced unfailingly upon each entering new physician or nurse–but clearly amenable to study and modification.

Before he or she writes orders for a patient in the ICU, the physician must first determine the patient's general and unique needs. This will enable him or her to write orders that promote productive activities of nursing care rather than orders which create activity seemingly suitable to a busy ICU but actually wasting this precious resource. An efficient method to determine needs is to classify the patient according to the primary objectives of ICU care: monitoring/observation; extensive nursing requirements; constant medical care (see Chap. 1, "Setting Objectives: Perspectives for Care").

We must restrict the allocation of nursing care in the monitoring/observation patients so that these patients can continue to receive this necessary quantum of care in the ICU but not waste resources by too many routine orders. Patients who need extensive ICU nursing care are stable physiologi-

TABLE 15-2. Comparison of Patient Populations and Nursing Care

	1976	1984
TOTAL NURSING HR/PATIENT	19.6 ± 4.8	11.9 ± 3*
TISS	27.6 ± 7.9	23.9 ± 10.2
APACHE II	11.9 ± 5.2	13.7 ± 8.3
DEATHS	6(46%)	17(26%)
LABOR COSTS ($)	994,358	1,102,642
PATIENT DAYS (PDs)	2431	3152

* Significant difference $p < 0.05$.

cally, and physicians need to curtail their enthusiasm for long lists of orders for "completeness" or other perceived reasons; because they are stable physiologically, their needs will be met by independent nursing functions. In the case of the patient who is physiologically unstable and requires constant physician attention, the nursing care engendered will be voluminous and contain both dependent (orders and interventions) as well as independent nursing interventions. We will use this classification to describe and give examples of the relation between type of patient and implied care required, thus, defining the scope and boundaries of required physician's orders.

ORDERS FOR MONITORING/OBSERVATION PATIENTS

The monitoring/observation class generally consists of patients who are admitted to the ICU usually for one day and ultimately survive. In our ICU, these patients typically need less than 12 hours of care in a 24-hour period and, therefore, can easily be "doubled" with a more demanding patient for the nursing assignment.[10] In our ICU, these patients make up approximately 20% of the population[5] and are primarily elderly patients undergoing major elective surgery with a known risk of postoperative complications and often have (many) risk factors such as preexisting cardiovascular disease, chronic obstructive pulmonary disease, or diabetes mellitus.[14] These high-risk patients are at risk to develop potentially devastating complications which cannot be cared for on a general ward.[14-16] They are often admitted to the ICU preoperatively, primarily for invasive hemodynamic monitoring and then, postoperatively, for observation and anticipatory care. If we remember this need and restrict other activity and laboratory testing, they can be cared for properly and efficiently. If cared for appropriately, they represent about 30% of the patients but consume only 6% of the total PDs.[16] Our nursing protocol for this patient classification covers all the general nursing care categories listed in the Appendix including assessment of physiologic stability. Vital signs, measurements from invasive monitoring devices, temperatures, and surveillance measures are obtained on admission and then repeated intermittently while *rapidly and progressively lengthening the interval* between measurements. Table 15-3 outlines our current vital signs/measurements protocol. We quickly realized that observation *alone* of these physiologic parameters, mostly displayed continuously, was adequate *unless* changes occurred, at which time *recording* would be performed as well. Recording can usually be advanced to every 4 hours within 4 to 8 hours. Orders can specify the alarms for whatever monitoring devices are in use, such as mean arterial blood pressure, heart rate, intracranial pressure, continuous mixed venous oxygen saturation, and peripheral arterial oxygen saturation. Limits should be chosen by combining knowledge of the individual patient's physiology with the range for "normals." Thus, they serve as "early warning systems" or surveillance devices to signal change to the nurse and physician. No orders need be written for calibration in most ICUs. Usually, the pressure monitoring modules are externally calibrated before admission or insertion of the inva-

TABLE 15-3. Vital Sign/Measurement Protocol

NONINVASIVE	FREQUENCY
Apical heart rate/rhythm Respiratory rate/quality Peripheral pulse oximetry (arterial oxygen saturation)	q 15 min × 4 → q 30 min × 2 → → q 1 hr × 1–2 hr → q 4 hr
Temperature, rectal, PA or bladder	q 1–2 hr if abnormal; otherwise q 4 hr
Cuff blood pressure	On admission or when questioned or when arterial catheter questioned
INVASIVE	
Mean arterial pressure Systolic/diastolic arterial pressure Pulmonary artery (PA) mean pressure PA occlusion pressure (PAO) Central venous pressure (CVP) Intracranial pressure (ICP) PA mixed venous O_2 saturation ($S\bar{v}_{O_2}$)	As above: rapidly advance if patient stable

Alarms for each patient's predicted and acceptable variability can be set to provide constant surveillance with the exception of the following intermittent measurements: cuff blood pressure, rectal and PA temperature, and PAO pressure.

sive catheter and once each shift thereafter. Anytime we suspect that a pressure measurement is inaccurate, recalibration will be done. The practice of repetitive balancing and calibration are holdovers from earlier eras of drifting monitors and transducers.

Fluid intake in parenteral or enteral form is also recorded in a manner designed to reduce repetitive, inefficient–and potentially inaccurate–charting. Each individual site of infusion is assigned to a column and the rate as well as total solution infused are recorded once per nursing shift (every 12 hours) unless the rate or type of solution changes (Fig. 15-1). To indicate when a new container of infusate is begun, an arrow is placed in that column, and the initial volume is entered. The total for each fluid infused is calculated by multiplying the hours of infusion times the rate (usual products for common rates quickly learned), and the grand total is calculated by crossadding all column totals. This is recorded once a shift. The amount of urine output is *observed* while in the collection chamber of a urimeter or on the display of an electronic device every 1 to 2 hours but measured and recorded hourly only if the amount is near or below the unit's "worry" limit (50 ml/hr, 0.5 ml/kg, or whatever). Depending on the stability of the patient's fluid balance, urine volume is *recorded* every 4 hours for most patients to even once per shift when there are no actual or anticipated problems. All other fluid outputs such as gastric secretions and fluid from surgically placed drains are generally measured and recorded every 12 hours although observation alone is more frequent (Fig. 15-2).

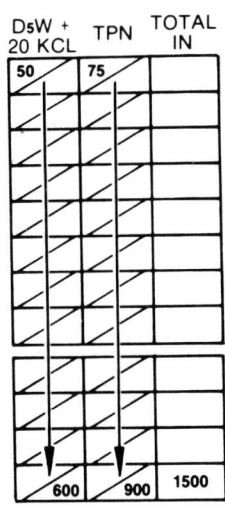

FIGURE 15-1. Comparison of the recording of IV intake. We previously kept hourly linear and cumulative totals, never used by either nurses or physicians in stable patients. We agreed to record rate and use an arrow to indicate the hours at that rate. In these examples, 60 entries and 34 calculations were replaced by 5 entries and 1 calculation. The information contained is the same. The hour-by-hour totals can be calculated, if need be (though need never seems to be). The 55 omitted entries and 33 unnecessary calculations were only possibilities for error.

Routine respiratory care of the monitoring/observation patient should include auscultation and recording of breath sounds. Suction of the endotracheal tube may be done on admission, but is usually done only when necessary because of accumulated or excessive secretions. If the patient appears hypoxemic or hyercapnic, the chest is auscultated. If the patient is extubated, breath sounds are auscultated as just described, and face mask oxygen usually provided. Incentive spirometry and coughing are taught to the patient and provided every 4 hours. We no longer use prophylactic chest physiotherapy or routine suctioning, again, shortening the list of older "standing" orders.

Most ICUs have defined protocols for dressing for invasive monitoring devices and other apparatus and wounds. These protocols, while differing to some degree, are usually formulated from general published guidelines or the policies of the hospital infection control and ICU committees. Needless to say, each new fellow or resident need not waste time or ink in writing his or her own preferences. Examples can be found in Chapter 16, "Preventive Care: Poorly Appreciated and Undervalued."

Bowel sounds are auscultated and recorded every 12 hours. Because of the relationship between stress ulcers and gastric pH, most ICUs monitor and treat pH in a uniform manner. Hygienic measures which include a bath,

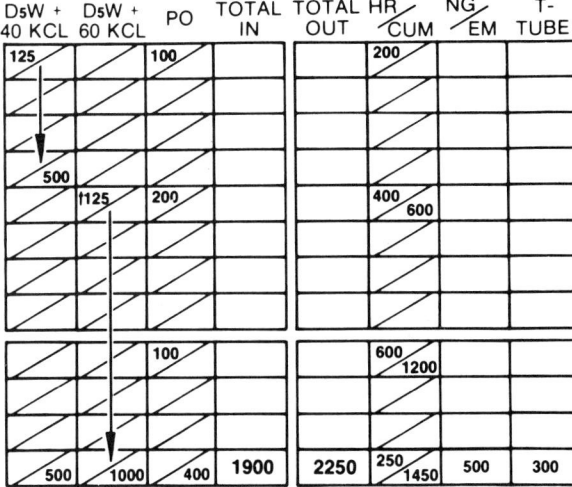

FIGURE 15-2. Intake and output according to the described simplifications. Only the essential information is included. In stable patients, urine volumes are measured only intermittently, although hourly observation is continued. Tube drainages are measured only once each shift unless volumes are large, or unless total intake and output figures should be calculated more frequently in the rare patient with clinical instability justifying more detail.

mouth care, Foley care, back or skin care, comfort measures, and cleaning the patient when incontinent are all, we believe, independent nursing functions and do not require written orders. Mobilization or activity is begun by turning and positioning the patient from side-to-side every 2 hours. Ambulation is usually done in collaboration with the physician (both in terms of orders and help)!

In summary, then, the physician's orders for the monitoring/observation patient should include the following: each—and only—specific laboratory test used to detect an expected complication, for example, an hematocrit to detect suspected hemorrhage; orders to wean ventilatory support and extubate as well as for any arterial blood gas required; alarm limits for continuous monitoring devices and ranges for clinically monitored parameters; intravenous fluid therapy; changes in the basic regimen as the patient's physiologic condition changes, for example, an order for a fluid bolus if the physician suspects hypovolemia; and medications.

ORDERS FOR PATIENTS WITH EXTENSIVE NURSING REQUIREMENTS

Extensive nursing requirement patients, by definition, are stable physiologically but consume more nursing care hours than those in the monitoring/

observation class. This type of patient makes up approximately 60% of our ICU population and remains in the ICU about 5 days (though 7% remained for more than two weeks) with a mortality rate of 11%.[5] Clinical examples of patients in this class include a former monitoring/observation patient who has developed complications such as infection or failure of one or more organ systems; the long-term patient with multitrauma; or a readmission to the ICU for treatment of complications. The role of physician orders is primarily anticipatory. Some clinical examples include assessment and treatment of the malnourished state; detection and treatment of the source(s) of infection; detection and treatment of organ system(s) failure; and ventilatory support. Specific orders could include adjustments in the composition or rate of parenteral nutrition infusion; a directed evaluation for fever; chest physiotherapy every 6 hours for a specific abnormality (*i.e.*, an atelectatic right upper lobe); an order for a 2-hour urine creatinine clearance to evaluate suspected renal dysfunction; and an order for an increase in the level of positive end expiratory pressure (PEEP) with subsequent physiologic evaluation in a patient with respiratory failure.

The nursing role in this class is more than extensive in just a temporal sense; it is independent, involving the active treatment of current problems and active prevention of further complications. Since these patients are reasonably stable physiologically, vital signs and measurements need only be recorded every 2 to 4 hours, using observation and the assistance from the monitoring alarms as in the monitoring/observation group. Sudden elevation in temperature is a common occurrence. If the patient has an indwelling Foley catheter for urinary drainage, the physician should consider using a catheter which also measures bladder temperature to obtain continuous core temperature measurement and to eliminate the frequent measurement of rectal temperatures to detect elevations or while cooling the patient.

Respiratory care of these patients is essentially the same, although because of a higher prevalence of moderate respiratory failure and pulmonary secretions, auscultation of breath sounds because of suspected hypoxemia, indicated endotracheal suctioning for secretions, and the assessment of the effectiveness of bronchodilator therapy are more frequent. Intake and output procedures are also handled in a similar manner to the monitoring/observation patient. More infusions or more complicated drainage systems, generating some of the increased nursing care, result in the patient's classification in extensive nursing care.

Hygiene and daily care activities such as the dressing changes are the same as those previously described. However, these interventions become of higher priority and are time-consuming. Mobilization and ambulation may be especially difficult in the patient with complicated wounds and many tubes, and especially if the patient is weakened by a long illness, this category often becomes a priority of care.

Although patient education and discharge planning are a part of the routine nursing care of the monitoring/observation patient, this category assumes much more importance in the extensive nursing requirement patient because of the longer ICU stay. Particular emphasis is placed on those procedures in which the patient can be an active participant. Discharge planning which involves other services such as the nutritional support team or the social worker are begun as soon as possible.

In general, the need for nursing care in this category still is less than 12 hr/PD, but more than needed for the monitoring/observation patient. A 1:2 nurse:patient ratio can be used; this assignment, however, may approach the limit of 24 hours of care per PD and the nurse may need support as well as assistance from the physician, the charge nurse, and ancillary personnel.

ORDERS FOR PATIENTS NEEDING CONSTANT PHYSICIAN CARE

The constant physician care group, the final classification to be described, requires intensive intervention from the physician as well as the nurse but makes up only approximately 12% to 20% of our ICU population.[5] Examples of these patients would be those who developed major complications and are unstable, a multisystem trauma victim who has multiple physiologic abnormalities, or an emergency admission for bleeding varices or the adult respiratory distress syndrome. The nursing hours required by these patients range from 13 to 24 hours. Although the nurse:patient ratio generally remains 1:2, for this to succeed, an attempt must be made to pair this patient with one requiring minimal care. If this is not possible, if there is no "light" or very stable patient, a 1:1 ratio would be necessary.

The vital signs and measurements for these patients may be done hourly or even more often if changes are occurring acutely; however, the frequency may be decreased as physiologic stability is achieved. Again, this assessment of stability and observation in place of continued rote recording can reduce the total number of nursing hours expended.

Although the remaining nursing protocols for the "constant physician care" patients are similar to those already described, the instability of the patient, resulting in more and different interventions, increases both the frequency and complexity of nursing care. As the need for dependent role functions increases (response to orders for medications), so, too, does the independent nursing function for the unstable patient require a multiperspective assessment to avoid critical oversights. Those patients will generate the most written orders by the physician, most related to changing interventions necessary to achieve physiologic stability, such as the type and rate of vasoactive infusions, and testing necessary to evaluate the etiology of the patient's problems, such as a chest radiograph to rule out pneumothorax.

To summarize, the physician must create general orders as in the previous categories. The physiologic instability which results in constant attention will create specific orders. Though these patients receive the largest number of nursing care hours, careful clinical decision-making and information processing resulting in excellent chart documentation will bring order to potential chaos and improve the likelihood of successful outcome. Harmonious interaction within the ICU team is a decidedly positive side effect.

CONCLUSION

The physicians, instead of believing that the length of the order sheet is somehow a good reflection of the thoroughness and ultimate value of "medical" care, can learn the role that order writing plays in confusing activity with productivity.

Intensive care is a limited resource; the principal limitation is the availability of excellent nursing care. The physician can develop understanding of both dependent and independent nursing role functions. By superimposing this understanding on a simple system of patient classification, order writing can enhance efficiency in the unit. The relationships among patient, disease, nurse, and physician are complex. With comprehension of independent nursing functions and the concept of collaborative practice, the physician can serve to enhance and expand nursing care, the factor limiting care in most ICUs today.[4] The approach herein described is intended to stimulate reassessment of our present practices, usually rooted in "antiquity" (circa 1960 in ICU terms). Structuring our goals through patient classifications and designing efficient care patterns to achieve the identified goals result in real fulfillment since tasks which were useless and time-consuming have been eliminated. The ultimate results are improved understanding and communication, diminishing stress and frustration, and improving the general mental health in the ICU.

REFERENCES

1. Morgan A, Daly C, Murawski B: Dollar and human costs of intensive care. *J Surg Res* 1973; 14:441
2. McKibbin RC, Brimmer PF, Galliher JM, et al: Nursing costs & DRG payments. *Am J Nursing* 1985; 12:1353
3. Schroeder RE, Rhodes AM, Shields RE: Nurse acuity systems: Cash vs. grasp (A determination of nurse staff requirements). *Nursing Forum* 1984; 21:72
4. Cullen DJ: Surgical intensive care: Current perceptions and problems. *Crit Care Med* 1981; 9:2905
5. Civetta JM, Husdon–Civetta JA: Maintaining quality of care while reducing charges in the ICU: 10 ways. *Ann Surg* 1985; 202:524
6. Cullen DJ, Civetta JM, Briggs BA, et al: Therapeutic intervention scoring system: A method for quantitative comparison of patient care. *Crit Care Med* 1974; 2:57
7. Dossey BM: The nursing process. In Kenner CV, Guzzetta CE, Dossey BM (eds): *Critical Care Nursing, Body—Mind—Spirit*, Little, Brown & Co, Boston, 1981
8. Sullivan S, Breu C: Survey of critical care nursing practice. Part IV. Staffing and training of intensive care unit personnel. *Heart Lung* 1982; 11:237
9. Hudson J, Caruthers T, Lantiegne K: Intensive care nursing requirements: Resource allocation according to patient status. *Crit Care Med* 1979; 7:69
10. Hudson–Civetta JA, Civetta JM, Weppler D, et al: Improved nursing efficiency and productivity. *Crit Care Med* 1987; 15:351

11. Knaus WA, Draper EA, Wagner DP, et al: APACHE II: A severity of disease classification system. *Crit Care Med* 1985; 13:818
12. Knaus WA, Wagner DP, Loirat P, et al: A comparison of intensive care in the U.S.A. and France. *Lancet* 1982; 62:642
13. Civetta JM: The inverse relationship between cost and survival. *J Surg Res* 1973; 14:265
14. Civetta JM, Hudson–Civetta JA. Cost effective use of the ICU. In Eiseman B (ed): *Cost Effectiveness in Surgery*. Philadelphia, WB Saunders, 1987; 3:13
15. Critical Care Medicine, Consensus Development Conference Summary, National Institutes of Health, 1983; 4(6)
16. Civetta JM, Hudson–Civetta J, Nelson LD: Costly care: Data, problems, and proposing remedies. *Crit Care Med* 1986; 14:357

APPENDIX: CATEGORIES OF NURSING CARE

		Activity and Description	Time
I.	**Vital Signs and Measurements**		
	A. Basic Vital Signs		
	1. Routine	1. Cuff blood pressure, pulse rate and rhythm, respiration rate and quality, temperature (rectal or PA), hypo/hyperthermia	8 min
	2. Individual	2. Above, separately	2 min
	B. Vascular Assessment	1. Presence/absence of peripheral pulses, color, temperature, movement, sensation, and comparison: all extremities	5 min
	C. Monitoring		
	1. Transducer setup	1. Assemble components of the transducer pressure monitoring system with sterile technique and initial external calibration	10 min
	2. Calibration	2. External system to verify accuracy of pressure measurement	2 min
	D. Arterial Catheter		
	1. Measurement	1. Include routine catheter maintenance and irrigation, systolic/diastolic pressure and mean arterial pressure, balance to patient position, assess waveform, set alarm limit	1.5 min/set of measurements

(Continued)

APPENDIX: CATEGORIES OF NURSING CARE (Continued)

I. Vital Signs and Measurements	Activity and Description	Time
2. Insertion	2. Assemble insertion tray, evaluate circulation to extremity, prepare limb restraint device, assist with procedure, verify tracing, apply sterile occlusive dressing and date and time, patient teaching regarding purpose and safety precautions, clean antimicrobial solution off patient's skin	15 min
E. Central Venous Pressure (CVP)		
1. Measurement	1. As above for arterial line except CVP includes only mean pressure	1.5 min each
2. Insertion	2. Assemble insertion tray, assist with explanation of procedure and positioning of patient, assist with procedure, verify waveform; apply sterile, occlusive dressing, date and time; patient teaching regarding purpose and safety precautions; clean antimicrobial solution off patient's skin	20 min
F. Pulmonary Artery Catheter		
1. All measurements	1. Includes routine catheter maintenance and irrigation; measurement of mean PA, PAO, CVP pressures, PA temperature, and mixed venous O_2 saturation; one ON/OFF PAO measurement on all intubated patients on PEEP/shift; assessment of waveform, set alarm limits	1.5 min set
2. PAO only	2. Mean pressure, waveform assessment	1 min

APPENDIX: CATEGORIES OF NURSING CARE (Continued)

I.	Vital Signs and Measurements	Activity and Description	Time
	3. Insertion	3. As above with CVP catheter as well as catheter preparation and testing prior to insertion, and obtaining a venous blood sample to calibrate the oximetry device *in vivo*	30 min
G.	Neurologic Vital Signs	1. Examination/assessment of pupil size, shape, equality and reactivity to light, accommodation; level of consciousness, movement of extremities, reaction to stimuli	8 min
H.	Intracranial Pressure (ICP)		
	1. Measurement	1. Includes routine catheter maintenance, measurement of mean pressure, assessment of waveform	1.5 min
	2. Insertion	2. Assemble insertion tray, assist with explanation of procedure and positioning of patient, assist with procedure, verify waveform; apply sterile, occlusive dressing, date and time; patient teaching regarding purpose and safety precautions; clean antimicrobial solution off patient's skin	Variable
I.	Medical Antishock Trousers (MAST)		
	1. Application	1. For both preoperative evaluation of cardiovascular function and treatment of hemorrhage, includes explanation to patient, turning patient to apply; assembling flowmeter, pressure monometer, and valve system	15 min
	2. Maintenance	2. Pressure checks, adjustments to flow, circulation checks to feet, assess skin integrity when removed	6 min/set of checks

(Continued)

APPENDIX: CATEGORIES OF NURSING CARE (Continued)

		Activity and Description	Time
II.	**Respiratory Care**		
	A. Blood Gases		
	1. Arterial	1. Drawn from arterial catheter: disinfect sample port, clear and flush catheter, complete laboratory voucher information, deliver to secretary, interpret results	4 min
	2. Mixed venous	2. Drawn from distal lumen PA catheter: as above, arterial, except sample to clear lumen and specimen must be drawn no faster than 1ml/20 sec	8 min
	B. Intubated Patient		
	1. Ventilator (respiratory therapist on duty in the ICU or if available by radio page: assume primary responsibility for ventilator function)	1. Patient teaching purpose and procedure; aware of support levels: IMV rate, PEEP level, pressure support, tidal volume; aware of patient parameters: PIP, spontaneous tidal volume; and immediate response to ventilator malfunction or alarm: manual insufflation with 100% O_2	4 min/shift
	2. Suctioning/insufflation	2. Patient teaching purpose and procedure; intermittent suction with instillation of normal saline and sterile technique; manual insufflation with 100% O_2; monitor for symptoms of hypoxia; assess amount, color, viscosity, and odor of secretions	8 min
	3. Auscultation of breath sounds	3. Position patient, explain purpose and procedure; auscultate side-to-side all lobes and compare: equality, adventitious sounds—wheezes, rales, or ronchi; check seal of endotracheal tube balloon	2 min

APPENDIX: CATEGORIES OF NURSING CARE (Continued)

II. Respiratory Care	Activity and Description	Time
4. Change endotracheal tube tape	4. Patient teaching purpose and procedure; suction mouth; check seal of balloon; change tape with assistance; mark position of tube; recheck seal of balloon	9 min
5. Intubation procedure	5. Arrange for a mechanical ventilator to be set up; preoxygenate the patient with face mask at 100% O_2; explanation to patient with restraint as necessary; assemble equipment; assist with positioning of patient, procedure, and taping of tube; auscultate and assess equality of breath sounds and seal of balloon	15 min
6. Chest physiotherapy	6. Assist respiratory therapist when necessary, includes suction and auscultation of breath sounds	15 min
C. Nonintubated Patient		
1. Supplemental O_2	1. Maintain reservoir of sterile water for humidity, assess function of flow device, maintain tubing free of excess condensation	2 min/shift
2. Incentive spirometry	2. Patient positioning; patient teaching of purpose and procedure; splint patient; auscultate chest before and after procedure; assess amount, color, viscosity, and odor of sputum produced	10 min
3. Auscultation of breath sounds	3. As above, intubated patient	2 min

(Continued)

APPENDIX: CATEGORIES OF NURSING CARE (Continued)

		Activity and Description	Time
II.	**Respiratory Care**		
	4. Nasotracheal suctioning	4. Explain procedure to patient; preoxygenate with face mask 100% O_2; intermittent suction with clean technique; auscultate breath sounds before and after procedure; assess secretions for amount, color, viscosity, and odor; monitor patient for symptoms of hypoxia	4 min
	5. CPAP mask (respiratory therapist as above, ventilator)	5. Explain procedure to patient, monitor seal on mask	2 min shift
	6. Chest physiotherapy	6. Explain procedure to patient, assist respiratory therapist in positioning patient when necessary	15 min
	D. Tracheostomy Care	D. Clean inner cannula, sterile technique; change and retie tapes; examine wound; note condition, drainage; change dressing; pad skin under tie if necessary	15 min

		Activity and Description	Time
III.	**Intake/Diet**		
	A. IV Fluid with Buretrol	A. Preparation of infusion, labeling, infusion rate and intake calculations; monitor rate of infusion	3 min for each
	B. IV Colloid Infusions	B. Preparation including patient and solution identification checks; infusion; observation for side effects	4 min/infusion
	C. IV Total Parenteral Nutrition	C. Check content of solution, monitor and chart infusion rate, monitor for side effects	2 min/infusion
	D. IV Drips, includes constant infusion pump		
	1. Preparation	1. Test and set up volumetric pump infusion device; prepare medication and add to infusion; monitor accuracy of infusion pump	6 min/infusion

APPENDIX: CATEGORIES OF NURSING CARE (Continued)

III. *Intake/Diet*	*Activity and Description*	*Time*
2. Record calculations	2. Monitor for side effects of infusion and prescribed rate; adjust infusion	4 min/calculation
E. Tubing Change	E. Includes all infusion and buretrols from solution to patient with sterile technique and labeling	4 min/solution
F. Nasogastric/ Gastrostomy Tube Feeding	F. Mixing powder packets with sterile water; label, date, and time solution; add dye for marker; add any medication; adjust and monitor infusion rate on volumetric pump; monitor patient for aspiration; test for residual feeding in the stomach; assess position of feeding tube	8 min/infusion
G. Oral Feedings	G. Assist patient as necessary; set up and position patient for maximum independence; may include caloric count documentation	15 min
H. Weight	H. Balance and preparation of the sling to be placed under patient; explanation to patient; transfer of the patient on and off the sling/stretcher	19 min
IV. *Output/Drainage* A. Foley Catheter	*Activity and Description*	*Time*
1. Routine catheter care	1. Clean around insertion site; monitor for erythema, exudate; maintain dependent closed drainage system; monitor for sediment, color and clarity	2 min/shift
2. Insertion straight catheterization	2. Assembly of insertion tray; explanation to patient; insertion with sterile technique; measurement of initial amount of urine; assess color and clarity of urine; clean antimicrobial solution off of patient's skin	12 min

(Continued)

254 Part II: People

APPENDIX: CATEGORIES OF NURSING CARE (Continued)

	Output/Drainage	*Activity and Description*	*Time*
IV.	3. Recorded outputs	3. Close visual inspection for color, clarity, and presence of sediment; measurement and disposal of urine; any mathematical calculation	2 min each
	4. Manual irrigation	4. Preparation and disposal of irrigation equipment; explanation to patient	2 min each
	5. Continuous bladder irrigation	5. Preparation of infusate; monitor and control rate of infusion; maintain patency, function, and sterility of three-way system; assess patient for any side-effects of therapy	10 min/shift
	B. Nasogastric Tube		
	1. Maintenance	1. Check placement each shift or when questionable; maintain security of placement; maintain function of low constant suction and patency of tube; reposition if necessary; may include periodic irrigation	8 min/shift
	2. Insertion	2. Explain procedure to patient; assemble suction/drainage equipment; insert tube, check placement, and secure position of tube	9 min
	3. *p*H	3. Measured q 6 hr routinely; aspiration of gastric contents; reconnection of suction	3 min/measurement
	4. Iced normal saline (GI bleeding)	4. Intermittent irrigation until blood return cleared if possible; medication may be added to irrigation	Variable
	C. Bowel Sounds/Abdominal Assessment	C. Auscultate rate and quality all four quadrants, percussion and palpation if bowel sounds absent and/or distention apparent	2 min

APPENDIX: CATEGORIES OF NURSING CARE (Continued)

		Activity and Description	Time
IV.	Output/Drainage		
	D. Chest Tubes		
	1. Routine	1. Assess integrity of closed underwater seal drainage system; assess amount and function of suction system; disconnect from suction and assess for presence/absence of air leak, strip chest tube to insure patency	4 min/tube/time if all checks made
	2. Insertion	2. Set up underwater seal drainage system; set up insertion tray; assist physician with explanation; assist with procedure; apply sterile, dry, occlusive dressing; auscultate breath sounds; perform routine checks, as above; clean antimicrobial solution off patient's skin	30 min
	3. Dressing	3. Remove old dressing and assess for drainage amount, type, color, and consistency; apply dry sterile gauze dressing and tape securely; routine every 48 hr or when soiled, saturated, or disturbed; assess stability of suture and chest tube's apparent position; date and time dressing	15 min
	E. Major Gastrointestinal Drainage (>2 tubes)	E. Includes maintenance of drainage system; assessment of patency and function; assess amount, type, color, odor, and consistency of drainage	11 min/shift
	F. Ostomies	F. Includes assessment of stoma viability and condition of surrounding skin; assess amount, color, odor, and consistency of drainage; application of drainage device as necessary; consult enterostomal therapist as need assessed; patient instruction in collaboration with standard care plan	12 min/bag change; 5 min/shift maintenance

(Continued)

APPENDIX: CATEGORIES OF NURSING CARE (Continued)

IV.	Output/Drainage	Activity and Description	Time
	G. Penrose Drains		
	1. Dressing change	1. Remove old dressing and assess for amount, color, type, consistency of drainage; apply dry, sterile gauze dressing and date and time; routine every 24 hr and when soiled, saturated, or disturbed	5 min each
	2. Change drainage bag	2. Assess for amount, type, color, and consistency of drainage	12 min if bag changed
	H. Sump Drains	H. Maintain and assess suction system; assess amount, color, consistency, type, and odor of drainage; maintain patency and elevation of drains	5 min/shift
	1. Dressing changes	1. As above for Penrose drains	5 min each
	2. Continuous irrigation	2. Prepare infusate and label; monitor/control rate of irrigation; assess function of suction device	4 min/infusion/shift
	I. Use of Bedpan	1. Assist patient with placement and with position; assess stool for amount, consistency, color, and hematest; measure if appropriate	8 min/use
	J. Sengstaken–Blakemore Tube	J. Pad helmet before application; explain device to patient and instruct with safety precautions; maintain traction and balloon; check and maintain tube patency; assess drainage for amount, type, consistency, and odor	30 min/shift

APPENDIX: CATEGORIES OF NURSING CARE (Continued)

IV.	Output/Drainage	Activity and Description	Time
	K. Peritoneal Dialysis	K. Prepare, warm, and label solution; administer solution; calculate dialysis fluid balance with each run; measure drainage and assess color, type, consistency, odor, and turbidity of drainage; monitor for side-effects of therapy such as electrolyte imbalance, infection, fluid retention, or dehydration	15 min/run
	L. Hemodialysis	L. Done in the ICU with a registered nurse specializing in dialysis; basically only monitoring for side-effects such as electrolyte imbalance; hypovolemia	Unable to quantitate
	M. Jackson–Pratt Drains	M. Maintain and assess suction by recharging suction bulb; safety measures to prevent accidental discontinuation; empty and recharge as ordered or as necessary, assess drainage	4 min/shift
	1. Dressing	1. As above, Penrose drain	5 min

V.	Daily and PRN Care	Activity and Description	Time
	A. Bath and Linen Change	A. Includes complete bed bath with backrub and application of lotion; includes decubitus care, see below. Range of motion exercises to all extremities; removal and reapplication of antiembolic stockings; assessment of skin integrity, turgor, color, temperature; complete change of bed linen	38 min

(Continued)

258 Part II: People

APPENDIX: CATEGORIES OF NURSING CARE (Continued)

V.	**Daily and PRN Care**	*Activity and Description*	*Time*
	B. Mouth Care	B. Nasotracheal intubation or extubated patient; if intubated, check seal on balloon; brush patient's teeth if he or she is unable, or assist the patient; rinse and irrigate mouth with medicated mouthwash solution; assess the integrity of the oral mucosa and tongue, observe for unusual drainage and, if present, note color, odor, amount, and consistency; assess for presence of a thrush infection or bleeding; oral intubation: assess seal of endotracheal tube balloon; suction mouth; if possible change the endotracheal tube tape and switch tube to other side of mouth (once a day) and clean bite block; turn head to side. Irrigate mouth with mouthwash solution and rub teeth/gums with gauze soaked in the solution; assess and observe mucosa and drainage as above	2 min
	C. Shave Male Patients	C. Electric razor	5 min
		Blade and shaving cream	8 min
	D. Decubitus Ulcer Care Grades 1 to 4 (more severe requires collaboration with physician)	D. Clean skin with soap and water; dry area thoroughly; position patient on side so that area to be treated is exposed; if abraded, spray with Neosporin; expose to heat lamp for 10–20 minutes; apply Maalox, Travase or other treatments as ordered	8 min Time included with bath; if severe must add time

APPENDIX: CATEGORIES OF NURSING CARE (Continued)

V. Daily and PRN Care	**Activity and Description**	**Time**
E. Dressing Changes		
1. Dry dressing, closed wound	1. Apply dry, sterile dressing noting date and time; observe old dressing for drainage. If present, note color, consistency, amount and odor; observe edges of suture/staple line for color, temperature, erythema, tenderness, and exudate	6 min
2. Wet to dry, minor open wound	2. Remove old dressing and assess as above; observe wound and wound edges as above; use karaya powder as indicated; observe for granulation tissue and bleeding; apply sterile, fluffed, wet gauze; label with date and time; set up sterile field with items needed and topical solutions/irrigations nearby	15 min
3. Major packing open infected wound	3. Remove old dressing and assess as above; observe wound and wound edges as above; preventive skin care as indicated; apply new dressings as ordered, label with date and time	20 min
4. Central/arterial/ICP line	4. Assemble prepackaged kit and solutions; don mask; remove old dressing; assess skin at insertion site for erythema or exudate (assess color, amount, odor, consistency); don gloves, palpate insertion site for warmth and tenderness; assess integrity of suture if used; cleanse skin as prescribed; apply antimicrobial ointment; reapply sterile, occlusive dressing; label with date and time	15 min

(Continued)

APPENDIX: CATEGORIES OF NURSING CARE (Continued)

V. Daily and PRN Care	Activity and Description	Time
F. Cultures	F. Includes completing laboratory voucher and delivery to secretary	
1. Peripheral blood by venipuncture	1. Assemble and label culture media; open kit and prepare kit and then patient's skin; withdraw blood; change needle; inject blood into media	5 min/culture
2. Tracheal aspirate	2. Insert secretion trap into sterile suction equipment. Instill sterile saline into endotracheal tube; hyperinflate lungs with 100% O_2, suction intermittently until specimen is obtained	8 min
3. Urine	3. Apply antimicrobial solution to specimen port of closed urinary drainage system; aspirate 1 ml urine; expel urine into culture media	4 min
4. Wound	4. Usually done while dressing is being changed; swab wound drainage and insert into media; anaerobic cultures are usually aspirated by the physician in CT suite or the operating room	4 min
5. Intracutaneous catheter cultures specimen obtained by physician	5. If catheter is to be discontinued: assist with procedure; don gloves if you need to handle the catheter segment; roll segment across agar plate; label plate; if done with guidewire change of catheter, done during catheter insertion procedure: see PA catheter insertion	4 min
G. Roto-Rest Bed Routine Rotating	G. Maintain bed rotating; stop only for procedures; air back of patient once a shift; remove and replace side cushions during patient's bath	60 min/shift

APPENDIX: CATEGORIES OF NURSING CARE (Continued)

		Activity and Description	Time
V.	**Daily and PRN Care**		
	H. Linen Change for Incontinence	H. Clean patient; assess skin integrity; turn patient, change linen; apply appropriate topical substance to buttocks	15 min
VI.	**Medications/Enemas**	*Activity and Description*	*Time*
	A. Medications	A. IV, IM, subcutaneous, nasogastric routes: prepare medication; administer medication; monitor patient for adverse reactions or effectiveness/result, record on flow sheet	2 min/medication
	B. Enemas	B. Preparation; administration; assess results; assist patient with bedpan	30 min
VII.	**Laboratory/Radiography**	*Activity and Description*	*Time*
	A. Laboratory Specimens	A. Clear catheter to be used; withdraw specimen; label for secretary; document and assess results	4 min/specimen
	B. Radiographs	B. Assist technician with position, patient, and plate; adjust bed; document test	8 min each
	C. Sugar and Acetone Urine Testing	C. Prepare specimen port with antimicrobial solution; withdraw specimen; perform test; document and assess results	4 min
	D. Dextrostix	D. Clear catheter to be used; withdraw 0.5 ml blood; flush catheter; perform test; document and assess results	4 min

(Continued)

APPENDIX: CATEGORIES OF NURSING CARE (Continued)

		Activity and Description	Time
VIII.	**Turning or Assisted Activity**		
	A. Turning	A. Turn and position patient with pillows; usually involves change of drainage pad; safely re-restrain extremity with arterial line	4 min
	B. Ambulation	B. Includes dangling patient's legs before ambulation; disconnect monitoring devices; ambulate a few steps to chair; rebalance monitoring devices; return patient to bed; monitor for adverse reactions to ambulation	12 min Additional ambulation variable time

		Activity and Description	Time
IX.	**Documentation/ Communication**		
	A. Shift Report	A. Systems review of patient from off-going nurse to on-coming nurse; after nurse has organized and begun patient shift care, a short summary version of report is given to the other nurse working in the room (4-bed, open patient care areas; assignment usually 1:2, nurse:patient)	15 min
	B. Admission/ Discharge Interview	B. Preprinted form completed and patient's problems, current and potential, are identified; major problems transcribed to nursing care plan at bedside	15 min
	C. Care Plan Update	C. Review of problems and priority as well as plan of patient care for each problem; changes are made as needed; done routinely once every 24 hr	5 min
	D. ICU Team Rounds	D. Work rounds at the bedside (patient-to-patient) with the fellow, junior residents, charge nurse, and bedside nurse; develop plan of care/ activities for day	10 min/patient

APPENDIX: CATEGORIES OF NURSING CARE (Continued)

IX.	***Documentation/ Communication***	***Activity and Description***	***Time***
	E. Systems Assessment	E. This charting is basically included in other areas, for example, neurologic status or vascular assessment	Incorporated into other categories
	F. Beeper Page/Phone Use	F. Includes time spent acquiring a free line; responding to answer	Variable, usually approximately 5 min
	G. Staff Meetings/ Education	G. Staff meetings are generally scheduled before and after work hours and the nurses receive overtime pay for attendance. Educational offerings may be scheduled as leave day with pay or are done as 45–60 min lectures and are scheduled as staff meetings	
	H. Emergency Cart Checks (intubation, cardiac arrest)	H. Assigned to nurses on a rotational basis to maintain everyone's familiarity with the equipment; a preprinted check list is used	5 min/cart
X.	***Transport***	***Activity and Description***	***Time***
	A. Admission of Preoperative Patient	A. Includes instruction regarding postoperative care and patient's role; check all bedside equipment for function; transcription of written orders, written plan of care developed for problems identified on interview; reading chart, discussion with physician and patient to obtain history which is written on the nursing care plan	50 min
	B. Admission of Patient	B. As above, patient is usually under anesthetic or an emergency and instruction often delayed	30 min

(Continued)

264   Part II: People

APPENDIX: CATEGORIES OF NURSING CARE (Continued)

		Activity and Description	*Time*
X.	**Transport**		
	C. Intraunit Transfer	C. Patient, all equipment, and supplies are moved from one room to another for ease of assignment or presence/absence of infection; includes gathering personnel required	30 min
	D. Transport to CT Scan	D. May include assembly of emergency equipment for transport; assemble transport monitor and attach to patient. Nurse must accompany and stay with patient during scan	140 min
	E. Discharge of Patient	E. Unless it is an interunit transfer or intermediate care, the nurse does *not* accompany the patient; patient must be detached from monitoring devices and transferred to a stretcher or wheelchair with supplies/medications; report must be given via telephone; ICU nurse to accepting ward nurse; unused medications must be credited and discarded, equipment disposed of or sorted for cleaning	30 min
	F. Postmortem Care	F. Body must be bathed and prepared with identification and protective devices; transfer to stretcher	30 min

APPENDIX: CATEGORIES OF NURSING CARE (Continued)

		Activity and Description	Time
XI.	*Psychosocial Interventions*		
	A. Family	A. Any time spent with the family members alone, in the patient's presence, or over the telephone; this time may include instruction, comfort measures, information sharing, crisis intervention, or needs assessment; may require an interpreter and thus increase time spent	Variable
	B. Social Services/ Spiritual Support Services/Dietary Services	B. Time spent obtaining a consult as well as actual interaction and problem identification with the assigned case worker; as above for priest, minister, rabbi; these services can be initiated by a need identified by or for the patient or family	Variable
	C. Patient Teaching	C. Included in all activities of patient care; on long-term patients may also generate the need for a multidisciplinary patient care conference	Variable

Preventive Care: Poorly Appreciated and Undervalued

Deborah Weppler
Joseph M. Civetta

16

The term "intensive care" usually creates an initial image of dramatic crises, minute-to-minute interventions, and the highest technology. Subconsciously, we tend to view the level of technology, severity of illness, and complexity of interventions as the major determinants of intensive care and, perhaps, as the only issues to be considered. To achieve success in the greatest number of patients, a different viewpoint must be cultivated. Although crises certainly exist and necessitate emergency interventions, these patients eventually stabilize and often receive prolonged care. Other patients never develop profound physiologic abnormalities but spend weeks or months in the intensive care unit. In such cases, many less spectacular and even uninteresting details assume an increasingly important role in determining the success or failure of treatment, as well as creating a major demand for the increasingly scarce resource of patient care.

Fundamental nursing care plays an important role in improving the patient's sense of well-being, avoiding lingering complications such as decubiti, which may markedly prolong hospitalization, and lessen the patient's sense of loss of control and overwhelming feelings of dependency. The team concept of intensive care fosters the practice of individual specialties monitoring themselves (*i.e.*, nurses monitoring nursing care and physicians monitoring medical care); however, care is most efficient when all components are truly understood and highly valued by all members of the team.

Continuity of care, the establishment and maintenance of routines, and the integrity of the unit rest primarily on nursing functions. Patients change, most of the physicians change, and the permanent bond depends not only on nursing actions but on the nurses themselves. The physician's knowledge of intensive care must not be restricted to pathophysiology and the choice of therapeutic interventions. A more complete understanding of the nature of total care and the specific bedside components is also important.

In this chapter, we discuss common bedside problems and activities along with useful corrective measures in order to provide the physician with the knowledge necessary to create a harmonious care plan. The effects of these problems on the functioning of the unit and the well-being of patients and families are, in our opinion, markedly underestimated. "An ounce of prevention is worth a pound of cure": at today's prices for intensive care, we cannot afford to be ignorant of these fundamental aspects of intensive care.

SKIN AND SUBCUTANEOUS TISSUES

There must be simple protocols for managing wounds; the skin surrounding drains, stomas, or open wounds; stomas and drains; decubitus ulcers; and superficial yeast infections. Each unit develops its own preferences, but the following recommendations are based on reasonably general principles.

WOUNDS

Wounds are closed in most clean cases and in some clean-contaminated cases. The skin is approximated with sutures or staples. It is usually covered with a dry sterile dressing for the first 24 to 48 hours, the time necessary for the wound to seal. Thereafter, the dressing may be changed or the wound may be left open to the air if no drainage is present. A light dressing may be used for comfort and convenience and to prevent bedclothes from catching on the sutures or staples. Routine nursing actions include observing and characterizing any drainage (color, odor, amount, consistency). The wound is observed for erythema around the sutures or staples and collections of fluid or pus around individual sutures or under the line of incision (which may indicate a loculated infection).

Contaminated wounds are usually managed in an "open" fashion. Typically, the fascia is closed but the subcutaneous tissues and skin are not approximated to avoid superficial wound infections. Occasionally, particularly after multiple dehiscences, the fascia itself is left open and abdominal contents are visible in the base of the wound. Many types of dressings are used. Dressings may be applied wet and removed after they have dried; this fosters superficial debridement, removes infected and necrotic material, and promotes a healthy granulating base. To be effective, dressings must dry; thus, they usually are not changed more often than two or three times a day. The wound may be packed completely with sponges soaked in normal saline, Betadine, diluted Dakin's solution, or diluted acetic acid solution. Ordinarily, one-fourth to one-half strength dilutions are used. These dressings are changed every 4 to 12 hours, depending on the amount of secretions and the degree of inflammation. Nurses generally select the specific hours for dressing changes. The physician should arrange to be called or should find a convenient time so that he or she and the nurse can examine the wound together. The wound is examined for pockets or loculated collections (Fig.

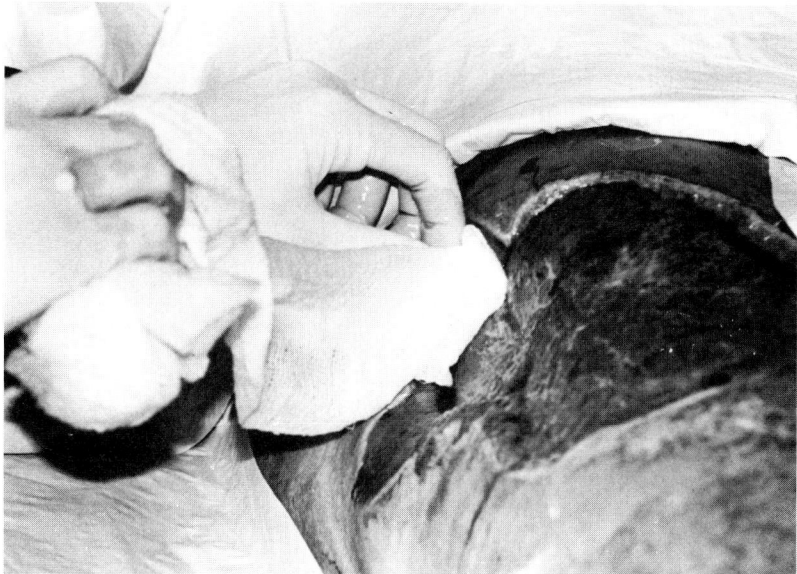

FIGURE 16-1. A wet-to-dry saline dressing for an undermined granulating wound of the thigh resulting from a pedestrian-auto accident. The nurse tucks moist gauze under the edges of the wound for debridement and to avoid creating closed pockets where pus might accumulate.

16-1). All tracts are packed open to ensure both drainage and debridement. Again, the characteristics of the drainage are noted. In addition, the characteristics of the tissue or organs are noted (*e.g.*, pink, pale, dusky, necrotic, shaggy).

SKIN SURROUNDING WOUNDS, DRAINS, OR STOMAS

Bodily secretions and some of the solutions used to dress wounds may be caustic and damage the surrounding skin. Dry dressings are used for protection. If wounds require frequent changing, removal of the tape may cause excoriations. In these situations, Montgomery straps are applied; when the dressing is changed, the straps are tied together, thus eliminating frequent removal of the adhesive tape.

STOMAS

The stoma itself is observed for viability. Instead of a pink and healthy color, edema, dusky mucosa, and even frank necrosis may be observed. The temperature of the mucosa can be estimated by touching with the finger. In the presence of an adequate blood supply, the mucosa is usually warm to the touch. Dusky mucosa that is cold probably has insufficient blood supply and will become necrotic. The skin surrounding the stoma is very susceptible to breakdown. Duodenostomies or jejunostomies secrete fluids that are more irritating than those secreted by ileostomies or colostomies. All stomas must be framed with a karaya ring, which should be approximately ¼ inch larger than the stoma. The ring is covered with a protective collection device (an ostomy bag). This appliance should be changed only if leakage develops, rather than on a routine basis. Skin breakdown occurs from frequent removal of adhesives as well as from the direct effects of the drainage. Characteristics of the drainage are usually noted as well. Excoriation can be severe, and simple measures may not permit application of a tight seal. Karaya gum powder can be "dusted" on the excoriated skin to provide a base for the karaya ring. An enterostomal therapist (if available) may be able to provide helpful strategies if difficult problems arise.

DRAINS AND FISTULAS

Both open and closed drainage systems are currently used. Closed drainage systems are used to prevent external contaminants from traveling into the drainage tract, resulting in internal contamination. These drains are usually connected to a suction apparatus and the amount of drainage is recorded daily. Other characteristics are noted as well. If open drains are used, the use of dry dressings and frequent changes may be sufficient if the amount of drainage is small. However, an ostomy bag can be used if an opening is tailored to surround the exit wound (Fig. 16-2). This helps to prevent skin

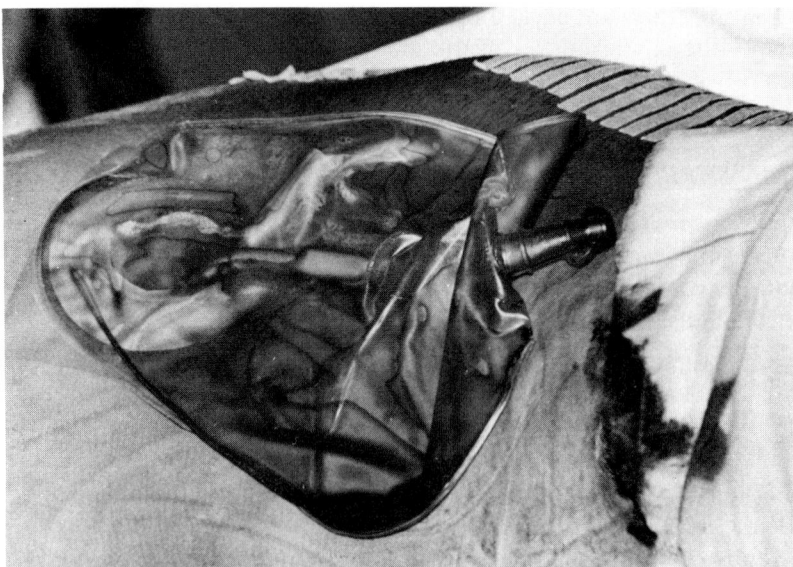

FIGURE 16-2. Catheter-Penrose drain, placed above a liver laceration, is enclosed in an ostomy bag. The opening has been tailored to leave little exposed skin, for protection; by capturing the drainage, the number of dressing changes may be reduced and the amount of drainage measured.

excoriation and provides a method of quantitating the amount of drainage. Patients may have many drains or fistulas (Fig. 16-3). Whenever possible, individual ostomy bags should be used for each, with both characteristics and amounts of drainage noted individually, and a labeled diagram should appear in both the chart and the nursing care plan.

Fistulas, particularly upper enteric fistulas, may pose perplexing management problems. The drainage may be very irritating, and if the tract or site is irregular it may be difficult to secure any appliance to protect the skin and to quantitate the drainage (Fig. 16-4). Again, an enterostomy therapist may know certain "tricks" to help in this situation.

DECUBITUS ULCERS

We tend to associate decubitus ulcers with long-term patients in nursing homes who do not receive ideal nursing care. However, decubitus ulcers may develop in the ICU. They are caused by pressure exerted on the subcutaneous tissue and skin when compressed between the weight of the body and a mattress or chair. The pressure affects capillary perfusion and interrupts the blood supply, producing ischemia and preventing the removal of cellular waste. When this pressure is unrelieved, cell necrosis may occur. The patient in shock or with cardiovascular instability has a marked decrease in cuta-

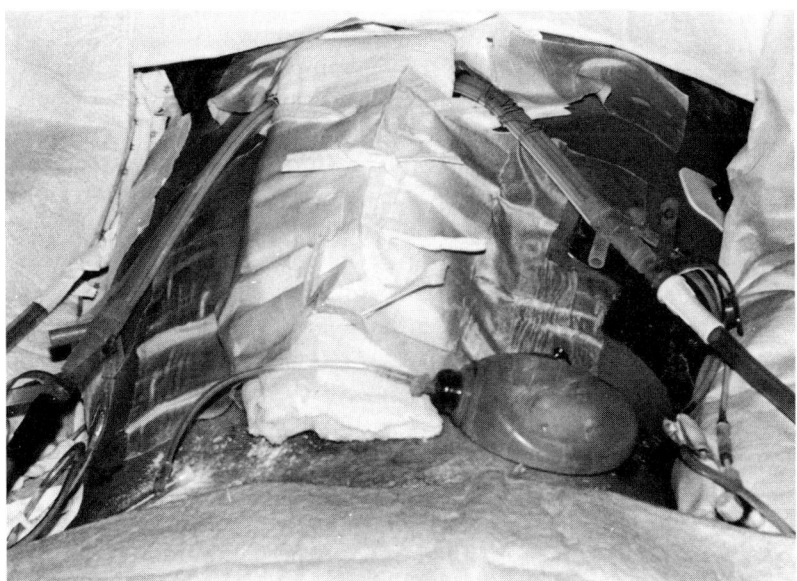

FIGURE 16-3. *Complicated abdominal wound containing two sumps to an esophagojejunal fistula (post-total gastrectomy), four CT-guided percutaneous catheters, and an open wound. Montgomery straps are used for the central wound. Sumps are connected to constant irrigation/suction systems. Percutaneous catheters use bulb suction devices.*

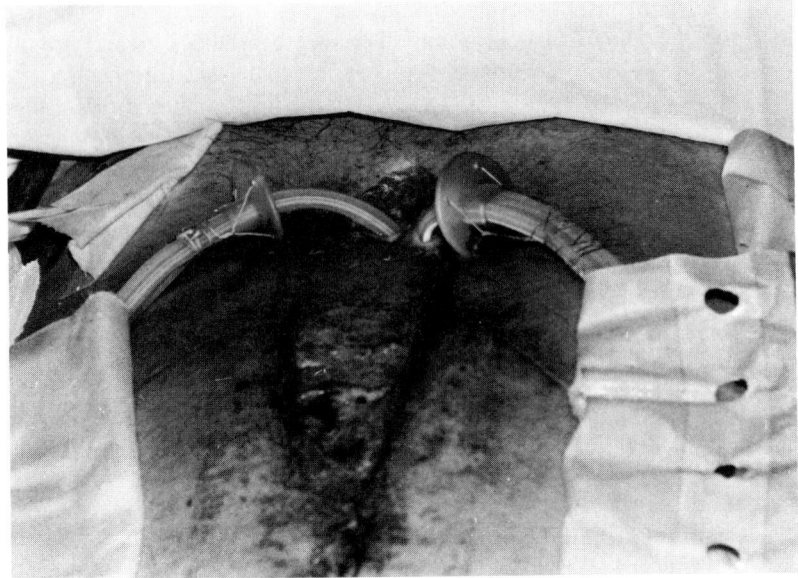

FIGURE 16-4. *This abdominal wound was left open following a third laparotomy for drainage of abscess. Despite the number of drains, amount and types of drainage, and complexity of dressing, the wound is granulating well and there are no signs of irritation in the surrounding skin—a tribute to nursing skill and ingenuity.*

neous blood flow, initiated by primary compensatory mechanisms. Although events seem to occur on a minute-to-minute basis, many hours may elapse while monitoring devices are inserted and interventions are initiated in sequence. If the patient is not turned and the pressure is not relieved because of "instability" or because there are "too many other things to do," pressure necrosis may occur, despite the fact that the patient was surrounded by numerous physicians and nurses delivering the "best" type of care.

Decubitus ulcers can be classified as superficial or deep. Superficial ulcers may be subdivided into four stages that are useful in planning effective treatment.

Stage I—The skin is erythematous but unbroken. Redness fades quickly when the pressure is relieved.

Stage II—There is a break in the epidermis, either a superficial ulcer or a blister (Fig. 16-5). The edges are distinct and blend into an area of indistinct redness, heat, and induration. The redness does not disappear when pressure is relieved. Drainage or pain may be present.

Stage III—The ulcer involves the dermis and subcutaneous tissue. The wound depth is thus greater than in stage II. Drainage and pain are often present. A hard eschar or necrotic tissue may be present in the wound.

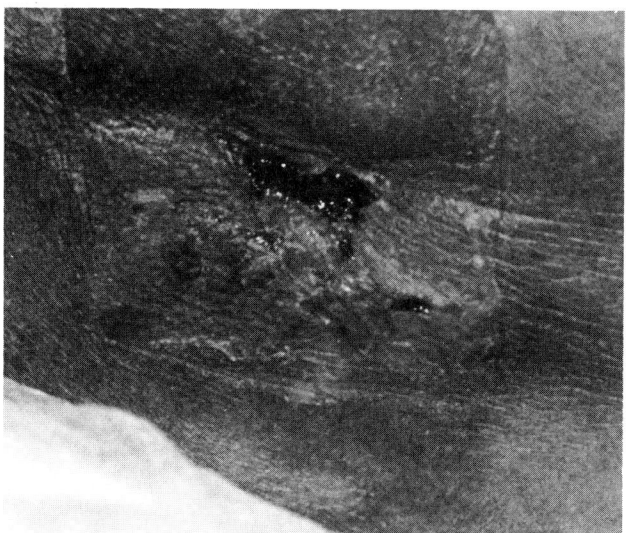

FIGURE 16-5. *Stage II decubitus ulcer with a 3-cm area of superficial skin breakdown. This patient had been in the ICU for 75 days following a motor vehicle accident.*

Stage IV—The lesion may extend into the muscle and down to bone (Fig. 16-6). Sinus tracts, necrosis, and drainage may be present, although pain may be absent at this stage.

Deep pressure ulcers develop in tissues under the skin and tend to occur in response to shearing forces. Necrosis begins beneath the skin rather than in the epidermis, as described in the development of superficial decubitus ulcers. Deep ulcers may present initially as blisters, which change into eschars. The lesion itself may be well developed before any signs are visible. Classic signs include a hard mass under the skin and purplish discoloration of the skin area subjected to pressure. The amount of tissue damage is usually much more extensive than indicated by the amount of skin area involved.

Patients susceptible to decubitus ulcers include those who are bedridden, elderly, or immobile. Other potentially predisposing characteristics include hyperactivity, obesity, cachexia, poor nutritional status, neurologic disease, conditions that impair sensation (*e.g.,* peripheral vascular disease or diabetes mellitus) and orthopedic problems. Patients who are physiologically unstable tend to be left immobile, and those with a multitude of obvious "crises" may receive less attention to fundamental position changes.

In addition to sites in the sacral area, decubitus ulcers in ICU patients may develop on the back of the head, behind the ear, and over the scapular spines, iliac crest, heels, and elbows. Preventive measures start with the recognition of susceptible patients. Then, it is necessary to ensure that change of position, good body alignment, and proper skin care are part of the initial

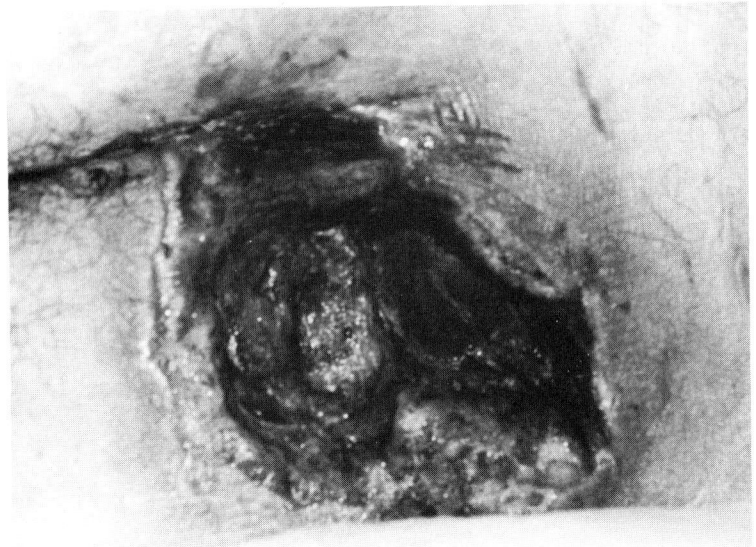

FIGURE 16-6. A Stage IV lesion with necrosis, extending to the sacrum. This lesion developed in a patient with profound cardiovascular instability that persisted for 3 weeks following acute myocardial infarction. The patient was treated with dopamine, dobutamine, amrinone, nitroprusside, and nitroglycerin in varying doses. Agitation or even movement precipitated marked venous desaturation (0.30) and increased pulmonary artery occlusion pressures (> 40 mm Hg) despite continuous infusion of morphine, 18 mg/hr. The compromised cardiovascular function produced decreased skin perfusion. The underlying instability worsened with movement, making position changes hazardous and resulting in this serious decubitus.

medical care plan, even in patients with cardiovascular instability. The "egg crate" mattress, "bunny boots," and elbow protectors should be used, especially in patients with peripheral vascular disease or diminished sensation.

Treatment

Prevention is clearly the best treatment. Improving nutritional status and ensuring frequent position changes are fundamental. Susceptible areas should be observed frequently to detect any signs of pressure, especially during their earliest stages. For stage I lesions (reddened area), use of the egg crate mattress and good skin care should suffice, since the redness will disappear when the pressure is eliminated. In stage II lesions, an actual break in the skin has occurred. In addition to the previously mentioned measures, a heat lamp may be used four times a day, Maalox may be applied to help dry up any drainage, karaya gum may be placed over the area, and an absorbable gelatin sponge can provide an artificial layer to absorb pressure over a bony prominence. The involved area itself can be surrounded by support so that there is no direct pressure. Stage III is a deeper ulcer. Wet-to-dry dressings or enzymatic ointments (Travase) may be used for debridement. In cases of thick, shaggy, necrotic tissue, surgical debridement may also be necessary. Local wound measures as described above may then be used.

Stage IV lesions usually require extensive surgical debridement, with local measures used to provide a clean granulating base. Often, formal operations, including resection of bony prominences and creation of a skin flap, are necessary. In the ideal situation, these lesions should never develop while a patient is in the ICU. Prolongation of hospitalization and increased expense, in addition to the need for major operative procedures and the risk of invasive sepsis, are horrifying consequences of these complications of ICU care.

TOPICAL YEAST INFECTIONS

Patients who receive long-term broad-spectrum antibiotics and those who are immunocompromised are the two groups at risk for topical yeast infections. The lesions are characterized by erythema, scale formation, peripheral papules, and pustules and are often pruritic. They commonly occur under skin folds in the neck, abdomen, thigh, axillae, and under the breasts. Therapeutic measures include keeping the area cool and dry and applying topical mycostatin powder each 12 hours or clotrimazole cream every 6 to 12 hours. Thrush is the term used to describe a candidal infection in the oral cavity. A thick white scaly coating is noted over the tongue and in other areas of the mouth. Nystatin (Mycostatin) liquid, 5 to 10 ml, is used as an oral rinse ("swish and swallow") four to six times a day. Patients who develop superficial yeast infections should be evaluated for more serious yeast infections in the wound, urine, or blood.

MUSCULOSKELETAL SYSTEM CONSIDERATIONS

COMPARTMENT SYNDROMES

Patients who have suffered crush injuries or have conditions producing vascular interruption may develop compartment syndromes, commonly in the lower leg. The injury itself or the ischemia induced by vascular interruption results in increasing tissue edema; the pressure within the compartment, limited by bone and fascia, then rises above venous and then arterial pressure. At this point, necrosis of the entire compartment contents occurs. Early signs and symptoms may be difficult to elicit in patients who have suffered multiple injuries and may not be fully responsive because of a closed head injury or the continued effects of sedatives or anesthesia. Pain, numbness, and loss of sensation are common findings. Swelling of the compartment may be noted, as well as limb paralysis and sensory deficits.

Any extremity subjected to trauma or ischemia should be monitored for all of these signs and symptoms; the diagnosis must be made early enough so that, when the pressure is relieved surgically (by fasciotomy), function can return (Fig. 16-7). This will not be the case if ischemic necrosis has occurred.

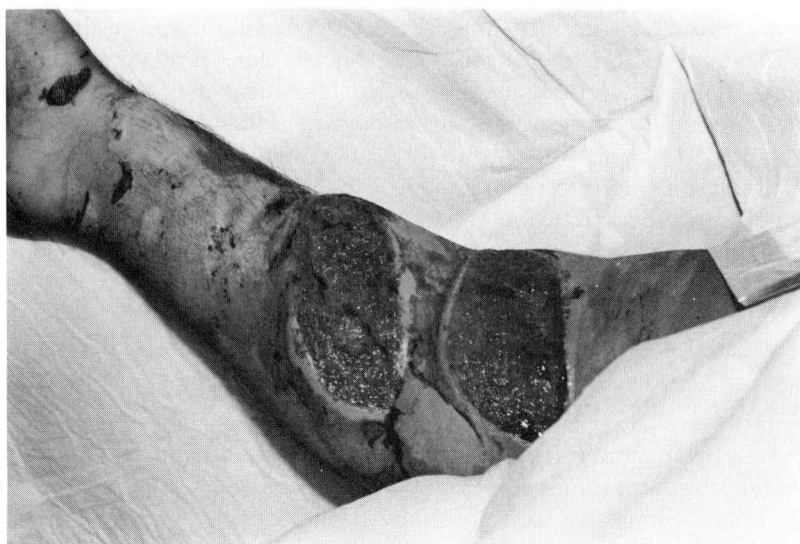

FIGURE 16-7. *A compartment syndrome in the forearm following fractures of radius and ulna, treated by fasciotomies. The wound edges separated and the bases are granulating. Split-thickness skin grafts may be necessary to close large defects.*

LOCALIZED ISCHEMIA

There are three clinical settings that lead to the development of patchy or localized ischemia. First, the edges of a wound, particularly in flap reconstructions, may have insufficient vascularity, and circumscribed areas of ischemia and necrosis may occur. Second, in association with generalized septicemia, emboli may lodge in end arterioles of the skin. These septic emboli may progress to produce an infected necrotic area. The third cause, ischemia secondary to vascular cannulation, is probably the most common. The frequency of this complication depends on several factors, including size and type of catheter, site selected, coexisting vascular disease, duration of catheterization, and the external pressure monitoring system. Color, sensation, muscle function, and temperature must be evaluated during each nursing shift. This problem must be recognized promptly so that the catheter may be removed before tissue necrosis occurs. Small emboli may break off from an indwelling arterial catheter and produce a localized patchy area of necrosis in one or more digits. If the artery itself has become thrombosed and there is insufficient collateral circulation (no matter how carefully the circulation was evaluated at the time of insertion), the viability of the hand, foot, or even the entire extremity (depending on the site of insertion) may be in jeopardy.

Most ICUs adhere to a protocol for the types of catheters inserted and the conditions of insertion. The best method to prevent ischemia is to use the smallest catheter, made of the least reactive substance, in the largest artery, and for the shortest period of time. If there are any signs of ischemia or changes in color, temperature, or sensation, the line must be removed as quickly as possible. If the artery is not fully thrombosed, this may provide a small increase in flow that is sufficient to reverse the ischemia. If ischemia persists, a sympathetic block should be performed, monitoring temperature in the digits before and after injection to document efficacy. Repeated sympathetic blocks with long-acting agents may provide a sufficient increment in blood flow through collateral circulation to maintain viability. Direct surgical repair has also been effective. Thrombectomy and reconstruction should be considered before the damage becomes irreversible. Thrombolysis may also be considered. Unfortunately, frank necrosis is a recognized complication. In these situations, amputation is delayed as long as necessary to allow the most distal demarcation possible.

CONTRACTURES

Elderly patients who remain immobilized for long periods of time and patients with neurologic impairment may develop contractures while in the ICU. Our attention, again, is usually focused on "life-threatening" and "attention-grabbing" pathophysiologic changes, such as acute hypotension or hypoxia. These long-term patients, who seem to make little or no discernible improvement, may actually be slipping away from a potentially functional life if contractures develop. Mobilization of such patients, with their many monitoring lines, tubes, and ventilators, is a difficult task that is sometimes easier left undone. However, early and repeated mobilization is an important method to forestall the development of contractures. Usually, the physicians in the unit must provide physical assistance in the process of mobilizing these patients. "Bunny boots" provide relief of pressure points; there is also an external device that can be adjusted to provide dorsiflexion in an attempt to prevent foot drop. Range of motion exercises should be performed by a nurse or technician on each shift to avoid contractures. This is usually done with the hygienic care.

If a patient is considered to be at high risk for developing musculoskeletal problems, the physical therapist should be consulted early, before problems occur. In addition to supervising exercises to prevent contractures, the physical therapist may be of inestimable value in helping to motivate these long-term patients, who often seem to prefer to "slip away." The experience gained in motivating difficult patients during long-term rehabilitation makes the physical therapist an invaluable asset to the ICU team.

SUBTLE INFECTIOUS PROCESSES

Usual sources of postoperative fever or sepsis in the ICU patient are well known. There is sepsis related to the primary problem, such as peritonitis, and a relatively short list of other sources, such as urinary tract or wound infection and nosocomial pneumonia. Some sources are less obvious and may be overlooked, especially in the long-term patient.

Phlebitis, especially in a previous IV site, is quite common. It may be merely sterile inflammation caused by irritating substances in the intravenous solution. If the inflammation is septic, it can produce both local and systemic problems. Local infection, including purulence, is the most common manifestation; septicemia may be persistent and septic emboli may also occur. The incidence of phlebitis increases markedly after 48 to 72 hours of peripheral intravenous infusion. Lines that were placed under adverse circumstances (*e.g.*, during emergency resuscitation or in a crowded emergency room) may have a higher incidence of phlebitis. To prevent phlebitis these lines should be removed as soon as replacement sites can be cannulated. The dressings over existing peripheral intravenous catheters are usually done according to hospital standards. Most protocols prescribe daily care and limit duration of infusion to 72 hours.

If the site becomes reddened or painful, the IV should be removed and warm compresses applied. Elevation of the extremity will help resolve edema. If the patient shows signs of systemic infection or if pus can be expressed from the needle entry site, surgical exploration is indicated. Proper therapy consists of opening the skin and removing the entire section of involved vein. Antibiotic therapy may be necessary if septicemia has developed.

Central venous catheters are usually inserted under sterile conditions and are cleansed every 48 hours, including the use of an antimicrobial ointment. The nurse assesses the site for any early signs of infection. Duration of catheterization varies according to the type of catheter and hospital procedure. When "line sepsis" is suspected, changing the catheter using a guidewire makes it possible to obtain a section of the intracutaneous segment of the catheter for culture. If the removed segment is positive on culture, the catheter inserted by guidewire is then removed and a new insertion site chosen. Local signs of infection, such as purulence or redness surrounding the catheter, indicate an advanced infection and should rarely be encountered if technique and assessment are of good quality. In addition to removing the catheter, it is important to review insertion and maintenance procedures to identify and correct potential "breaks in technique" that may have resulted from human error, from not knowing or understanding the policy, or even from a faulty protocol. However, in most positive catheter segment cultures, there are no external signs of infection.

SINUSITIS

Inflammation and infection of one or more paranasal sinuses are often related to tubes passed through the nares. Although nasotracheal intubation may often be the easier route in patients with head injury, the incidence of sinusitis is high and there is a general preference to avoid prolonged nasal intubation. Feeding tubes, nasogastric tubes, or other enteric tubes may be a sufficient stimulus to induce the edema that occludes the ostium of the sinus and, thus, creates the conditions for sinusitis. Generally, the most common symptom is pain; however, this is difficult to evaluate in an intubated or unconscious

ICU patient. The diagnosis may be made if purulent drainage is observed around the indwelling tube. More commonly, however, sinusitis is diagnosed after specific tests have been ordered because the diagnosis was entertained. Sinus radiographs are difficult to obtain in the ICU and are of questionable value. Many cases of sinusitis occur in association with head injury, and the sinuses should be evaluated on the patient's computed tomography scans.

Indwelling nasotracheal tubes should be removed in all patients as soon as possible. In a patient with sinusitis, prompt removal is mandatory. An orotracheal tube or tracheostomy should be substituted for the nasotracheal tube. The nasogastric tube should be removed and replaced through the mouth, even though tubes in this position are often more difficult to maintain and may be less comfortable for the patient. Systemic and local vasoconstrictive agents may reopen the ostia, and antibiotic therapy may be used. When spiking temperatures persist, if air–fluid levels are seen by radiograph, the sinus can be aspirated to obtain a culture specimen. An antral window may be necessary to promote better drainage.

PERINEAL INFECTIONS

Although they are more commonly associated with the emergency room, perirectal abscesses may occur in ICU patients, particularly those at prolonged bedrest. Incision and drainage with subsequent packing are necessary after the abscess has matured.

Epididymitis is an infrequent and often unsuspected cause of sepsis in males with long-term indwelling Foley catheters. Physicians in the ICU tend to examine the heart and lungs and surgeons examine the abdomen, but perineal examinations are "deferred"—hence, both perirectal abscesses and epididymitis are easily overlooked because they are not looked for.

COMPLICATIONS ASSOCIATED WITH ICU DEVICES

Whenever we violate the patient's physical integrity during monitoring and therapy, specific complications may result in disfiguring cosmetic problems that will persist long after the "lifesaving" ICU care is but a dim memory. Pressure from indwelling tubes may produce local ischemia that may progress to necrosis if this possibility is not considered and preventive and therapeutic measures are not part of the daily care plan.

Endotracheal Tubes

It is often difficult to secure an endotracheal tube so that its distal tip remains in a constant position in the trachea, neither too close to the vocal chords nor progressing into the main-stem bronchi. These tubes must be taped securely around the head (Fig. 16-8). It is essential to avoid local pressure induced by the method of taping or angulation or by excessive weight when the tube is attached to the ventilator circuit. The tip of the nose, the alar

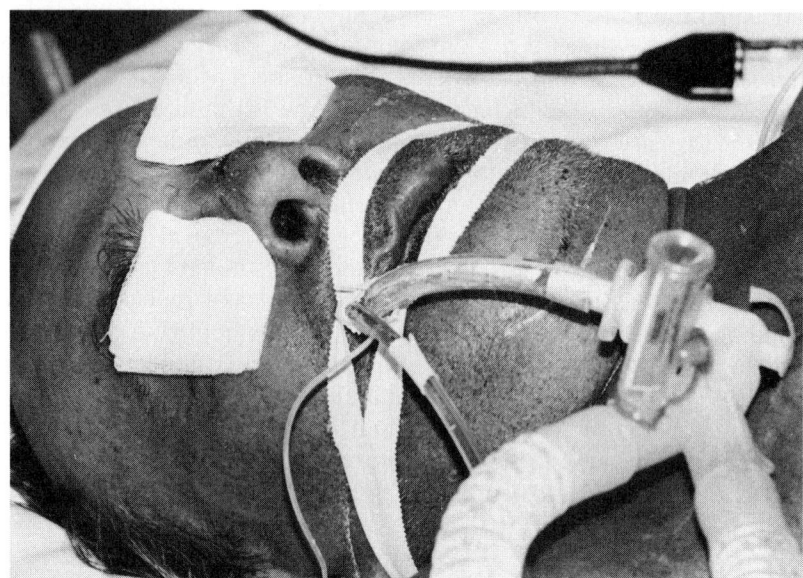

FIGURE 16-8. The oral endotracheal tube has been secured with tape passing around the patient's neck and across the upper and lower lips. This patient with a closed head injury had undergone emergency nasotracheal intubation but developed fever; maxillary sinutis was diagnosed by CT scan. Note that both the endotracheal tube and the tube for gastric decompression exit through the mouth.

cartilage, and the corner of the mouth are particularly vulnerable. We prefer to alternate sides of the mouth every 24 to 48 hours to avoid prolonged pressure. If nasal tubes are employed, it is extremely important to avoid angulation and pressure at the tip of the nose. Again, nasotracheal intubation, often preferred on the basis of the increased patient comfort and ease of fixation, has a significant complication rate in terms of pressure necrosis and sinusitis.

Nasogastric and Feeding Tubes

Nasogastric and feeding tubes should be taped so that neither angulation nor pressure can occur. Often, the tubes may be taped in a position that does not cause pressure, and then after suction apparatus or feedings are attached, the tube is angulated, resulting in unwanted and unexpected pressure (Fig. 16-9).

Tracheostomy Tapes

Umbilical tapes are often used to secure tracheostomy tubes in place. These should be tied snugly, but there should be space for one finger to fit between the patient's neck and the tape itself. If excoriation occurs under the tape or

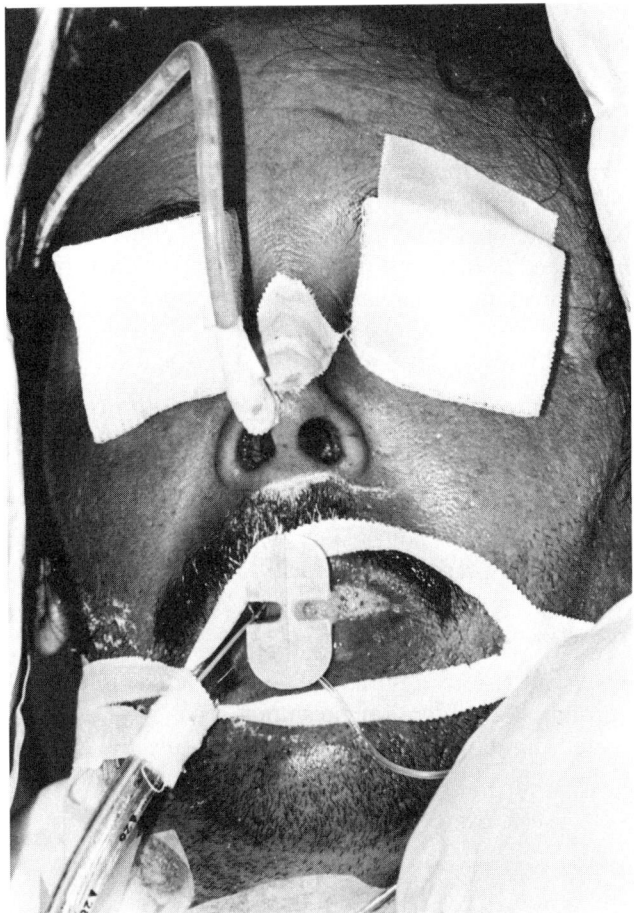

FIGURE 16-9. *This nasogastric tube was placed and taped with the tubing in line with the arc entering the nose. For illustrative purposes, the tube was angulated when connected to the suction apparatus. If the tube was left in this position, pressure would be placed on the tip of the nose at the angle formed by the septum and alar surface. Ultimately, necrosis would result.*

near the stoma, the neck should be padded with plain gauze pads before the ties are secured.

Traction Helmet

Bleeding esophageal varices are life-threatening and difficult to control. Inflation of the gastric and esophageal balloons of the various tubes used often is insufficient to control bleeding unless traction is added. Pulley systems and weights at the end of the bed are extremely difficult to use for protracted periods of time. The development of a traction helmet permitted constant traction to be maintained relatively easily. However, if this traction is applied too forcefully, necrosis of both the forehead and cheeks can occur. Large areas of full-thickness skin necrosis on the face are far too common. After the patient survives hospitalization, disfiguring scars will remain. This complication may be prevented if the helmet is secured with all three of the straps so that there are no shearing pressures. Abdominal combine dressings may be used to provide additional padding between the helmet and the patient's face. Despite the need to maintain traction, the affected areas of the skin must be examined to preclude ischemia and necrosis.

Arterial Catheter Armboard

To facilitate the placement of a radial artery catheter, the hand is usually fixed with the wrist extended, the fingers are secured, and padding is placed beneath the dorsum of the hand. Excoriations, ischemia, and breakdown may occur. The tapes may need to be loosened, especially if edema develops. The armband position can usually be adjusted so that the character of the arterial tracing is unchanged but pressure is avoided (Fig. 16-10).

Military Antishock Trousers

Military antishock trousers (MAST) were originally designed for prehospital use in patients with profound hypotension presumed secondary to acute blood loss. The anticipated duration of such use included only the time to move the patient from the scene of the accident to the emergency room and,

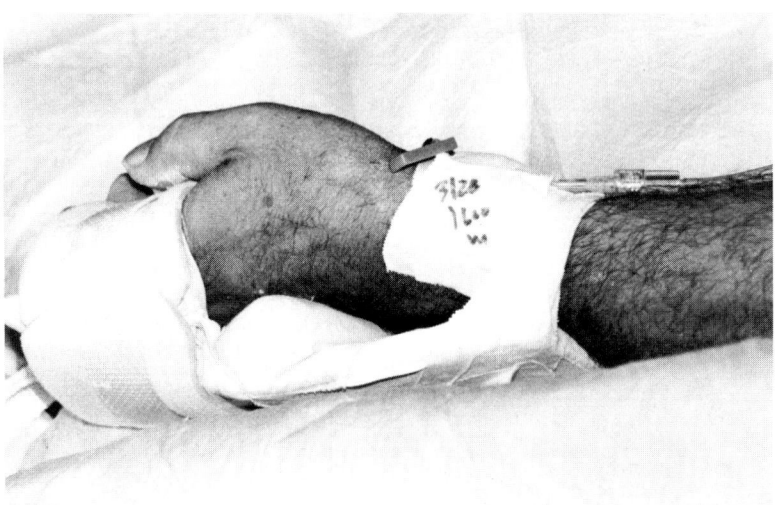

FIGURE 16-10. The hand containing a radial artery catheter is padded, fixed to an armboard, and restrained. Angulation and pressure have been minimized while maintaining function of the catheter and fixation.

subsequently, to the operating room. However, external compression has also been used in an attempt to control bleeding from pelvic fractures and in association with dilutional or hypothermic coagulopathies in patients who have received multiple blood transfusions. Patients treated in this manner may remain in the MAST for 24 to 48 hours. Pressure is usually maintained at approximately 30 to 40 mm Hg, which is sufficient to create two potential complications. The first complication, more serious but fortunately rarer, is a compartment syndrome similar to that described earlier in this chapter. Patients maintained in the MAST must, therefore, have frequent assessments of color, temperature, motion, and sensation in the feet to detect changes before rising compartment pressures produce ischemic and irreversible changes. The second complication, which is almost universal in patients who are in the MAST for 24 to 48 hours, consists of blistering of the skin that was covered by the garment. Management is similar to that of blisters induced by thermal injury. We generally pad the inside of the MAST with towels and pillowcases to distribute the pressure as evenly as possible, to pad protuberances, and to minimize blister formation.

MISCELLANEOUS CONDITIONS

MISSED EXTREMITY FRACTURES

In the initial assessment of the multitrauma patient, life-threatening injuries must be the primary focus. Emergency operative intervention may often be necessary, and evaluation can be completed only after admission to the ICU. The symptoms that would be of use in evaluating an alert patient in the emergency room include pain, limited range of motion, or actual deformity. Postoperative or unconscious patients cannot be assessed in this manner. In addition, complications of extremity fracture, such as compartment syndrome or vascular compromise, must be detected by repetitive examinations of color, temperature, muscular function, sensation, and pulses. An area that is deemed suspicious should be further evaluated by a radiograph.

ALTERATIONS IN BOWEL FUNCTION

Constipation *per se* is not a common ICU problem. Ileus secondary to retroperitoneal hemorrhage (following emergency aortic aneurysmectomy or fracture of the lumbosacral spine), peritonitis, or gastrointestinal surgery may be expected to be of protracted duration. Many "nostrums" are used to stimulate "bowel function," but none has proved useful in the ICU setting.

The most common problem in the ICU is diarrhea, which can be particularly distressing for the patient and the entire staff; it may be difficult to control, creates unpleasant chores for the caregivers, and increases the patient's dependency and discomfort. It is commonly associated with the administration of antacids to prevent stress gastrointestinal bleeding and the use of enteral feedings. Diarrhea may also be a side effect of many antibiotics and medications, such as lactulose. It can also occur during resolution of protracted ileus.

Treatment is most successful if the cause can be eliminated. Antacids containing aluminum seem to be less diarrheagenic than those containing magnesium. Enteral feedings should not be advanced too rapidly in either rate or concentration. Patients seem to differ in their tolerance of different formulas; therefore, a process of trial and error may be necessary. The addition of sodium chloride often decreases diarrhea. Antidiarrheal medications seem to be more effective if given at normal doses at specified intervals rather than by adding a similar total quantity to the enteral feeding mixture. Medications that may be of some value include diphenoxylate, 10 ml every 6 hours as necessary, or loperamide, 2 mg every 6 hours. Lactobacillus can be used to reestablish normal bowel flora and is given in doses of about one package every 8 hours.

Persistent diarrhea is certainly psychologically demeaning to the patient and frustrating to the nursing staff. In some instances, we resort to the use of a rectal tube to ameliorate the situation temporarily while other measures are "juggled" to achieve more permanent control. A 30-Fr Foley catheter with a 30-ml balloon is inflated in the rectal ampulla and attached to gravity drainage. The balloon should be deflated and the tube repositioned during each shift to prevent pressure necrosis. There are often strong feelings about the use of rectal tubes. Especially in cases of lower pelvic surgery, this approach should be discussed with the surgical team before it is used. The rectal tube should be withdrawn as soon as diarrhea is controlled. If the amounts are voluminous they should be incorporated in the intake and output measurements. Good skin care with the use of ointments may be of value in preventing or treating excoriation.

ALTERATION IN BLADDER FUNCTION

The duration of Foley catheterization has been clearly demonstrated to correlate with the incidence of urinary tract infection. If a closed system is used and maintained, the incidence of nosocomial urinary tract infection is no higher in the ICU than in the general wards. However, Foley catheters, the almost ubiquitous monitoring device, are often left in place in ICU patients far longer than is necessary for monitoring purposes or even hygienic reasons. Elimination of constant bladder drainage is a high priority because urinary tract infections are the most frequent iatrogenic infectious complications in this country. A highly dramatic resuscitation and operation may "save" a patient with a ruptured liver, but the same patient may later die of septic shock following nosocomial urinary tract infection. An external "Texas" catheter is an option for males. However, once the catheter is removed, the patient must be evaluated for overflow incontinence or inability to void. Recommendations for the long-term management of paraplegics and quadriplegics include intermittent straight catheterization rather than the use of continuous drainage by a Foley catheter.

Yeast may often be identified in urinalysis or in urine cultures in long-term ICU patients. Most often, there is no systemic evidence of pyelonephritis. If catheterization must be continued, we often use continuous bladder irrigation (50 mg amphotericin B in 1000 ml sterile water per day) through a three-way Foley catheter. An alternative is an infusion of one-quarter strength acetic acid at approximately the same rate (40 ml/hour). This is usually continued for about a week; after it is stopped, urinalysis is obtained to check again for the presence of yeast.

VARIOUS TYPES OF ICU BEDS

The usual ICU bed is of low-leakage construction so that the patient is protected from external sources of electricity that might be transmitted by means of the invasive monitoring catheters. It is usually adjustable for the comfort of the patient and to accommodate commonly used treatment positions, such as the Trendelenburg position. As mentioned previously, however, pressure sores can develop in ICU patients, who may be difficult to move about or position because of their size, requirements for immobility, or the paraphernalia used in treatment. Other types of beds have been introduced to counteract these problems.

ROTOREST KINETIC TREATMENT TABLE

The Rotorest Kinetic Treatment Table (Kinetic Concepts, Inc., San Antonio, TX) is a device permitting side-to-side rotation that would otherwise be difficult or impossible, particularly in patients with injuries of the spinal canal (Fig. 16-11). The patient is initially placed on the flat surface, supports are inserted on both sides of the head and torso, and all extremities are immobilized and secured to the bed frame. The patient can be rotated manually or automatically while a constant alignment is maintained. This continuous side-to-side rotation, in conjunction with secure mobilization, is certainly an easier and safer method for management of patients with paraplegia and quadriplegia in the acute stages. Further, the changes in position—which are much greater in magnitude and easier to maintain compared to the use of pillows in the usual ICU bed—prevent prolonged pressure over prominences or in specific skin areas because the patient is in constant motion. This should diminish skin complications. Also, position changes are commonly advocated to prevent pulmonary complications and deep venous thrombosis and can be increased in both amplitude and duration using this device.

In general, the Rotorest bed is indicated for patients at high risk for these specific complications who require immobilization; patients who are difficult to mobilize or to maintain in side-to-side rotations can also benefit. The latter patients usually include those in coma and those with spinal cord injuries, multiple trauma, and pulmonary problems (particularly those which are unilateral).

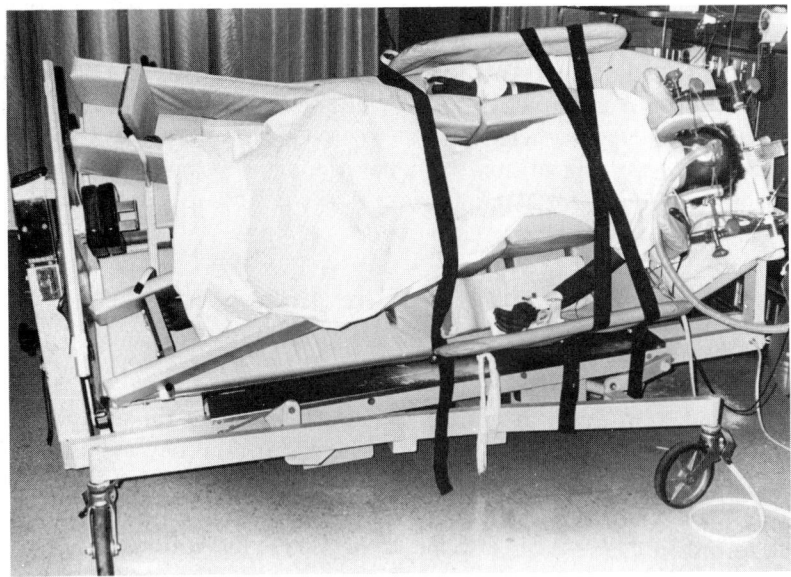

FIGURE 16-11. *A patient who suffered a C3 vertebral injury has been placed in the Rotorest Kinetic Treatment Table. The patient is immobilized, the spine is maintained in alignment using tongs, and side-to-side rotation is used continuously.*

CLINITRON BED

The Clinitron bed (Support Systems International, Columbia, SC) is a therapeutic surface designed for patients who have or are at risk for skin breakdown. The surface in contact with the patient is composed of silicon beads covered by a material permeable to both air and liquids. The "sand" is "fluidized" by forcing air through the bed matrix. This surface can conform to the patient's exact body contours extremely efficiently, resulting in maximal weight distribution and, therefore, minimal pressure to any one area. The Clinitron bed is indicated for long-term bedridden patients in whom reduced pressure and increased comfort are considered important goals. It is also useful for patients with large open abdominal wounds.

KINAIR BED

The KinAir bed (Kinetic Concepts, Inc., San Antonio, TX) is, like the Clinitron, designed for patients for whom skin care and comfort are major considerations (Fig. 16-12). Its support surface is composed of 24 cushions that are individually attached to an air pressure source. The surface can be made to conform to the patient's body by selectively regulating airflow to the various segments, making them firmer or softer as necessary. The overall indications for the KinAir bed are similar to those for the Clinitron bed except that positions other than supine can be structured, which is useful when

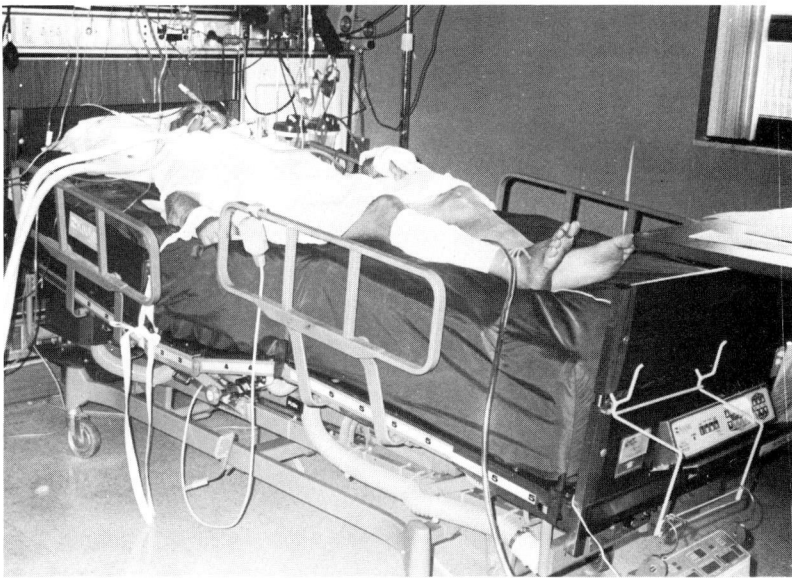

FIGURE 16-12. Both position and support can be tailored to the patient's specific needs in the KinAir bed. This is useful for providing differential pressure for the treatment of existing skin lesions and permits the use of different positions in patients who are usually treated in a supine position only.

position changes are desirable or when patients will be mobilized from the bed regularly.

BURKE BED

The Burke bed (Burke, Inc., Mission, KS) is an extra-wide bed suitable for the extremely obese patient.

CONCLUSION

The prominent and even sole focus on profound physiologic abnormalities and lifesaving interventions that generally forms the initial concept of intensive care must be discarded. Attention to the details of daily bedside care makes a tremendous difference in the comfort and mental state of the patient, in the easing of unglamorous but overwhelming nursing tasks, in the cost and outcome of the entire care process, and, thus, on the overall ICU milieu. There is no question that knowledge of these problems and of their prevention and treatment enhances the physician's ability to improve the care that is given and the result that is obtained.

Accepting a New Admission 17
Mihae Yu

*I*ntensive care units were first developed for high technology crisis-oriented reactions where rapid resuscitation could be achieved, but it has subsequently become a place where various levels of care are being provided—from acute life-threatening resuscitation to the chronic care of patients needing prolonged life support.

This chapter discusses the logistics of admitting ICU patients and initiating appropriate levels of care.

BEFORE TRANSFER

Very few patients are admitted without some degree of warning, and one of the duties of the ICU physician is to evaluate the candidates before transfer. Initial assessment on the floor, emergency room, or operating room can be brief, but needs to answer two questions: Does this patient need "intensive" care and, if so, is it safe to transfer the patient in his/her present condition? The need to bring a patient into ICU is a joint decision by both the referring and receiving physicians. It is hoped that there is some degree of verbal communication between the two to identify the major problem(s), outline initial diagnostic and therapeutic maneuvers, and assess urgency of transfer.

PATIENT CATEGORIZATION

Although we all have our own way of assessing the severity of patients' illnesses, it is important to quantify clinically the ICU patients based on accepted methods. Therapeutic Intervention Scoring System (TISS)[1] and Acute Physiologic and Chronic Health Evaluation (APACHE) score[2,3] allow quantitation of the patient's illness and are useful for organizing an appropriate level of care. Comparison of ICU patients for studies on clinical course and outcome, as well as on allocation of cost and resources, is another objective.

These various methods of patient categorization are discussed in more detail in Chapters 2 and 9. They all have similar themes, and the patient needing intensive care admission generally falls into one of the following three categories relating to the patient and one "situational" category:

1. Those with life-threatening problems that require emergency attention: hypotension, severe respiratory distress, cardiac arrest. These patients usually need continuous physician intervention.
2. Those with recent major insult but relative physiological stability, yet intensive nursing input: the bleeding or trauma patient, those with unstable myocardial infarction with multiple arrhythmias.
3. Those with high risk of complications or those with low probability of complication, but the complication, if it does occur, could be devastating: stable myocardial infarction, upper gastrointestinal bleeding, status post vascular surgery requiring pulse checks.
4. Finally, patients admitted for nonmedical reasons owing to desire of the attending physician or family, possibly owing to limited observation on the floor; other social and medicolegal realities sometimes make ICU admission operationally a near necessity, independent of the physiological particulars.

PATIENT ASSESSMENT

Seeing the patient is the quickest and most valuable source of information and is essential in determining whether the patient may be safely transported in his present condition. A protective conservative approach is used until the patient has reached the safe haven of the ICU.

If the patient is in severe respiratory distress, now is the time to intubate, not inside the elevator. If blood pressure is marginal, a dopamine drip should be prepared and transported with the patient, ready for use. Portable EKG monitor, suction device, and oxygen tank may all be part of the necessary equipment. If a circuitous route to the ICU is taken (*e.g.*, via the x-ray department for further diagnostic tests), there are other considerations such as the life of the battery pack in the monitor or capacity of oxygen tanks.

The ICU physician must also explain to the patient and family why the transfer is necessary to allay the anxiety of being whisked away to a busy and frightening environment. The patient is forewarned of strange noises from various mechanical devices, ventilator noise, alarms from monitors, and different personnel who might be involved in their care. Ignorance nurtures fear, whereas knowledge of what to expect has a calming effect. The family should also be reassured that visitors are allowed in the ICU and that taking their beloved ones to the unit does not mean prolonged separation.

PREPARING THE ICU

Even before the definite decision to admit the patient is made, it is crucial to warn the unit of a possible admission. Bed and nursing staff are not always instantly available, and early communication with adequate preparation on the receiving end makes for a smooth transfer. In a busy, full ICU, skill is needed to select a patient for immediate discharge and to arrange patients according to available nursing care.

If special equipment will be needed on arrival, this information is related to the charge nurse—it takes time to set up ventilators, prepare transducers for arterial lines, mix medications, and have enough infusion pumps ready.

ADMISSION INTO INTENSIVE CARE

Intensive care patients are treated similarly to trauma victims in that priority is given to the most life-threatening problem first. The traditional approach of taking a complete history and physical examination is discarded—stabilization is the goal, then evaluation. There are several phases of initial evaluation.

THE EMERGENT ADMISSION

A patient may be admitted in critically unstable condition. The ICU physician takes charge: simultaneous therapeutic maneuvers and urgent diagnostic testing can be accomplished simultaneously if tasks are divided and allocated to the right personnel. This organized division of labor makes the difference between quick effective resuscitation and chaos.

Initial resuscitation of a severely hypotensive unfamiliar patient is, again, analogous to resuscitation of a trauma victim.

1. Immediately call for help if adequate, experienced personnel are not available.
2. Get control of the airway followed by adequate oxygenation and ventilation. It is better to be overcautious by elective early intubation than to have an obtunded hypotensive patient aspirate or become hypoxic because of cardiovascular collapse.
3. Obtain venous access and use fluids or pressors, or both, to support blood pressure until the cause of hypotension can be ascertained.
4. When blood pressure is acceptable, further procedures that help in the management of that patient can be performed: arterial line, pulmonary artery catheter insertion. Do not delay therapy while attempting to monitor the patient.
5. Laboratory work is sent, and immediately available results are used to adjust initial patient therapy.

INITIAL EVALUATION: PART I

Fortunately, most patients are not critically unstable, allowing time for nursing staff to "hook up" the patient to various monitors. Much information can be gathered and treatment started by being at the patient's bedside. Now is the best time to glean further information from the transporting physician, whether the anesthesiologist, emergency room doctor, surgeon, or house officer on duty. It is surprising how much is missing from the often scanty initial written record of an emergency admission.

General important points to review are pertinent medical history, recent episodes of hypertension and hypotension, fluid and blood products given, pressor or antihypertensives used, and record of dysrhythmias. In the postoperative patient, additional information is sought on length of surgery, choice of anesthetics, estimated blood loss, dose and time of last narcotic dose, and the reason why the patient is still intubated *or* extubated.

Technical aspects of surgery that might play an important role in the future course of the patient should be discussed with the surgeon. Was the abdomen "wet" when closed, raising the possibility of postoperative bleeding? Was the abdominal exposure wide with significant amount of insensible fluid loss (about 1 liter loss per hour)? Was there spillage of gastrointestinal content (especially colonic), with possibility of late sepsis? The surgeon might also discuss particular intraoperative difficulties or problems and the indications for and placement of tubes and drains.

INITIAL EVALUATION: PART II

After the busy work of settling the patient has been completed and while laboratory results are pending, a more orderly and complete history, physical examination, and chart review can be done. It takes skill to pull out the pertinent facts from a distressingly thick chart, but it pays to start at the very beginning with the emergency room admission sheet or initial history and physical examination to get a perspective of the patient's hospital course. Initial blood pressure, respiratory rate, and admitting laboratory test results may reveal baseline information before the illness started, although in an acute severe illness this information might not reflect the real norm for that patient.

Review of renal and liver function, nutritional status, baseline arterial blood gas, and EKG are all necessary information to care adequately for the patient.

Attention is then focused on the most recent events (*i.e.*, progress notes, nursing notes), current medication sheet, consultant's assessments, and operative record.

A thorough physical examination—paying attention to catheters, drains, and tubes—must be done within the first few hours of admission. This will serve to judge future progress or deterioration and, with clear written documentation, can be used by other physicians involved in the patient's care.

Systems review should include assessment of metabolic derangements such as temperature and electrolyte abnormalities.

Neurologic function can be followed objectively by using the Glasgow Coma Scale.

Careful observation of respiratory rate followed by auscultation of lungs, assessment of arterial blood gas, and chest radiograph gives an idea of the patient's pulmonary function. Position of endotracheal tube is noted. In an average adult, the 22- to 24-cm mark should be at the level of the teeth, but it should be 1 to 2 cm further in if a nasotracheal intubation was done. If a chest tube is present, check for proper suction, leaks in the connections, and whether the tube is functioning or has become occluded with clots.

Cardiovascular examination starts with observing the EKG monitor for rhythm and rate, measurement of blood pressure, auscultation of heart, palpation of peripheral pulses, and evaluation of neck veins.

Equipment used in the hospitals, like any machinery, is fraught with error. Even obtaining a simple arterial blood pressure is now complicated and confused by inadequacies of our electromechanical transducers and the way we measure pressure. It is well documented that there is poor correlation between indirect measurement of blood pressure, which is based on measurement of flow under an occluding cuff, and direct pressure measurement via an intravascular catheter.[4] Further, direct pressure measurement is significantly effected by the frequency and damping of external measurement system (transducers and tubings with varying resonant frequency).[4-6] Treating underdamped or overdamped pressure with antihypertensives and pressors, respectively, can be dangerous. Until further studies are done to establish what the most accurate method of blood pressure measurement is, occlusion pressure is a reasonable way of approximating systolic pressure.

It is also desirable to read pressure measurements directly off the wave form on a scaled display monitor rather than to rely on digital readouts. Digital displays are inaccurate because even the most sophisticated computerized system with built-in algorithms cannot truly learn to discard respiratory and motion artifacts. Water manometers have no role in the ICU; water has too low a frequency response to reflect accurately the biologic system. When there is any doubt about the validity of the number, always rezero the system to atmospheric pressure and recalibrate to a known pressure.

In assessment of gastrointestinal function, history of bowel movement is significant, as is presence or absence of bowel sounds (pitch, quantity), degree of abdominal distension and tenderness, and inspection of wounds. A nasogastric tube is in the stomach in an average adult if the end exits from the nares at the second black mark. Make sure all drains are connected and functioning properly.

Examine the skin for areas of phlebitis, breakdown, and rash, and note the degree of edema.

A good head and neck examination, inspection of back and extremities, and a rectal examination with stool guaiac test completes the examination.

INITIAL EVALUATION: PART III

After a complete history and physical examination, the third phase of patient admission starts; this consists of follow-up, both short- and long-term to tidy up the current problems.

If present information is inadequate, other sources are sought: [a] old charts, including a call to the record room of another hospital; [b] talking to family members, other physicians; [c] getting more laboratory work and diagnostic x-ray studies; or [d] doing further diagnostic procedures such as insertion of pulmonary artery catheters.

Short-term follow-up consists of compulsive and frequent checks on the patient as well as learning the results of laboratory work, treating immediate problems, and re-evaluation until a coherent picture of the patient, the diagnosis, and the treatment has evolved. Do not rely on the nursing staff to call you with subtle signs that might be harbingers of major problems. No news is *NOT* good news!

Long-term follow-up can also be initiated. Work-up of hypertension and endocrine problem (thyroid disease) can be started; psychiatric support for suicide vicitims and the start of nutritional support all help to complete the patient care.

GIVING REPORT

The final task consists of communicating all the hard work to the critical eyes of your colleagues.

Like the newspaper headlines, the first few sentences should capture the essence of the problem and tune in the listener to the appropriate area of focus. A long round-about history leading to why the patient was admitted and dwelling upon unrelated medical history not only bores the listeners, but also distracts them from the main issue.

Give the who–why–when–where–what routine: [a] Briefly explain *who* the patient is (name, age, sex, attending); [b] *why* the patient got into trouble; [c] *when* and *where* it happened; and [d] *what* happened and *what* was done. The report is not complete without the presenter's assessment of the problem(s), plans for the day, and expectant course of the disease process (prognosis).

Be ready to explain and defend each therapeutic maneuver, but be willing to change the treatment plan if better ideas are expressed by your colleagues.

We quickly learn that all it takes is admission of one sick patient to effect the tempo of the whole unit. It then becomes a busy, active, and educational place.

REFERENCES

1. Cullen DJ, Civetta JM, Briggs BA, et al: Therapeutic intervention scoring system: A method for quantitative comparison of patient care. *Crit Care Med* 1974; 2:57
2. Knaus WA, Zimmerman JE, Wafner DP, et al: APACHE—Acute Physiologic and Chronic Health Evaluation: A physiologically based classification system. *Crit Care Med* 1981; 9:591
3. Knaus WA, Draper EA, Wafner DP, et al: APACHE II: A severity of disease classification system. *Crit Care Med* 1985; 13:818

4. Bruner JMR, Krenis LJ, Kunsman JM, et al: Comparison of direct and indirect methods of measuring arterial blood pressure. *Med Instr* 1981; 15:11
5. Bruner JMR, Krenis LJ, Kunsman JM, et al: Comparison of direct and indirect methods of measuring arterial blood pressure: Part II. *Med Instr* 1981; 15:97
6. Bruner JMR, Krenis LJ, Kunsman JM, et al: Comparison of direct and indirect methods of arterial blood pressure: Part III. *Med Instr* 1981; 15:182

Index

Page numbers followed by *f* indicate figures; page numbers followed by *t* indicate tables; page numbers followed by *n* indicate footnotes.

ABGs (arterial blood gases), standing orders for, 143–144
Acquired immune deficiency syndrome (AIDS), autonomy principle and, 45
Act-utilitarianism, 39
Acute Physiology Score and Chronic Health Evaluation (APACHE), 30, 160t–161t, 162, 163t, 164. *See also* APACHE II
Admission to ICU, 289–294
 assessment of patient in, 290, 291–294
 categorization of patient for, 289–290
 for constant physician care, 9
 criteria for, 3–7
 decision-making and outcome predictions in, 28–29. *See also* Decision-making; Outcome predictions
 distribution of limited care and, 10–12
 of elective patients, 27t, 27–28, 28t
 emergency, 25–27, 26t, 291
 for extensive nursing care, 8–9, 243–245
 on first-come-first-served basis, 11–12
 for monitoring and observation, 8, 240–243, 241t, 242f, 243f
 preparation of ICU for, 290–291
 reporting on, 294
 in terminal illness, 6–7
Age. *See* Children; Elderly patients; Infants
Agitation, 227–229. *See also* Delirium
 haloperidol in, 225t
 treatment of, 228–229, 229t
AIDS, autonomy principle and, 45
Akathisia, 224, 229
Albumin, serum levels of, in outcome prediction, 27
Alcoholism, delirium in, 224
Alprazolam (Xanax), 229t
Amphotericin B, bladder irrigation with, 285
Antianxiety agents, 228–229, 229t
Antibiotics, topical yeast infections due to, 275
Antidepressants, 230
Antidiarrheal agents, 284
Antipsychotic drugs
 in delirium, 224–225, 225t
 in patient refusal to cooperate, 231
Antishock trousers, complications associated with, 282–283
Anxiety. *See also* Fears; Stress
 and agitation, 227–229
 treatment of, 228–229, 229t
APACHE (Acute Physiology Score and Chronic Health Evaluation), 30, 160t–161t, 162, 163t, 164
APACHE II, 30, 31, 31t, 164, 165t, 166
 in long-term ICU patients, 168, 169t
Apathy, in ICU patients, 229–231
Apraxia, construction, in delirium, 218
Arm. *See also* Extremities
 compartment syndromes of, 275, 276f

297

Arterial blood gases (ABGs), standing orders for, 143–144
Arterial catheter armboard, complications associated with, 282, 282f
Assessment procedures. *See also* Decision-making; Diagnostic evaluation
  initial, on admission to ICU, 291–294
  before transfer to ICU, 290
Assisted activity, nursing care allocation for, 262
Ativan (lorazepam), 228, 229t
Attending personnel
  ICU, 178, 195–196
  surgical, 193–194
Authority and responsibilities of ICU staff, 14–15, 183–190
Autonomy of patient
  and informed consent, 67–68
  as medicomoral principle, 45

Baby Doe case, 102–104
Baby Jane Doe case, 104–106
Barber case, 53–54, 55–56, 82
Bartling v. Superior Court, 47, 51
Beds, types of, 285–287
  Burke, 287
  Clinitron, 286
  KinAir, 286–287, 287f
  Rotorest Kinetic Treatment Table, 285, 286f
Bedsores (decubitus ulcers)
  prevention of, 271–274, 273f, 274f
  treatment of, 274–275
Behavioral disturbances, 215–233. *See also* Psychological considerations
  agitation, 227–229, 229t
  apathy, 229–231
  delirium, 217–225. *See also* Delirium
  dependency, 232
  depression, 211–212, 229–231, 230t
  hostility, 232
  incidence in ICU of, 215
  initial evaluation of, 216f, 216–217, 217t
  refusal to cooperate, 231–232
Beneficence principle, 44–45
  and informed consent, 66–67

Benzodiazepines, in anxiety treatment, 228–229, 229t
Bladder function, alterations in, 284–285
Blood gases, standing orders for, 143–144
Blood pressure
  delirium and, 224
  measurement of, 293
Blood transfusions, religious objections to, 100
Bone. *See* Musculoskeletal system
Bouvia, Elizabeth, refusal of therapy by, 57
Bowel function
  alterations in, 283–284
  and APACHE score, 160t
Brain death
  criteria for, 87
    Harvard, 85–86, 86t
  statutory definition of, 86–87
Broad-spectrum antibiotics, topical yeast infections due to, 275
Brophy v. New Eng. Sinai Hosp., 77n
Burke bed, 287
Butyrophenones, for delirium, 224–225, 225t

California Natural Death Act, 51, 95
Candidal infection
  oral, 275
  superficial, 275
  urinary catheterization and, 285
Cannulation
  and arterial catheter armboard, 282, 282f
  infections associated with, 278
  localized ischemia and, 276–277
Cardiopulmonary resuscitation (CPR)
  and do-not-resuscitate orders, 80–81, 97–98
  and outcome prediction, 154t
Cardiorespiratory variables, in outcome prediction, 27–28, 28t, 147–151, 148t–149t, 152t, 153t
  APACHE scores and, 160t, 163t, 165t
CARE = CURE philosophy, 40–42
Catheterization. *See also* Cannulation; Drainage systems
  rectal, 284
  urinary, 284–285

CCU. *See* Intensive care unit (ICU)
Central nervous system injury, irreversible
  with brain death, 85–87, 86t
  without brain death, 88–91
Central venous catheterization, infections associated with, 278
Centrax (prazepam), 229t
Charting procedures, documentation in. *See also* Documentation
  legal considerations of, 125–131. *See also under* Malpractice suits
Child Abuse Prevention and Treatment Act, and withdrawal of therapy from infants, 105–106
Children, withdrawal of therapy from, 100–102
Chlordiazepoxide (Librium), 229t
Chlorpromazine (Thorazine), for delirium, 225
Cimetidine, benzodiazepines and, 228
Circulation, Respiration, Abdomen, Motor, and Speech (CRAMS) score, 25, 26t
Clinical decision-making, 19–35. *See also* Decision-making
Clinitron bed, 286
Clonazepam (Clonopin), 229t
Clorazepate (Tranxene), 229t
Clotrimazole, for topical yeast infections, 275
Collaboration, among team members, 180–181. *See also* Critical care team
Coma, 88–91
  irreversible, 85–87, 86t
Commonwealth v. Golston, 87
Communication
  with behaviorally disturbed patients. *See* Behavioral disturbances
  breakdowns in, malpractice claims and, 117, 118–125
    conflicting opinions in, 121–124
    false expectations in, 119–120
    inconsistent statements in, 120–121
    lack of rapport in, 118–119
    lost information in, 124–125
  about death and dying, 228
  nursing care allocation for, 262–263
  problems of, for ICU patients, 211
  among staff members, 198–201

Compartment syndromes, 275, 276f
Competency
  determination of, 98, 99t
  lack of. *See* Incompetent patients
Compliance with therapy, problems in, 231–232. *See also* Refusal of therapy
Complications Impact Index, 151
Condition Index Score, 151, 153t
Confusion, delirium and, 218
Conroy, Claire, court case involving, 78n, 92–93
Consent for treatment, informed, 59–69. *See also* Informed consent
Consequentialist ethics, 39
Constipation, 283
Construction apraxia, in delirium, 218
Consultants, 196–197
  requests for, frequency of, 226t
Contractures, 277
Control, sense of
  in family, 205–206
  in patient, 209–210, 231–232. *See also* Autonomy of patient
Cooperation of patient, problems in, 231–232. *See also* Refusal of therapy
Cost of medical care, 4–5, 133–134
  admission to ICU and, 7
  annual increase in, 4
  containment of, efforts in, 139–140
  and cost effectiveness, 136f, 136–137
  efficiency and, 13–14
  ethical considerations and. *See* Distributive justice
  payment systems for, 4, 136–137
  and quality of care, 4, 5
Court decisions. *See* Judicial involvement; Legal issues; *specific cases*
CPR. *See* Cardiopulmonary resuscitation
CRAMS (Circulation, Respiration, Abdomen, Motor, and Speech), 25, 26t
Crisis. *See* Emergency care
Critical care team, 175–181. *See also* Staff; *specific members, e.g.,* ICU fellow
  collaboration among, factors contributing to, 180–181
  expectations of, related to surgeon, 200
  functions of, 176–177

Critical care team (*continued*)
  information lost in transition and, malpractice claims and, 124–125
  interrelationships of, 191–202
    communication in, 198–201
    in limitation or refusal of therapy, 50t, 53–57
    members of, 192f, 192–193
    organizational factors in, 177–178
    roles of, 178–180, 193–198
    stress in, 175–176
    surgeon's expectations of, 199–200
Critical care unit. *See* Intensive care unit (ICU)
Criticism of treatment by others, malpractice claims and, 121–124
Custody of a Minor, 102

Daily care activities, nursing care allocation for, 257–261
Dalmane (flurazepam), 229t
Death and dying. *See also* Brain death; Life support measures; Mortality
  and anxiety, 227–229
  concepts and definitions of, 5
  ethical considerations of. *See* Ethical considerations
  in long-term ICU patients, variables in, 32–33, 33t
  reactions of patients and families to, 212–213, 227–229
  and refusal of therapy. *See* Refusal of therapy
  right to. *See* Right to die
  sanctity versus quality of life and, 6. *See also* Quality of life
  societal values and goals of medicine in, 9–10
  and withdrawal of therapy. *See* Withdrawal of therapy
Decision-making, 19–35
  acquisition of new information affecting, 23
  on admission to ICU, 28–29
  after assessment, 22–23
  for continued care, 30–31
  decision trees in, 144–145, 146t, 147t
  in diagnostic evaluation, 21–22. *See also* Diagnostic evaluation
  in discharge from ICU, 33–34
  for emergency versus elective patients, 25–28, 26t, 27t, 28t
  ethical considerations in, 37–58. *See also* Ethical considerations
  on health care status of patient, 20–21
  and iatrogenesis, 111–112
  judicial involvement in. *See* Judicial involvement; Legal issues
  on likely therapeutic effects, 22
  for long-term care, 23, 32–33, 33t
  on newly acquired diseases and complications, 21
  outcome definition in, 23–24
  outcome predictions in, 21. *See also* Outcome predictions
  for short-term outcome, 23, 29–30, 31t
  time influence on, 24, 25t
Decision trees, in selection of laboratory tests, 144–145, 146t, 147t
Decubitus ulcers
  prevention of, 271–274, 273f, 274f
  treatment of, 274–275
Defense mechanisms, 209
  concepts behind, 203–206
Delayed-type hypersensitivity, in outcome prediction, 27
Delirium
  causes of, 220–221, 222t, 223t
  clinical features of, 217t, 217–218
  differential diagnosis of, 219–221
  drug-induced, 220, 222t
  EEG in, 219
  immediate concerns in, 216–217
  laboratory tests in, 221, 223t
  mental status examination in, 219, 220f–221f
  treatment of, 224–225, 225t
Dementia, 219
  reversible. *See* Delirium
Denial, as defense mechanism, 204
Deontological ethics, 39
Dependency, 232. *See also* Control, sense of
  rebellion against, refusal to cooperate as, 231–232
Depression
  clinical features of, 230, 230t
  drug-induced, 231
  in ICU patients, 211–212, 229–231
Device-related complications, 279–283, 280f, 281f, 282f
Dextroamphetamine, for apathy, 230

Diagnosis related groups (DRGs), 4, 5, 136–137
Diagnostic evaluation. *See also* Decision-making; Outcome predictions
  in behavioral disturbances, 216f, 216–217, 217t. *See also* Behavioral disturbances; Delirium
  and iatrogenesis, 111, 112–113, 113t
  nursing care allocation for, 261
  selection and sequencing of, 21–22
Diarrhea, 283–284
Diazepam (Valium), for anxiety, 228, 229t
Diet. *See* Nutrition
Dinnerstein, Shirley, court case involving, 80, 94–95
Diphenoxylate, for diarrhea, 284
Discharge from ICU, decision-making and outcome predictions in, 33–34
Disclosure, standards of, informed consent and, 59–60
Disorientation, in delirium, 218
Distributive justice
  as medicomoral principle, 45–47
  in resource allocation, 10–12
  society's interest in, 56–57
Documentation
  ICU fellow's responsibilities for, 189–190
  legal considerations of, 125–131. *See also under* Malpractice suits
  nursing care allocation for, 262–263
  of patient assessment on admission, 294
Do-not-resuscitate orders, 80–81, 97–98
Drainage systems
  nursing time required for, 253–257
  skin care with, 269, 270f, 270–271, 271f, 272f
DRGs (diagnosis related groups), 4, 5, 136–137
Droperidol (Inapsine), for delirium, 224–225
Drugs. *See also specific drug or type of drug*
  administration of, nursing care allocation for, 261
  in anxiety treatment, 228–229, 229t
  in apathy treatment, 230–231
  delirium caused by, 220, 222t
  in delirium treatment, 224–225, 225t
  depression caused by, 231
  diarrhea caused by, 283–284
Durable power of attorney, Natural Death Acts and, 97
Dying. *See* Death and dying
Dysgraphia, 218

Economics of medical care. *See* Cost of medical care
Education. *See* Training
Edwin Smith Surgical Papyrus, The, 3
EEG (electroencephalogram), in delirium, 219
Ego problems, and critical statements, malpractice claims and, 122–124
Elderly patients
  ageism toward, and informed consent, 69
  contractures in, 277
  delirium in, 219. *See also* Delirium
  treatment of, 224
Elective procedures, decision-making and outcome predictions in, 27t, 27–28, 28t, 154t
Electroencephalogram (EEG), in delirium, 219
Emergency care
  decision-making and outcome predictions in, 25–27, 26t, 154t
  ICU admission for, 291
  ICU fellow in, 186
  informed consent and, 60–61
Emotional factors. *See* Behavioral disturbances; Psychological considerations
Endotracheal tubes
  complications associated with, 279–280, 280f
  position of, 292–293
Enema administration, nursing care allocation for, 261
Enteral nutrition, and diarrhea, 284
Epididymitis, 279
EPS (extrapyramidal syndromes), drug-induced, 224, 229
Equipment. *See also* Monitoring; *specific type of equipment*
  errors and, 293
Esophageal varices, traction helmets for, complications associated with, 281–282

Ethical considerations, 37–58
  critical care team approach and, 53–57
  definitions of terms used in, 38–39
  deontological approach to, 39
  in informed consent, 65–68
    preventive ethics and, 64–65
  in limitation or refusal of therapy, 47–53, 48t–50t
    critical care team's role in, 54–57
    family's role in, 52–53
  medicomoral principles and, 39–47
    application of, 46–47
    autonomy, 45
    justice, 45–46
    nonmaleficence, 44–45
    potential for salvageability, 42–44
    preservation of life, 44
  in right to die. See Right to die
  utilitarian approach to, 39
Euthanasia. See Right to die
Evaluation. See Assessment procedures; Decision-making; Diagnostic evaluation
Expectations
  false, malpractice claims and, 119–120
  staff, uncommunicated, 199–201
Extrapyramidal syndromes (EPS), drug-induced, 224, 229
Extremities
  compartment syndromes of, 275, 276f
  fractures of, missed, 283

Family, 204
  control in, sense of, 205–206
  in cooperation problems, 231
  of delirious patient, 225
  denial reaction of, 204
  of dying patient, 212–213
  fears of, 204–205
  ICU fellow's interactions with, 186
  of incompetent patient
    and informed consent, 63–64
    as surrogate, 78–79
  in limitation or refusal of therapy, 49t, 52–53
  relationship with nurses of, 179
  staff involvement with, 206–209
  unreceptive, 209
Fears
  of family, 204–205
  of patient, 209–210
    and agitation, 227–229

Feeding tubes. See Nasogastric tubes
Fellowship in ICU. See ICU fellow
Financing. See Cost of medical care
Fistulas, preventive care for, 270–271, 271f, 272f
Florida, Natural Death Act in, 95–96
Flurazepam (Dalmane), 229t
Folstein's Mini-Mental State examination, 219, 220f–221f
Fractures, extremity, missed, 283
Funding. See Cost of medical care

Gases, arterial blood, standing orders for, 143–144
Gastrointestinal function, alterations in, 283–284
Gastrointestinal variables, in APACHE score, 160t
Green, In re, 102

Halazepam (Paxipam), 229t
Halcion (triazolam), 229t
Half-life of antianxiety agents, 228, 229t
Hallucinations, in delirium, 218
Haloperidol
  for anxiety, 229, 231
  for delirium, 224, 225t
Harvard brain death criteria, 85–86, 86t
Health care costs. See Cost of medical care
Helmets, traction, complications associated with, 281–282
Hematologic variables, in APACHE scores, 161t, 165t
Hospital Prognostic Index, 27, 27t
Hostility, of patient, 232
Humanitarianism, and limitation of therapy, 55
Hydration, artificial, withdrawal of, 82
Hypersensitivity, delayed-type, in outcome prediction, 27

Iatrodemics, 109, 112
Iatrogenesis, 109–115
  in arterial catheterization, 282
  in central venous catheterization, 278
  and clinical care evaluation, 115
  decision-making process in, 111–112

device-related, 279–283, 280f, 281f, 282f
diagnostic errors and, 111
diagnostic evaluation and, 112–113, 113t
incidence of, 109
outcome definitions and, 114–115
prehospital patient status and, 110
therapeutic interventions versus manipulations in, 113–114
types of, 109–110
ICU. *See also* Intensive care unit
ICU attending personnel, role of, 178, 195–196
ICU fellow, 14, 183–190. *See also* Physician(s)
communication responsibilities of, 198–199
documentation responsibilities of, 189–190
emergency care by, 186
goals and objectives of, evolution of, 185–186
initial adjustment of, 183–184
organizational tasks of, 186–187
orientation of, 184–185
prioritization by, 187–188, 189t
relationship with nurses of, 179
rewards of, 190
roles and responsibilities of, 178–179, 186–187
stress of, 189–190
and surgical team, 196
Illness–Injury Severity Index (IISI), 25, 26t
Immobilization
and contractures, 277
and decubitus ulcers, 271–275, 273f, 274f
Rotorest Kinetic Treatment Table in, 285, 286f
Immune deficiency, acquired, autonomy principle and, 45
Immune function
assessment of, 27, 27t
compromised, topical yeast infections due to, 275
Inapsine (droperidol), for delirium, 224–225
Incompetent patients
family decisions for, 63–64, 78–79
and informed consent, 62–64
legal decision-making for, 77–80, 91–95
and refusal of therapy, 77–79

court proceedings for, 79–80
surrogates for, 77–79
Infants, withdrawal of therapy from, 102–106
Infections
subtle, 277–283
device-related, 278, 279–283, 280f, 281f, 282f
perineal, 279
phlebitis, 278
sinusitis, 278–279
yeast
topical, 275
urinary catheterization and, 285
Informed consent, 59–69, 99–100
autonomy principle in, 67–68
beneficence principle in, 66–67
in continuing care
with expected recovery, 61
with poor prognosis, 61–62
in crisis intervention, 60–61
degrees of disclosure and, 59–60
documentation of, 129–130
elements of, 59
ethical foundations of, 65–68
for incompetent patients, 62–64
obtainment of, strategies for, 60–62
preventive ethics and, 64–65
psychological considerations in, 68–69
Informed refusal, 99–100. *See also* Refusal of therapy
Intensive care, goals of, 7–9
outcome prediction and, 140–145, 143t, 144t, 146t, 147t
Intensive care psychosis, 210–212. *See also* Behavioral disturbances
Intensive care unit (ICU)
admission criteria for, 3–7. *See also* Admission to ICU
attending personnel of, 178, 195–196
discharge from, decision-making and outcome predictions in, 33–34
environment of, psychological reactions to, 209–212
fellowship in, 14. *See also* ICU fellow
iatrogenesis in. *See* Iatrogenesis
interrelationships in, 14–15, 191–202
length of stay in, mortality and, 140
scheduling in, 187–188, 189t
staff of. *See* Critical care team; Staff; *specific type, e.g.,* Nursing staff
Intestines. *See* Gastrointestinal *entries*

Intubation. *See specific type*
Ischemia, localized, 276–277

Jehovah's Witnesses
    and informed refusal, 100
    and parental refusal of therapy, 102
John F. Kennedy Hosp. v. Bludworth, 96
Judicial involvement, in treatment decisions, 71–84. *See also* Legal issues; *specific cases*
    and emerging legal consensus, 75–83
    public debate about, 72–75
Junior staff members
    ICU, 197
    surgery team, 197–198
Justice
    distributive, 10–12, 56–57
    as medicomoral principle, 45–47

KinAir bed, 286–287, 287f
Koop, C. Everett
    on right to die, 90
    on withdrawal of therapy from minors, 101

Laboratory tests
    in behavioral disturbances, 221, 223t
    management principles and, 142–143, 144t
    nursing care allocation for, 261
    repeated, no orders for, 145, 147t
    selection of, structured decision trees in, 144–145, 146t, 147t
    standing orders for, 143–144
    unnecessary, reduction of, 112–113, 113t, 141–145, 144t, 146t, 147t
Lactobacillus, for diarrhea, 284
Law. *See* Legal issues
Leach v. Akron General Medical Center, 79
Leg. *See also* Extremities
    compartment syndromes of, 275
Legal issues, 85–106. *See also* Judicial involvement
    and avoidance of legal problems, 117–131. *See also* Malpractice suits
    in brain death, 85–87, 86t

in care of incompetent patients, 77–80, 91–95. *See also* Incompetent patients
    documentation, 125–131, 189–190
    do-not-resuscitate orders, 80–81, 97–98
    and durable power of attorney, 97
    ethics and, 38. *See also* Ethical considerations
    informed consent, 99–100. *See also* Informed consent
    in irreversible central nervous system injury
        with brain death, 85–87, 86t
        without brain death, 88–91
    in limitation of therapy, 48t–50t, 55–56. *See also* Refusal of therapy
    Living Wills, 51, 95–97
    malpractice suits, 117–131. *See also* Malpractice suits
    Natural Death Acts, 51, 95–97
    questionable competency and, 98, 99t
    refusal of therapy, 99–100. *See also* Refusal of therapy
    in withdrawal of therapy, 75–83, 99–100
        from infants, 102–106
        from minors, 100–102
Librium (chlordiazepoxide), 229t
Life support measures
    definitions of, 4, 5
    ethical considerations of, 47–53, 54–57. *See also* Ethical considerations
    humanitarian concerns in, 55
    patient refusal of. *See* Refusal of therapy
    and quality of life. *See* Quality of life
    and right to die. *See* Right to die
    societal objectives and, 10
    withdrawal of. *See* Withdrawal of therapy
Limitation of therapy. *See also* Refusal of therapy
    ethical considerations in, 47–57
Litigation. *See* Legal issues; Malpractice suits
Living Wills, 51, 95–97
Localized ischemia, 276–277
Loperamide, for diarrhea, 284
Lorazepam (Ativan), 228, 229t
Lower extremity. *See* Extremities; Leg

Malpractice suits
  and documentation of charts, 125–131
    fraudulent or lost records in, 128
    general nature of, 130–131
    informed consent in, 129–130
    legibility in, 126
    notes on reasoning process in, 125–126
    repetition in, 127–128
    untoward events in, 129
  precursors to
    conflicting opinions, 121–124
    false expectations, 119–120
    inconsistent statements, 120–121
    lack of rapport, 118–119
    lost information, 124–125
Manipulation, therapy versus, 22
  iatrogenesis and, 113–114
Manometers, 293
MAST (military antishock trousers), complications associated with, 282–283
Medical care, cost of. *See* Cost of medical care
Medical director, roles and responsibilities of, 178
Medical ethics. *See* Ethical considerations
Medications. *See* Drugs; *specific drug or type of drug*
Medicolegal issues. *See* Legal issues
Medicomoral principles, 39–47. *See also* Ethical considerations
  application of, 46–47
  autonomy, 45
  justice, 45–46
  nonmaleficence, 44–45
  potential for salvageability, 42–44
  preservation of life, 44
Mellaril (thioridazine), for delirium, 225
Mental status. *See also* Incompetent patients
  in delirium, 219, 220f–221f
  and informed consent, 68
  intensive care psychosis and, 210–212
  in outcome prediction, 154t
Metabolic variables, in APACHE scores, 161t, 165t
Methylphenidate (Ritalin), for apathy, 230
Midazolam (Versed), 229t
Military antishock trousers (MAST), complications associated with, 282–283
Mini-Mental State (MMS) examination, 219, 220f–221f
Minors, withdrawal of therapy from, 100–102
MLR (multiple logistic regression), in outcome prediction, 151–152, 154t, 156
MMS (Mini-Mental State) examination, 219, 220f–221f
MOFS (multiple organ failure syndrome), 139, 168
Monitoring
  admission to ICU for, 8, 29–30
  in initial evaluation, 291–293
  nursing care allocation for, 240–243, 241t, 242f, 243t, 247–252
  physician's orders for, 240–243
  of vital signs, 247–249
    frequency of, 240–243, 241t, 242f, 243f
    in nursing care index, 166–167, 167t
Morality. *See also* Ethical considerations
  definition of, 38
Mortality. *See also* Death and dying
  length of ICU stay and, 140
  observed, outcome predictions and, 170, 170f
Motor response
  in agitation, 227
  in delirium, 218
Multiple logistic regression (MLR), in outcome prediction, 151–152, 154t, 156
Multiple organ failure syndrome (MOFS), 139, 168
Muscle tone, in delirium, 218
Musculoskeletal system, preventive care for, 275–277
  in compartment syndromes, 275, 276f
  in contractures, 277
  in localized ischemia, 276–277
  missed extremity fractures and, 283
Mycostatin (nystatin), for topical yeast infections, 275

Nasogastric tubes
  complications associated with, 280
  positioning of, 280, 281f
  and sinusitis, 279

Nasotracheal tubes, and sinusitis, 279
Natural Death Acts, 51, 95–97
Neuroleptics
  for anxiety, 228–229
  side-effects of, 229
Neurologic variables, in APACHE scores, 161t, 165t
Neuropsychiatric signs, in delirium, 218
No-code orders, 80–81, 97–98
Nonmaleficence, 44–45
  and informed consent, 66–67
Nursing assistants, 181
Nursing care
  allocation of, 8–9, 235–246
    and classification of patients by nursing care hours, 236–240, 237t, 239t
    for daily and PRN care, 257–261
    for documentation and communication, 262–263
    and elimination of nonessential tasks, 238
    for intake and diet activities, 252–253
    for laboratory and radiography activities, 261
    for medications and enemas, 261
    nurse:patient ratio in, 236, 237, 238, 245
    for output and drainage activities, 253–257
    for patients requiring constant physician care, 245
    for patients requiring extensive nursing care, 243–245
    for patients requiring monitoring/observation, 240–243, 241t, 242f, 243f
    for psychosocial interventions, 265
    for respiratory care, 250–252
    shortage of nurses affecting, 238
    for transport of patients, 263–264
    for turning or assisted activity, 262
    for vital signs monitoring, 247–249
    in outcome predictions, 166–167, 167t
  preventive. See Preventive care
Nursing staff. See also Critical care team; Staff
  involvement with families of, 206–209
  professional status of, 53
  ratio to patients of, 8, 236, 237, 238, 245
  relationship with physicians of, 175–176, 180–181, 235–236
  roles and responsibilities of, 179–180, 198, 235–236
    dependent and independent of physician orders, 235–236
Nutrition
  artificial, withdrawal of, 82. See also Right to die; Withdrawal of therapy
  assessment of, 27, 27t
  enteral, and diarrhea, 284
  staff responsibilities in, 252–253
Nystatin (Mycostatin), for topical yeast infections, 275

Objectives of critical care, 3–16. See also Intensive care; Intensive care unit (ICU)
Observation. See Monitoring
"On call" schedule, 188
Orientation, for ICU fellow, 184–185
Outcome definition, 134–135
  in decision-making, 23–24
  iatrogenesis and, 114–115
Outcome predictions, 21, 134f, 134–135. See also Decision-making
  acquisition of new information affecting, 23
  on admission to ICU, 28–29
  APACHE scores in. See APACHE; APACHE II
  and brain death, 87
  for continued care, 30–31
  and cost containment, 139–140
  and cost effectiveness, 136f, 136–137
  on discharge from ICU, 33–34
  for emergency versus elective patients, 25–28, 26t, 27t, 28t
  and false expectations, malpractice claims and, 119–120
  and informed consent, 61–62
  for long-term ICU patients, 32–33, 33t, 168–170, 169t
  nursing care index in, 166–167, 167t
  observed mortality and, 170, 170f
  patient-disease interactions in, 147–156, 148t–149t, 152t, 153t, 154t

physician perceptions in, 155t–161t, 156–166, 163t, 165t
and potential for salvageability, 42–44
and resource utilization, 137, 139
severity of illness and, 137, 138t
short-term, 29–30, 31t
time influence on, 24, 25t
TISS in. *See* Therapeutic Intervention Scoring System (TISS)
values and limitations of indices in, 168t, 168–171, 169t, 170f
Oxazepam (Serax), for anxiety, 228, 229t

Pain, agitation due to, 227
Parents, refusal of children's therapy by, 102
Patchy ischemia, 276–277
Patient's Bill of Rights, 47
Paxipam (halazepam), 229t
Payment. *See* Cost of medical care
Pediatric patients. *See* Children; Infants
Perceptual disturbances, in delirium, 218
Perineal infections, 279
Perphenazine (Trilifon), for anxiety, 228–229, 231
Personnel. *See* Critical care team; Staff; *specific type, e.g.,* Physician(s)
Pharmacology. *See* Drugs; *specific drug or type of drug*
Phlebitis, 278
Physician(s). *See also* Critical care team; Staff
 in allocation of nursing care. *See* Nursing care, allocation of
 authority of, 176–177
 bedside care by, 9
 communication responsibilities of, 198–201, 204
 consulting, 196–197
 ethical decision-making by, 40–42. *See also* Medicomoral principles
 ICU attending, 195–196
 ICU fellow. *See also* ICU fellow
  and surgical team, 196
 ICU juniors, 197
 interrelationships of, 14, 191–202
  with nurses, 175–176, 180–181, 198, 235–236

  with respiratory therapists, 198
  team members and, 192f, 192–193
 involvement with families of, 204, 205, 206–209
 lawsuits against. *See* Malpractice suits
 perceptions of, in outcome predictions, 155t–161t, 156–166, 163t, 165t
 preventive ethics and, 64–65
 roles and responsibilities of, 193–198
  patients with behavioral disturbances and, 226–227
  on surgery team, 191–192, 193–195, 197–198
  ICU fellow and, 196
Physician's orders
 for constant physician care patients, 245
 do-not-resuscitate, 80–81, 97–98
 for extensive nursing requirement patients, 243–245
 for monitoring/observation patients, 240–243, 241t, 242f, 243f
 nursing functions dependent and independent of, 235–236
Physiologic variables, in outcome predictions. *See* APACHE; APACHE II
Potential for salvageability, 42–44
Power of attorney, Natural Death Acts and, 97
Prazepam (Centrax), 229t
Prediction of outcome. *See* Outcome predictions
Preservation of life, 44. *See also* Life support measures
President's Commission for the Study of Ethical Problems in Medicine, 95, 96
 competency criteria of, 98, 99t
Pressure sores (decubitus ulcers)
 prevention of, 271–274, 273f, 274f
 treatment of, 274–275
Preventive care, 267–287
 bed types for, 285–287
  Burke, 286–287, 287f
  Clinitron, 286
  KinAir, 286–287, 287f
  Rotorest Kinetic Treatment Table, 285, 286f
 for bladder function alterations, 284–285

Preventive care (*continued*)
  for bowel function alterations, 283–284
  for missed extremity fractures, 283
  for musculoskeletal system, 275–277
    compartment syndromes in, 275, 276f
    contractures in, 277
    localized ischemia in, 276–277
  for skin and subcutaneous tissues, 268–275
    in area surrounding wounds, drains, or stomas, 269
    decubitus ulcers, 271–274, 273f, 274f
    drains and fistulas, 270f, 270–271, 271f, 272f
    stomas, 269–270
    topical yeast infections of, 275
    wounds of, 268–269, 269f
  for subtle infectious processes, 277–283
    ICU device-associated, 279–283, 280f, 281f, 282f
    perineal, 279
    sinusitis, 278–279
Preventive ethics, informed consent and, 64–65
Prioritization, by ICU fellow, 187–188, 189t
PRN care activities, nursing care allocation for, 257–261
Professional community standard of disclosure, informed consent and, 60
Prognosis. *See* Outcome predictions
Prognostic Nutritional Index, 27, 27t
Prospective payment systems, 4, 5, 136–137
Psychological considerations, 203–213
  in agitation, 227–229, 229t
  in apathy, 229–231
  defense mechanisms, 203–206
  in delirium, 217–225. *See also* Delirium
  in denial, 204
  in dependency, 232
  in depression, 211–212, 229–231
  in family reactions, 204–209
    to imminent death of patient, 212–213
  in fears
    family's, 204–205
    patient's, 209–210
  in hostility, 232
  in informed consent, 68–69
  in loss of control
    by family, 205–206
    by patient, 209–210, 231–232
  and nursing interventions, time allocation for, 265
  patient's symptoms relating to, 210–212
    hypothetical sequence of, 226, 227f
  in refusal to cooperate, 231–232
  in staff involvement with families, 206–209
  in stress
    of ICU patients, 211
    and informed consent, 69
    of staff, 175–176, 189–190
Psychosis, in ICU patients, 210–212. *See also* Behavioral disturbances

Quackenbush case, 98, 100
Quality of life. *See also* Right to die
  and alleviation of suffering, 39–42
  in clinical decision-making, 32
  and doctrine of substituted judgment, 88–91
  sanctity of life versus, 6
Questionable competency, patients of, legal decisions for, 98, 99t
Quinlan, Karen Ann, 71, 72, 73, 76, 79, 93
  and doctrine of substituted judgment, 88–91

Radial artery catheter, complications associated with, 282, 282f
Radiography, nursing care allocation for, 261
Rapport, lack of, malpractice claims and, 118–119
RAS (reticular activating system), in delirium, 218
Reasonable person standard of disclosure, informed consent and, 60
Rebellious behavior, 231–232
Recordkeeping. *See* Documentation
Rectal catheterization, for diarrhea, 284
Reflexes, in delirium, 218

Refusal of therapy. *See also* Right to die; Withdrawal of therapy
 as behavioral disturbance, 231–232
 and countervailing state interests, 75–77
 ethical considerations in, 47–52, 48t–50t
  critical care team and, 50t, 53–57
  family and, 49t, 52–53
  humanitarian decisions and, 55
  incompetent patient and, 77–79
  informed, 99–100
  judicial involvement in. *See* Judicial involvement
  and legal repercussions, 55–56
  parental, 102
  and society's impact, 56–57
Religion, and informed refusal, 100
Renal variables, in APACHE scores, 160t, 165t
Requena, Matter of, 77n
Resource allocation, 10–12, 14. *See also* Nursing care, allocation of
 cost effectiveness of, 136f, 136–137
 ethical considerations and, 46–47, 56–57
 outcome predictions and, 137, 139. *See also* Outcome predictions
Respiratory care, 250–252
 for extensive nursing care patients, 244
 for monitoring/observation patients, 242
Respiratory therapists, 181, 198
Respiratory variables, in outcome prediction, 27–28, 28t, 147–151, 148t–149t, 152t, 153t
 APACHE scores and, 160t, 163t, 165t
Restoril (temazepam), 229t
Resuscitation
 and do-not-resuscitate orders, 80–81, 97–98
 and outcome prediction, 154t
Reticular activating system (RAS), in delirium, 218
Right to die. *See also* Refusal of therapy; Withdrawal of therapy
 for incompetent patients
  Conroy case and, 78n, 92–93
  Dinnerstein case and, 94
  President's Commission on, 95
  Quinlan case and, 71, 72, 73, 76, 79, 88–91, 93

 Spring case and, 94–95
 Storar case and, 73, 92
 and Natural Death Acts, 51, 95–97
Risk factors. *See also* Outcome prediction
 for iatrogenic disorders, 111–112
Ritalin (methylphenidate), for apathy, 230
Roe v. Wade
 and right to die, 90
 and withdrawal of therapy from minors, 100–102
Roles of ICU staff, 178–180, 193–198. *See also* Critical care team; Staff; *specific staff members*
Rotorest Kinetic Treatment Table, 285, 286f
Rule-utilitarianism, 39

Saikewicz, Joseph, court case involving, 73, 76, 79, 91, 93
Salvageability, potential for, 42–44
Sanctity of life
 and alleviation of suffering, 39–42
 quality of life versus, 6. *See also* Quality of life
Satz v. Perlmutter, 77
Scheduling of ICU workday, 187–188, 189t
Secretaries, 181
Seiferth, In re, 102
Senior staff members, surgery team, 194–195
Sepsis, unusual sources of, 277–283
Sepsis-Related Mortality index, 27, 27t
Sepsis syndrome, 32–33
Septicemia, localized ischemia and, 276
Septic variables, in APACHE score, 161t
Serax (oxazepam), for anxiety, 228, 229t
Severity spectrum, outcome predictions and, 137, 138t. *See also* Outcome predictions
Severns v. Wilmington Medical Center, 93
Shift scheduling, 188, 189t
Sinusitis, 278–279
Skeletal system. *See* Musculoskeletal system
Skin and subcutaneous tissues, preventive care for, 268–275

Skin and subcutaneous tissues, preventive care for (*continued*)
  bed types and, 285–287, 286f, 287f
  in decubitus ulcers, 271–274, 273f, 274f
  in drains and fistulas, 270f, 270–271, 271f, 272f
  in stomas, 269–270
  in topical yeast infections, 275
  in wounds, 268–269, 269f
Sleep disturbances, in ICU patients, 210
  delirium and, 218
Societal objectives, 9–10
  and limitation of therapy, 56–57
Spring, Matter of, 73, 94–95
Staff. *See also* Critical care team
  communication responsibilities of, 198–201
  ICU attending, 178, 195–196
  ICU fellow, 183–190. *See also* ICU fellow
  involvement with families of, 204, 205, 206–209
  junior members of
    on rotation through ICU, 197
    on surgery team, 197–198
  malpractice claims and
    conflicting opinions and, 121–124
    inconsistent statements and, 120–121
    information loss through transition and, 124–125
  medical director, 178
  nursing. *See* Nursing staff
  physicians. *See* Physician(s)
  residents
    on ICU, 197
    on surgery team, 197–198
  respiratory therapists, 181, 198
  roles of, 178–180, 193–198
  scheduling shifts of, 188, 189t
  senior members of. *See also* ICU fellow
    surgery team, 194–195
  stress of, 175–176, 189–190
  on surgery team, 191–200
  unit secretaries, 181
Standing orders, deletion of, 143–144
State Department of Human Services v. Northern, 98
State of Kansas v. Shaffer, 86
Stelazine (trifluoperazine), for anxiety, 229

Stimulants, for apathy, 230–231
Stomas, preventive care for, 269–270
Storar, John, court case involving, 73, 92, 95
Stress
  in critical care team members, 175–176, 189–190
  in ICU patients, 211
  and informed consent, 69
Subcutaneous tissues. *See* Skin and subcutaneous tissues
Subjective standard of disclosure, informed consent and, 60
Subspecialty teams, communication with, 201
Substituted judgment doctrine, 88–91
Superintendent of Belchertown State School v. Saikewicz, 73, 76, 79, 91, 93
Surgeon(s), 191–192. *See also* Physician(s)
  attending, 193–194
  expectations of, about ICU, 199–200
  ICU fellow and, 196
  ICU team communication with, 199–201
  ICU team expectations of, 200
  junior, 197–198
  preventive ethics and, 64–65
  senior, 194–195
Surrogates, for incompetent patients, 77–79

Team approach. *See also* Critical·care team
  in ethical decision-making, 53–57
Temazepam (Restoril), 229t
Terminal illness. *See also* Death and dying; Life support measures
  admission to ICU in, 6–7
Therapeutic intervention(s)
  decision-making in, 22–23
    judicial involvement in, 71–84. *See also* Judicial involvement
  iatrogenesis and, 113–114
  and outcome predictions. *See* Outcome predictions
  patient refusal of. *See* Refusal of therapy
  withdrawal of. *See* Withdrawal of therapy

Therapeutic Intervention Scoring System (TISS), 30, 31, 31t, 155t–159t, 156–162
  in long-term ICU patients, 168, 169t
Thioridazine (Mellaril), for delirium, 225
Thiothixene, for anxiety, 229
Thorazine (chlorpromazine), for delirium, 225
Thrush, 275
TISS (Therapeutic Intervention Scoring System), 30, 31, 31t, 155t–159t, 156–162
  in long-term ICU patients, 168, 169t
Topical yeast infections, preventive care for, 275
Torres, In re, 80
Tracheostomy tapes, complications associated with, 280–281
Traction helmet, complications associated with, 281–282
Training
  by ICU fellow, 178
  of ICU fellow, 185–186
Tranquilizers, for anxiety, 228–229
Transfusions, religious objections to, 100
Transport of patients, nursing care allocation for, 263–264
Tranxene (clorazepate), 229t
Trauma. *See* Emergency care
Trauma Index, 25, 26t
Trauma Score, 25, 26t
Treatment. *See* Therapeutic intervention(s)
Tremor, in delirium, 218
Triage Index, 25, 26t
Triazolam (Halcion), 229t
Trifluoperazine (Stelazine), for anxiety, 229
Trilifon (perphenazine), for anxiety, 228–229, 231
Tubes. *See specific type*
Turning activities, nursing care allocation for, 262

Ulcers, decubitus
  prevention of, 271–274, 273f, 274f
  treatment of, 274–275

Untoward events, charting of, 129
Upper extremity. *See* Arm; Extremities
Urinary function, alterations in, 284–285
Utilitarianism, 39

Valium (diazepam), for anxiety, 228, 229t
Value history of patient, as guide for patient care, 63, 65, 66–67
Varices, esophageal, traction helmets in, 281–282
Vascular cannulation
  and arterial catheter armboard, 282, 282f
  infections associated with, 278
  localized ischemia and, 276–277
Versed (midazolam), 229t
Vital signs monitoring, 247–249
  frequency of, 240–243, 241t, 242f, 243f
  in nursing care index, 166–167, 167t

Withdrawal of therapy. *See also* Refusal of therapy; Right to die
  court proceedings for, circumstances necessitating, 79–80. *See also* Judicial involvement
  and criminal liability, 82–83
  legal standards in, 81–82. *See also* Legal issues
  infants and, 102–106
  minors and, 100–102
  nutritional, 82
Wounds
  localized ischemia of, 276
  preventive care for, 268–269, 269f

Xanax (alprazolam), 229t

Yeast infections
  topical, preventive care for, 275
  urinary catheterization and, 285